READER'S DIGEST

The COMPLETE
Manual of
FITNESS
and
WELL~BEING

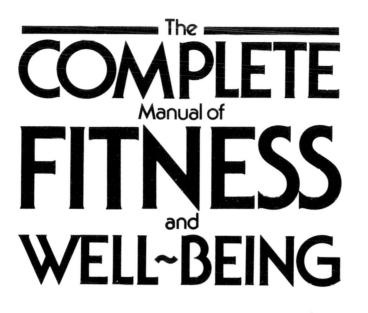

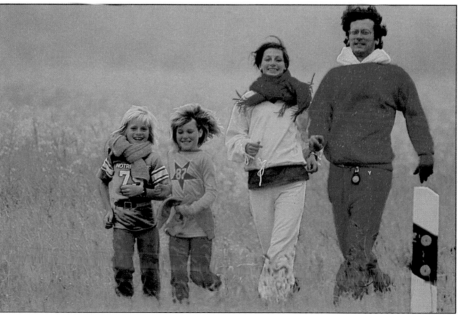

The Reader's Digest Association, Inc.
Pleasantville, New York/Montreal

Edited and designed by
Marshall Editions Limited, London

MANAGING EDITOR	Ruth Binney
EDITOR	Barbara Horn
COORDINATING EDITOR	Anne Kilborn
ART EDITOR	Simon Blacker
DESIGN ASSISTANT	Jonathan Bigg
PICTURE RESEARCHERS	Zilda Tandy
	Celia Dearing
	Mary Corcoran
INDEXER	Donald Binney
PRODUCTION	Barry Baker
	Janice Storr

READER'S DIGEST STAFF

EDITOR	Kaari Ward
ART EDITOR	Richard Berenson

READER'S DIGEST GENERAL BOOKS

EDITOR IN CHIEF	John A. Pope, Jr.
MANAGING EDITOR	Jane Polley
ART DIRECTOR	David Trooper
GROUP EDITORS	Norman B. Mack
	Joel Musler (Art)
	Susan J. Wernert

Based on the original edition of *The Complete Manual of Fitness and Well-being*,
Copyright © 1984 Marshall Editions Limited, London;
published in the U.S.A. by Viking Penguin, Inc.

Revised Edition

Library of Congress Cataloging in Publication Data

The Complete manual of fitness and well-being.

Reprint. Originally published: New York, N.Y.:
Viking, 1984.
Bibliography: p.
Includes index.
1. Health. 2. Physical fitness. I. Reader's
Digest Association. [DNLM: 1. Health. 2. Physical
Fitness—popular works. QT 255 C737 1984a]
RA776.C75 1988 613 87-9735
ISBN 0-89577-270-1

Printed in the United States of America
Second Printing, February 1989

General Medical Consultant
Jack D. Singer, M.D.

Consultants and Contributors
Carola Beresford-Cooke
Jane Cooper, C.S.W., M.Ed.
Sandra C. Durmaskin, M.A.
Johanna Dwyer, D.Sc., R.D.
Judy Garlick, B.A.
Gordon Jackson, M.B., M.R.C.P.
Marjorie Jaffe
Thomas C. Kelly, M.A.
Patricia Last, F.R.C.S., F.R.C.O.G.
Phillip Lee, M.D.
Elizabeth MacFarlane, M.B., B.S.
Tom Myers
B.R. Patterson, M.I.S.P.E.
Paulette Pratt
Carolyn Ritchie, Ph.D.
N.S. Sadick, M.D., F.A.C.P.
Arlene Sobel, M.A.
Keith Stoll, M.Sc., M.Phil., Ph.D
Shelley Turner, B.A.
Marc E. Weksler, M.D.
Clyde Williams, B.Sc., M.Sc., Ph. D.
Peter Williams, M.A., B.M., B.Ch.
H. Beric Wright, M.B., F.R.C.S., M.F.O.M.

CONTENTS

INTRODUCTION   8-9

HOW ARE YOU?   10-25

How fit are you really?   12
How's your diet?   16
What's your lifestyle?   18
How's your emotional health?   20
Can you cope?   22
How long might you live?   24

WHOLE-LIFE PROGRAMS   26-51

Growing up   28
Finding an identity   30
Young adults   32
Settling down   36
Mature and established   40
Into middle age   44
Adjusting to retirement   48
Old and graceful   50

EATING FOR HEALTH   52-93

Nutrients and foods   54
Food groups   56
Vitamins   58
Minerals   60
Making sure your diet is healthy   62
Eating habits   66
Energy and calories   68
The meaning of metabolism   70
What you should weigh   72
Keeping your weight in line   76
Reducing diets   80
Sample menus/1,200 calories   81
Sample menus/1,800 calories   82
Sample menus/2,400 calories   83
A high-fiber diet   84
A low-sodium diet   85
Vegetarian diets   86
Fluids   90
Food allergies and problems   92

GETTING FIT, STAYING FIT   94-159

What is fitness?   96
Aerobics   98
Fitness testing   100
Fitness goals   102
Rating a health club   104
Warm up, cool down   106
Choosing a program   108
Walking   109
Bicycling   110
Jogging and running   112
Swimming   116
Exercises in water   118
Indoor fitness   120
Home gym   124
Stretching   126
Special stretch program   128
Strengthening   132
Preventing injuries   136
The back   138
Back exercises   140
Exercises for the abdominals   142
Exercises for hips and thighs   144
Exercises for the upper body   146
Yoga   148
Family fitness   154
Keeping it going   156
Competition   158

HEAD TO TOE   160-183

Skin   162
Hair   168
Eyes   172
Ears   175
Teeth and gums   178
Hands and nails   180
Feet   182

YOUR SEXUALITY 184-211

Sexual development	186
Maturity	190
Improving your sex life	194
Contraception	196
Relationships under pressure	200
Premenstrual syndrome	202
Female health screening	204
Midlife transition	208
Male health screening	210

PREGNANCY AND BIRTH 212-235

Preparing for pregnancy	214
Prenatal care	217
Staying fit in pregnancy	220
Prenatal exercise program	222
Giving birth	228
Postnatal care	230
Exercises to do with baby	234

FEELING GOOD, STAYING YOUNG 236-259

Aging and attitude	238
Facing up to retirement	240
Retirement communities	244
Getting the most from retirement	246
Keeping fit	250
Fitness program 65+	254
Preventing accidents	256
A fit mind	258

COPING WITH STRESS 260-299

Personality	262
Your place in the world	264
Stress	266
Travel stress	270
Managing stress	272
Sleep and dreams	276
Stress and illness	278
Prescribed drugs	280
Nonprescribed drugs	282
Smoking	284
Alcohol	289
Coping with crises	294

TREATMENTS AND THERAPIES 300-337

Heat therapy	302
Home sauna safety	304
Hydrotherapy	306
Massage	308
Osteopathy and chiropractic	312
Alexander Technique	314
Rolfing	316
Acupuncture and reflexology	318
Shiatsu massage	320
Herbalism and aromatherapy	322
Sports psychology	324
Biofeedback	326
Zen and meditation	328
Hypnosis	330
Psychoanalysis	332
Behavior therapy	334
Cognitive therapy	336

Calorie charts	338
Index	342
Credits and acknowledgments	352

INTRODUCTION

Good health is difficult to define, but it is certainly more than just the absence of disease. It reflects a state of mental, social, and physical fitness and well-being, and is strongly influenced by lifestyle. THE COMPLETE MANUAL OF FITNESS AND WELL-BEING is a practical do-it-yourself guide to maintaining good health and achieving lifelong fitness and well-being.

Take the tests and answer the quizzes in "How Are You?" to assess your fitness now, then see what steps are recommended for your age and sex in the "Whole-Life Programs" that follow. Together these two chapters will guide you to a wealth of information and advice throughout the book.

"Eating for Health" explains how your body uses food, how a balanced diet works, and how you can keep your weight under control. This chapter also explains why you need vitamins and minerals, and shows where they can be obtained. It provides sample menus for 1,200-, 1,800-, and 2,400-calorie diets, and for vegetarian, high-fiber, and low-sodium diets as well.

Turn to "Getting Fit, Staying Fit" for information on how physical activity affects the body and improves well-being. You will find a variety of sports programs for getting in shape. If you are interested in aerobic stretching or strengthening exercises, you can choose from clearly illustrated routines for each activity.

"Head to Toe" shows you how to care for your body on a daily basis so that you will look as good as you feel. In addition, it provides advice about self-help and professional care.

A rewarding sex life is, for most adults, an essential of well-being. "Your Sexuality" describes the physical and emotional aspects of sexual development and behavior in men and women, and explains in a practical, commonsense way some of the problems of establishing and maintaining healthy and fulfilling sexual relationships.

Adopting a healthy lifestyle before a baby is conceived, and maintaining it during pregnancy and immediately after birth, will help to give a newborn child the best possible start in life. "Pregnancy and Birth" recommends how best to prepare for parenthood, and how to eat, exercise, and relax during pregnancy, and in the early weeks after a baby is born. It offers practical advice on getting ready for labor, and it explains many of the childbirth choices available to prospective parents.

As you grow older, your body, your relationships, and your lifestyle gradually change. "Feeling Good, Staying Young" examines these changes and shows how to prepare for them. It also provides practical suggestions for health screening and care throughout your life.

Your emotional health is just as important to your well-being as is your physical fitness. "Coping with Stress" and "Treatments and Therapies" offer many self-help programs and tell you about professional services that can guide you in overcoming problems.

By making an effort to become fit and stay fit, and by following a healthy lifestyle, you can prolong and improve the quality of your life.

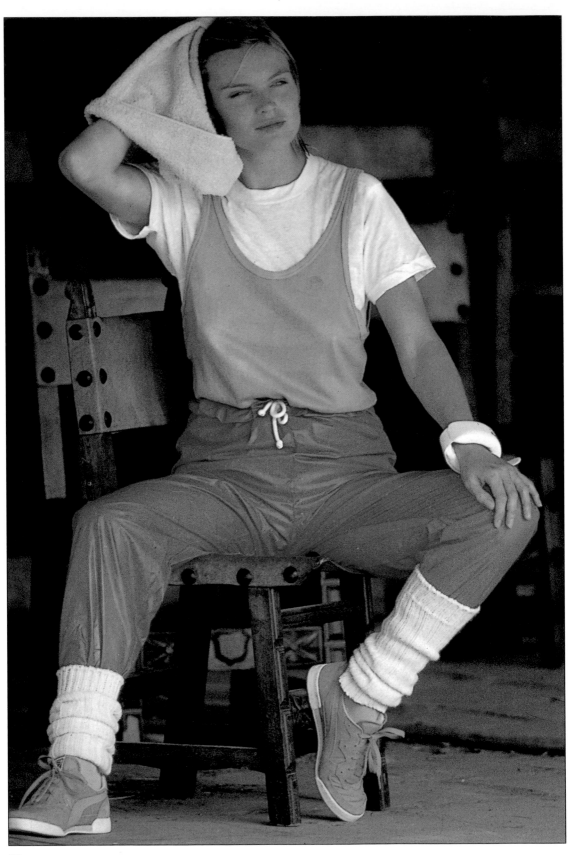

HOW ARE YOU?

Before you begin to think seriously about your fitness and well-being, there are a number of questions you must ask yourself. Do you know, for example, how fit you are, how well you cope with stress, or how well you take care of yourself? This chapter will not only help you to answer these and other questions about your physical and emotional health. More important, it will enable you to identify the changes you need to make to improve your chances of a healthier and a longer life.

However willing you may be to make changes in your daily routine, you are unlikely to arrive at the best solutions unless you first subject yourself to critical scrutiny. This preliminary self-assessment section offers a variety of tests by which you can measure yourself. The results will help you to define your levels of fitness and flexibility, of external and internal stress, of private and social vitality. They will allow you to study your diet and to estimate your life expectancy.

Through assessment of your current levels of achievement and of your attitude toward yourself, you will be able to use this book as fully as possible. As well as defining those parts of your life that would benefit from change, you will be able to identify those elements that cannot reasonably be changed and so begin to come to terms with them.

The tests that appear in this chapter and elsewhere in the book are intended only as a guide. If, for any reason, you feel anxious about your physical or mental health, consult a doctor. For a detailed analysis of your current state of fitness, you will need to undergo a complete physical examination that includes a medical screening of all your vital signs and body functions. Such a screening will provide scientific measurements of, for example, the working of your heart and respiratory system, will quantify your body fat percentage, and analyze your blood, and so give further insights into your metabolism and dietary needs.

Many people have an unrealistic idea of their level of fitness. Some do a lot of exercise without thinking about it, more do a little exercise and believe themselves ultrafit. Fitness is a combination of heart and muscle capacity to use oxygen for energy production. To find out how you rate, try the tests on these and the following pages. Your scores will immediately reveal those areas in which you need to improve your performance.

Turn to Chapter 4, "Getting Fit, Staying Fit" (pages 94–159) for information and exercise programs for developing your fitness. After six weeks, or halfway through an aerobic program, retake these tests. After another six weeks, or at the end of an aerobic program, try again—the results should be encouraging.

TEST 1
What is your resting heart rate?

Your resting pulse is a simple and accurate gauge of cardiovascular fitness. As your fitness level increases, your resting pulse rate will become slower, stronger, and more regular. It is best to take your pulse when you wake up in the morning because any form of emotional or physical exertion will affect it during the day. Individual rates vary but, as a rule, women have a slightly higher pulse rate than men.

Take your pulse at your wrist (at the base of your thumb) or by feeling the artery in your neck just below the ear and toward the jawbone. Now consult the chart to see how you rate.

Caution: If you find your resting pulse falls in the "Poor" category on the charts, call your doctor.

| RESULTS | Resting pulse rate | | | | | | | |
| | MEN | | | | WOMEN | | | |
	Excellent	Good	Fair	Poor	Excellent	Good	Fair	Poor
20–29	59 or less	60–69	70–85	86+	71 or less	72–77	78–95	96+
30–39	63 or less	64–71	72–85	86+	71 or less	72–79	80–97	98+
40–49	65 or less	66–73	74–89	90+	73 or less	75–79	80–98	99+
50+	67 or less	68–75	76–89	90+	75 or less	77–83	84–102	103+

TEST 2
What is your heart recovery time?

Try this simple step test to assess your aerobic fitness and stamina. The test reveals how efficiently your heart and lungs feed oxygen to your body by measuring the time it takes for your heart to slow down after it has speeded up for exercise. Do not attempt this test if your resting pulse rate is in the "Poor" category on the chart in Test 1.

Step on to a stair about 8 inches high, then step down again, moving one foot after the other. Repeat 24 times a minute for 3 minutes. Stop and take your pulse. After resting for 30 seconds, take your pulse again and consult the chart. Repeat this test after a few weeks of participation in an aerobic exercise program and see if your heart recovers more quickly. The heart's natural capacity declines with age, so beware of exceeding the safe limit as you grow older.

Caution: If at any moment you feel dizzy, nauseated or painfully breathless, stop immediately.

| RESULTS | Recovery pulse rate at 30 seconds | | | | | | | |
| | MEN | | | | WOMEN | | | |
Age	Excellent	Good	Fair	Poor	Excellent	Good	Fair	Poor
20–29	74	76–84	86–100	102+	86	88–92	93–110	112+
30–39	78	80–86	88–100	102+	86	88–94	95–112	114+
40–49	80	82–88	90–104	106+	88	90–94	96–114	116+
50+	83	84–90	92–104	106+	90	92–98	100–116	118+

TEST 3
What is your safe maximum pulse rate?

Your heart needs to pump more blood when you exercise. Take your pulse at intervals when you are doing any exercise and do not exceed these rates.

RESULTS	Safe maximum pulse rates			
Age	20–29	30–39	40–49	50+
Men	170	160	150	140
Women	170	160	150	140

TEST 4
How active are you?

This test will show how much physical activity you normally get, and whether you need to get more.

1. How often do you do physical activities (including fitness classes and sports) that make you out of breath?
a. Four times or more a week
b. Two to three times a week
c. Once a week
d. Less than once a week

2. How far do you walk each day?
a. More than 3 miles
b. Up to 3 miles
c. Less than 1 mile
d. Less than $\frac{1}{2}$ mile

3. How do you travel to work/the stores?
a. All the way by foot/bicycle
b. Part of the way by foot/bicycle
c. Occasionally by foot/bicycle
d. All the way by public transportation or car

4. When there is a choice which of the following do you do?
a. Always take the stairs—up and down
b. Take the stairs unless you have something to carry
c. Occasionally take the stairs
d. Take the elevator unless it is broken

5. What do you usually do on weekends?
a. Spend several hours gardening/decorating/ on home repairs/sports
b. Sit down only for meals and in the evening
c. Take a few short walks
d. Spend most of the time sitting reading/ watching TV

6. Which of the following do you do without a second thought?
a. Do the household chores after a day's work
b. Rush out to the store again if you have forgotten something
c. Get other people to run your errands
d. Telephone when you could make a personal visit

RESULTS:
Add up your score. Score 4 points for every **a** answer, 3 points for a **b**, 2 for a **c**, and 1 for a **d**.

20 or over
You are naturally very active and probably quite fit.

15–20
You are active and have a healthy attitude toward fitness.

10–15
You are only mildly active and would benefit from some more exercise.

Under 10
You are rather lazy and need to rethink your attitude toward activity. Try to reorganize your day to allow for some exercise.

TEST 5
What can you do without strain?

Answer any one of the questions below to assess your current level of fitness. **Without straining yourself**, how long does it take you to:

1. Walk 3 miles on level ground?
a. 75 min or more
b. 50 min to 75 min
c. less than 50 min

2. Swim 500 yds?
a. 25 min or more
b. 20 min
c. 10 min or less

3. Run 1 mile on level ground?
a. 15 min or more
b. 9–15 min
c. less than 9 min

RESULTS:
If you cannot score **a** on any question, you should begin a fitness program now. Other scores:

a. If you have covered the distance you have made a start. Now keep it up until the test feels easy.

b. You are moderately fit. If you want to improve, increase the distance and speed up gradually.

c. You have reached a good level of fitness and are ready to start a more vigorous fitness program.

Strength, flexibility, and proper weight are important elements of all-round fitness and good health. Weak and flabby muscles can lead to pain and injury. Obesity and lack of flexibility can seriously impair mobility, making exercise and even daily routine difficult. This condition creates a vicious cycle of inactivity, since lack of exercise results in further loss of suppleness and, possibly, further increase in weight. In addition, obesity is associated with a number of diseases, including diabetes, atherosclerosis, heart disease, gallbladder disease, and some forms of cancer.

The formula on page 73 shows you how to determine your body mass index and the tables on page 75 show your ideal weight.

The tests given here provide quick ways of finding out what kind of shape you're in. Retake these tests regularly and keep track of your progress. If you have followed a program of diet and exercise, you will see improvement as you look back at your early results.

The flexibility and strength tests on page 15 are spot checks of specific muscle groups; they do not evaluate your overall strength and flexibility.

TEST 1
Are you carrying excess fat?

Pinch yourself at the waist and on the upper arm, grasping as much flesh as possible between your forefinger and thumb.

RESULTS:
If you can pinch more than 1 inch of spare flesh, you probably need to shed some fat. To do so, you may need only to tone up—replace fat with muscle—or to lose weight. Every $\frac{1}{4}$ inch of fat beyond the 1 inch maximum represents about 10 pounds of fat.

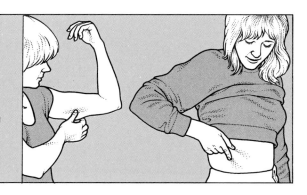

TEST 2
How are you changing?

Men and women tend to accumulate fat in different areas of their bodies. In men, flab generally builds up around the waist, shoulders, and upper arms. In women, excess fat usually accumulates around the waist, hips, thighs, upper arms, and breasts.

Check yourself with a tape measure. If you're a man, measure around your waist, upper arm, and hips. Breathe out, keeping your muscles relaxed; then measure your waist at the level of your navel. Next, breathe in and measure the circumference of your chest when your lungs are at their fullest.

If your waist measures more than your chest, you're carrying too much fat.

If you're a woman, measure around your waist, hips, thigh, upper arm, and bust. There is no quick calculation of overweight for women, but monthly measurements will show if you're reducing.

If you swim regularly, there's a way you can tell whether or not you're getting rid of fat. Float on your back, without using your hands to keep yourself up. Breathe out as much as you can. Using a clock or watch with a second hand, time how long it takes you to sink. As you lose excess fat, your buoyancy decreases and you sink faster.

TEST 3
How efficient are your lungs?

Accurate measurement of lung efficiency requires a laboratory test (see pages 100–101), but the following simple checks will prove a rough guide.

1. Take a deep breath and time how long you can hold your breath.

2. Breathe in and out as deeply as you can; measure your chest in each position.

RESULTS:
Your lungs are probably working with adequate efficiency if you can hold your breath for 45 seconds or more and if the difference between the two chest measurements is 2 to 3 inches or more.

TEST 4
How flexible are you?

Flexibility benefits all physical activities and helps prevent pain and stiffness after exercise. In general, women tend to be more supple than men.

To test your flexibility, lay a yardstick or a 3-foot length of tape on the floor and sit with your heels touching it. With legs straight and feet comfortably apart, slowly bend forward from the waist, reaching as far as you can without straining. Place a marker at the spot where your fingers touch the floor.

Measure the distance between your heels and the marker. If the marker lies beyond the yardstick, score a plus (+) 1 or 2, etc., for the number of inches it lies beyond; if the marker is in front of the yardstick, score a minus (−) 1 or 2, etc.

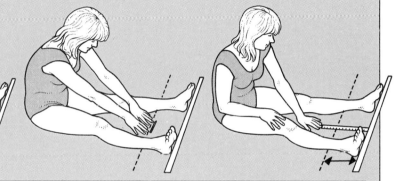

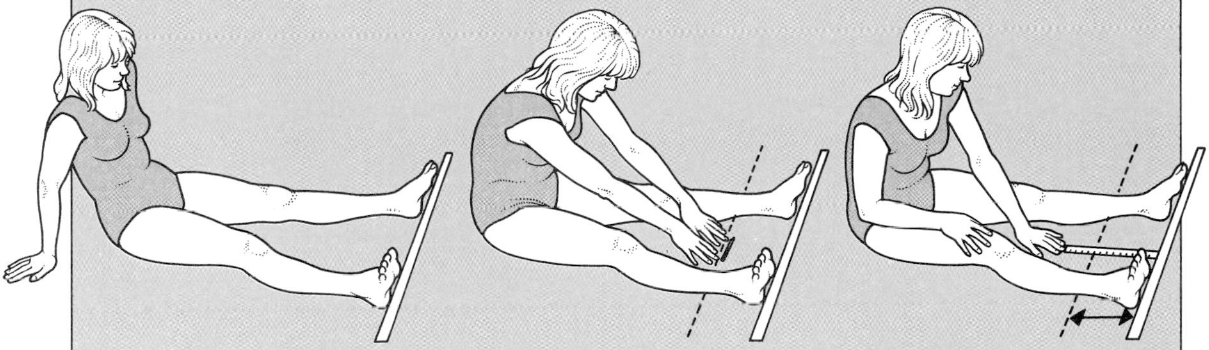

RESULTS	MEN			WOMEN		
Stretch rating	**Up to age 35**	**35–45**	**45+**	**Up to age 35**	**35–45**	**45+**
Excellent	+ 2½in.	+ 2in.	+ 1½in.	+ 3¼in.	+ 2¾in.	+ 2½in.
Good	+ 1¼in.	+ ¾in.	+ ¼in.	+ 2in.	+ 1½in.	+ 1¼in.
Fair	− 2in.	− 2in.	− 2½in.	− ½in.	− ¾in.	− 1¼in.
Poor	− 3¼in.	− 4in.	− 4in.	− 1½in.	− 2in.	− 2½in.

TEST 5
How strong are you?

Muscular strength and endurance are essential for fitness. To achieve aerobic fitness, your muscles must be able to sustain exercise without fatigue. One way to measure strength is by counting the number of sit-ups you can do.

Lie on your back with your ankles firmly wedged under a solid object or held by another person. Bend your knees and place your arms behind your head. Pull up to a sitting position, using the strength of your stomach muscles. Count the number of sit-ups you can do in 1 minute. Measure your results against the ratings in the chart below.

RESULTS	Strength rating					
	MEN			**WOMEN**		
Age	**Excellent**	**Good**	**Poor**	**Excellent**	**Good**	**Poor**
12–14	45	35	25	44	34	24
15–19	50	40	30	40	30	20
20–29	40	30	20	33	23	13
30–39	35	25	20	27	17	12
40–49	30	20	15	22	12	7
50–59	25	15	10	20	10	5
60–69	23	13	8	17	7	4

HOW'S YOUR DIET?

Eating is a pleasure and a necessity, but many people either eat more than they need and put on excess weight, or become diet fiends. The questions on these pages allow you to analyze your eating habits and assess whether they need improvement. To ensure that your answers are accurate, make a note of everything you eat—and the time and place—for a week. Remember, good eating habits will benefit the whole family, from the oldest to the youngest.

TEST 1
Does your diet pass the test?

Answer **a**, **b**, or **c** to the following questions.

1. How many meals do you eat each day as a rule?
   a. Three or more
   b. Two
   c. One

2. Do these meals include breakfast?
   a. Always
   b. Once or twice a week
   c. Rarely

3. If you have breakfast, does it consist of:
   a. Cereal and toast, plus a beverage?
   b. Fried foods, such as bacon and eggs?
   c. Just a beverage?

4. How many times a day do you eat snacks?
   a. Never or very rarely
   b. Once or twice
   c. Three or more times

5. How often do you eat red meat?
   a. Less than three times a week
   b. Three to six times a week
   c. More than six times a week

6. How often do you eat fresh fruit, vegetables, and salads?
   a. Three times a day
   b. Once or twice daily
   c. Three or four times a week or less

7. How often do you eat fried foods?
   a. Once a week or less
   b. Three or four times a week
   c. Most days

8. Do you add salt to your food?
   a. Sparingly, if at all
   b. Moderately
   c. Liberally

9. How often do you eat creamy desserts or chocolate?
   a. Once a week or less
   b. One to four times a week
   c. Most days

10. What spread do you use on bread?
    a. Soft margarine made from polyunsaturated vegetable oil
    b. A mixture of butter and margarine
    c. Butter only

11. How many times a week do you eat fish?
    a. More than twice
    b. Once or twice
    c. Once or less

12. How often do you eat whole-grain cereals or whole-wheat bread?
    a. At least once a day
    b. Three to six times a week
    c. Less than three times a week

13. Before cooking or eating meat, how much fat do you trim off?
    a. All the visible fat
    b. Some of the fat
    c. None of the fat

14. How many 8-oz cups of coffee or tea do you drink each day?
    a. Two or less
    b. Three to five
    c. Six or more

15. How many alcoholic drinks do you consume each day?
    a. One or less
    b. Two or three
    c. More than three

RESULTS:
Add up your score. Score 2 points for every **a** answer, 1 for a **b**, and 0 for a **c**.

25–30
You have an excellent diet, with little need for improvement.

20–25
You have a good diet, but it could improve a little.

15–20
You have only a moderately good diet, and improvement is needed in some areas.

0–15
You have a poor diet, which needs considerable improvement.

If your scores show that your diet and eating habits need improvement, and you want to find out more about healthy eating, turn to Chapter 3, "Eating for Health" (pages 52–93) and Chapter 9, "Coping with Stress" (pages 260–299), You will also find facts about food and diet in many other chapters of the book.

When you have revised your diet according to the guidelines given in these chapters, then take all the tests again.

TEST 2
How do you eat?

For you or your family, how many of the following statements are true?

1. Three-course meals are the rule.
2. Food is offered as a reward for good behavior
3. Candy, potato chips, and other similar snacks are always available in the house.
4. Food is given to compensate for misfortune or disappointment.
5. Going without food is a punishment for poor behavior.
6. Meals are eaten quickly, without conversation.
7. Eating results from tension or boredom.
8. Food is eaten standing up or "on the run."
9. Second helpings are the rule, not the exception.
10. Food cabinets are filled to overflowing.
11. Meals are served on large plates, amply filled.
12. The TV stays switched on during meals.

RESULTS:
If you answer "yes" to 3 or more of these points, then you and/or the members of your family are probably eating more than you need—and not sensibly. You may thus risk being overweight.

TEST 3
How much fat do you eat?

On average, how many of the foods listed below do you eat or use in cooking each day?

RESULTS:
If you regularly eat 3 or more of these foods each day, you are probably eating too much fat in your diet.

Butter	Bacon	Pastries/doughnuts
Margarine	Avocado	Cream
Cooking oil	Eggs	Potato chips
Sausages or frankfurters	Cakes	Nuts
Salami or other preserved meats	Cookies	Ice cream
Mayonnaise	Hard cheese	Tongue
Salad dressing	Cream cheese	Meat with fat
Fish canned in oil	Fried foods of any kind	Chocolate
	Pies	Pancakes

TEST 4
How much do you know about food?

Are the following statements true or false?

1. Potatoes, cereals, and bread are fattening foods.
2. All but the best diets need supplementing with vitamins.
3. Vegetables do not contain proteins.
4. Liver is the only good source of iron in the diet.
5. Eating apples helps to clean your teeth.
6. Eating sugar is the best way to get "instant" energy.
7. Skim milk contains less calcium and other minerals than whole milk.
8. Frozen vegetables are deficient in vitamins.

ANSWER:
All these statements are false.

WHAT'S YOUR LIFESTYLE?

Your lifestyle has a great influence on your health and sense of well-being. It also reflects your personality and philosophy of living. Of course, not all aspects of life, such as your place of work and your home, can be easily changed. However, you may be imposing unnecessary stresses on yourself by failing to recognize problem areas. Answer the questions on these pages to find out how much your way of life may be affecting your health and happiness.

For advice and ideas about improving your lifestyle and sense of well-being, turn to: Chapter 2, "Whole-Life Programs" (pages 26–51); Chapter 6, "Your Sexuality" (pages 184–211); Chapter 8, "Feeling Good, Staying Young" (pages 236–259); Chapter 9, "Coping with Stress" (pages 260–299); and Chapter 10, "Treatments and Therapies" (pages 300–337).

After you have consulted the relevant pages and decided which elements of your lifestyle you want to change and how to go about it, put your plans into action. Return to these quizzes after three months and see if your score and your lifestyle have improved.

TEST 1
Your working life

Many people appear to be oblivious to their work environment. However, since you probably spend about eight hours a day at your job, you need to consider the effect the workplace has on you. Ask yourself these questions to see how your environment measures up.

Do any of the following describe your workplace?

1. Subject to excessive noise
2. Cramped with too much furniture/equipment
3. Poorly lit
4. Inadequately heated/cooled and ventilated
5. Drab and depressing looking
6. Generally messy and dirty

RESULTS:
If you have answered "yes" to any of these points, consider how to improve the conditions. For example, try to rearrange the furniture to create more space and take better advantage of any natural light; cheer up the place with pictures and plants; and discuss improvements to basic systems with the people responsible.

TEST 2
Getting to work

Most people have to travel some distance to get to work and home again. Think about these questions to see if you are doing this in the best way.

1. Have you other options for getting to work?
2. Does your journey take more than one hour each way?
3. Can you reduce the cost, stress, and pollution of daily traveling?

RESULTS:
The most suitable method of transportation gets you to your destination fastest, with the minimum amount of stress and discomfort. Is it worth leaving home earlier to avoid the crowding and frustrations of rush hour? Can you bicycle to the station, or walk to the next bus stop to combine getting exercise with getting to work? Can you reduce your traveling time by changing your route? If you have to travel by car, can you arrange for a pool with colleagues?

TEST 3
Your home life

You may be so accustomed to your home surroundings that it does not occur to you to reassess them. Use these questions to help you see if you need to make improvements.

1. Are all the rooms well laid out for comfort and for efficient use?
2. Is the lighting adequate for reading, sewing, and relaxing?
3. Are the heating, cooling, humidifying, and ventilating facilities adequate?
4. Do the walls look clean and cheerful?
5. Are you free from excessive outside noise?
6. Does each member of the household have enough space and privacy?
7. Do your appliances operate efficiently?

RESULTS:
Answering "no" to any of these questions means that your home is producing a background of discomfort and tension, which has a negative effect on your general well-being. See what positive action you can take to remedy these ills. For example, perhaps you can reorganize the furniture to make the rooms more spacious, redecorate to give a more cheerful appearance, replace inefficient appliances.

TEST 4
Your emotional life

1. Do you have a good relationship with your children?
2. Is your sex life satisfying?
3. Do you have a well-rounded social life?
4. Do your loved ones feel loved?
5. Do you feel loved?

RESULTS:
Communication is the key to beginning to change any "no" answers to "yes." If you have answered "no" to any of these questions, first ask yourself why it is so. Then take the initiative in discussing the problem with the person or persons concerned. Remember that communication is also about listening, and that the solution to problems lies in taking positive action.

TEST 5
How do you use your leisure?

Are you aware that it takes an effort to use your leisure well; an effort of planning to create extra time and an effort of will not to lapse back into bad habits? More important, do you enjoy your leisure activities to the full? Count up "yes" answers only.

Do you:	Score
1. Watch TV for more than 2 hours, on 4 or more evenings a week?	0
2. See friends at least twice a week?	2
3. Take the family out for some fresh air and exercise at the weekends?	3
4. Go to museums, theaters, the movies?	2
5. Often wander around stores for lack of anything else to do?	1
6. Tinker around at home?	1
7. Make time for exercise more than 3 times each week?	4
8. Spend 4 or 5 hours a week on an active hobby?	4
9. Spend 4 or 5 hours a week on a sedentary hobby?	3
10. Play a team sport regularly?	4
11. Go out eating and drinking every night?	0
12. Go to a class or club every week?	3
13. Set aside time to relax/think/meditate alone?	3
14. Organize the rest of the family?	0
15. Do office work at home?	0
16. Not really have any leisure?	−4
17. Work on the home?	3
18. Enjoy your family?	3

RESULTS:
Add up your score.

30 or over
You have a healthy, balanced lifestyle and deserve a sense of well-being.

20–30
You have a positive attitude toward leisure, but might benefit from some more physical exercise.

10–20
You need to rethink your priorities. Your free time may not be evenly balanced, and you might benefit from introducing more variety and activity into your leisure time.

Under 10
You probably do not enjoy your free time much. If you often find yourself at loose ends, try to increase your circle of friends, do more exercise, and cultivate a new interest. If you never have enough time to yourself, try to reorganize your life.

TEST 6
Are your vacations good for you?

1. Do you often end up working instead of going away?
2. Do you forget to take all your days off?
3. Do you wait until it is too late to plan the most suitable vacation?
4. Do you usually return home feeling exhausted by the family?
5. Do you always go to the same place out of habit?
6. Do you avoid "active" vacations for the wrong reasons?
7. Do you spend your vacations working on your home?
8. Do you always end up with the vacation you don't want but which suits your family/partner/friends?
9. Would you really prefer to go away with someone else?
10. Do you rarely get what you want from a vacation?

RESULTS:
If you answered "yes" to any of the above, ask yourself why it is true. Learn from past mistakes, decide what you really want from a vacation, and explore all the possibilities. Discuss these with your intended companions and try to agree on a vacation that will give you all a massive injection of well-being.

HOW'S YOUR EMOTIONAL HEALTH?

However physically fit and healthy you are, you will not enjoy a sense of well-being unless you are emotionally healthy. The quizzes on these pages will help to clarify your attitudes toward yourself, your life, and other people.

To find out more about yourself and how to improve your self-image and lifestyle, turn to Chapter 2, "Whole-Life Programs" (pages 26–51); Chapter 6, "Your Sexuality" (pages 184–211); Chapter 9, "Coping with Stress" (pages 260–299);

TEST 1
How are your loving relationships?

1. Do you have sexual problems in your relationship?
2. Do you find it hard to talk to your partner about personal matters?
3. Do you often snap at your loved ones and then regret it?
4. Do you think your relationship/marriage is emotionally one-sided?
5. Do you avoid visiting your parents if at all possible?
6. Do you dread going home?
7. Do you spend too much time arguing about money?
8. Do you feel jealous of your partner?
9. Do you feel trapped in your relationship?
10. Do you feel your relationship is holding you back?
11. Do you wish you had a relationship?

RESULTS:
If any of these is true, either your relationships or your attitude toward them needs some thought and effort. Analyze the good and bad points of your situation and try to come to a realistic conclusion. Then try to identify the pattern that always leads to problems in your relationships. Use the following questions to help you do this. Discuss your answers with your partner or a close friend, and try to change that pattern.

Questions to ask yourself

1. Can I see things from my partner's/relative's point of view? What is my partner's view of life and of me? Why do we always end up on opposite sides?
2. How can we change this situation? It's a problem, not a battle.
3. Have some of the solutions we've employed in the past produced more problems?
4. What is it that I may be doing to keep the problems going? After all, some of the responsibility may be mine.

TEST 2
How are you coping with the world?

1. Do you find your emotions get out of control?
2. Do you try to avoid people and awkward situations?
3. Do you seek approval from everyone you meet?
4. Do you see yourself through others' eyes?
5. Do you dread being alone?
6. Do you feel unable to control your life pattern?
7. Do you think it is weak to feel grief, anguish, anxiety?
8. Do you think that a perfect relationship is possible?
9. Do you feel detached from the rest of the world?
10. Do you dislike yourself?
11. Do you feel depressed and lonely?
12. Do you feel you have nothing to contribute?
13. Do you feel persecuted and talked about?
14. Do you avoid contact with other people?
15. Do you harbor regrets and resentments?

RESULTS:
Add up your score. Score 1 point for never; 2 for rarely; 3 for sometimes; 4 for often.

Under 20
You seem to have a rational view of life. Perhaps it is too rational and those around you might feel that you are a stable force but that sometimes life with you lacks a little sparkle.

20–35
You are lucky, you have a healthy, balanced outlook. You could, however, make life slightly easier for yourself by questioning some of your beliefs and expectations.

35–50
You suffer, as most people do, from some doubts and dissatisfactions. Accept who you are and make the most of yourself.

50–60
Look at your good points and take things less seriously. It's time to improve your outlook.

and Chapter 10, "Treatments and Therapies" (pages 300–337).

Once you have identified any problems you may have, try to analyze the solutions, establish realistic courses of action, and make sure you see them through. After three months, take the quizzes again and see how you have changed for the better.

TEST 3
How strong is your self-esteem?

Answer as many questions as apply.
1a. Do you tend not to believe compliments?
 b. Do you feel most criticism of yourself is justified?
 c. Do you know yourself and see compliments as irrelevant?
 d. Do you feel compliments are your due?

2a. Do you constantly criticize yourself?
 b. Do you feel most criticism of yourself is justified?
 c. Do you welcome constructive criticism?
 d. Do you think a criticism is a jealous remark?

3a. Do you feel most at ease with people you consider inferior to you?
 b. Do you prefer to be with people like yourself?
 c. Do you enjoy meeting a variety of people?
 d. Do you prefer to mix with prestigious/powerful people?

4a. Do you need reassurance?
 b. Do you avoid disagreements?

 c. Do you trust your own judgment and capabilities?
 d. Are you always right?

RESULTS:
Add up your score. Score 1 point for every **a** answer, 2 points for a **b**, 3 for a **c**, and 4 for a **d**.

4
You seem to have an unnecessarily low opinion of yourself. Concentrate on your good points and try to take things less seriously. It's time to start doing things that will improve your self-confidence.

4–12
Start by selecting the aspect of yourself that you are least happy with and change it. Go on from there.

12–20
You are confident and seem to have a healthy and realistic view of yourself.

20–24
You probably disguise uncertainty behind arrogance. Try to find out how others see you and develop a greater understanding of yourself.

TEST 4
What is your attitude toward work?

Answer one question in each group.
1a. Do you feel overly tense at work?
 b. Do you see work as a means of self-fulfillment?
 c. Are you keen to get back to work after a break?

2a. Do you blame yourself for every small mistake and feel angry or inadequate?
 b. Do you take occasional failure in your stride?
 c. Do you blame others for any mistakes?

3a. Do you always feel you are struggling to complete your work and need to work overtime?
 b. Do you make sure you get enough breaks?
 c. Do you worry about tomorrow's tasks before you have completed today's?

4a. Do you work because you have to?
 b. Do you work to be useful/to learn/for mental stimulation/for enjoyment?
 c. Do you work for public recognition/prestige/power?

RESULTS:
Majority of a answers
You are either not coping with the workload or, alternatively, you may have placed too high a series of expectations upon yourself. Ask yourself whether it is you who demands the performance that you provide or whether it is your boss. If you want to stay on in your job, change your timetable or your standards—otherwise there is danger ahead.

Majority of b answers
You have a healthy, balanced attitude to work. You probably contribute a lot, derive satisfaction from your job and manage to lead a full life.

Majority of c answers
You are either an ambitious, but workaholic, employee, or you are extremely anxious about your performance. Be careful not to allow work to squeeze out your social life or your mental, physical and emotional well-being will suffer. Try to get your work into perspective.

CAN YOU COPE?

You will probably experience intense stress at certain periods of your life. It usually occurs at times of change and is caused by events over which you may not have any control. It is also possible to create your own psychological stresses, which, once identified, can be kept in check. Continual stress imposes a tremendous strain on the heart, channels energy in unproductive directions, and is extremely fatiguing. Resistance to disease, the ability to cope with even minor emotional and mental demands, and day-to-day performance are all severely impaired.

For more information on the causes, cures, and side effects of stress, see Chapter 9, "Coping with Stress" (pages 260–299). For other advice about ways in which you can reduce stress, turn to Chapter 10, "Treatments and Therapies" (pages 300–337), and Chapter 4, "Getting Fit, Staying Fit" (pages 94–159).

When you have pinpointed how best to control your own stress levels, put the ideas into practice. After three months, retake these tests to see how effective you have been in resolving problem areas. If your stress ratings have not improved and you have not recently lived through one of the significant life crises shown in Test 2, do not give up; turn again to the relevant pages and look for a different solution.

TEST 1
Is your personality stress-prone?

1a. Are you competitive and aggressive at work and in sports and games?
 b. If you lose a few points in a game, do you give up?
 c. Do you avoid confrontation?

2a. Are you ambitious and anxious to achieve a lot?
 b. Do you wait for things to happen to you?
 c. Do you find excuses to put things off?

3a. Do you like to get things done quickly and often become impatient?
 b. Do you rely on other people to spur you into action?
 c. Do you often rerun the events of the day and worry about them?

4a. Do you talk fast, loudly, and emphatically and interrupt a lot?
 b. Can you take "no" for an answer with equanimity?
 c. Do you find it hard to express your feelings and anxieties?

5a. Do you get bored easily?
 b. Do you like having nothing to do?
 c. Do you always accommodate other peoples' wishes, not your own?

6a. Do you walk, eat, and drink quickly?
 b. If you forget to do something, do you not bother?
 c. Do you bottle things up?

RESULTS:
Add up your score. For every "yes" answer to an **a** question: score **6**. For every "yes" answer to a **b** question: score **4**. For every "yes" answer to a **c** question: score **2**

24–36
You live at a high-stress pace and might be prone to coronary heart disease, ulcers, and other stress-related illness. For your own sake, slow down, take time to relax. Look at your philosophy of life and perhaps take up a non-competitive hobby in your free time.

12–24
You are relaxed and free from stress. However, a certain amount of stress is healthy and a spur to positive achievement. If you want to achieve more, consider being less apathetic.

0–12
You create stress by inaction. First try to relieve any symptoms of stress, then start a campaign to build up your confidence, self-esteem, and assertiveness. Make a list of your good points and concentrate on them.

Although there is a certain amount you can do to alter the way in which you react to situations and to people around you, it is difficult to change those aspects of your personality that have been present from an early age. It is not clear whether personality traits are determined by heredity or are a result of upbringing and environment, but if you want to change them, firmness of purpose is essential. It is well worth persisting in your attempts, especially if your personality puts your health at risk.

TEST 2
What is your stress score?

How many of the following life crises have you experienced in the last six months? Add up your score on this events table, worked out by Dr. Richard Rahe of Washington Medical School, to find out how much "stress cushioning" you need.

1.	Death of a spouse	100
2.	Divorce	73
3.	Marital separation	65
4.	Jail sentence	63
5.	Death of a close family member	63
6.	Personal injury or illness	53
7.	Marriage	50
8.	Losing a job	47
9.	Marital reconciliation	45
10.	Retirement	45
11.	Change in health of a family member	44
12.	Pregnancy	40
13.	Sex difficulties	39
14.	Gain of a new family member	39
15.	Business readjustment	39
16.	Change in financial state	38
17.	Death of a close friend	37
18.	Change to a different line of work	36
19.	More or fewer arguments with a spouse	35
20.	High mortgage or loan	31
21.	Foreclosure of mortgage or loan	30
22.	Change in responsibilities at work	29
23.	Son or daughter leaving home	29
24.	Trouble with in-laws	29
25.	Outstanding personal achievement	28
26.	Spouse beginning or stopping work	26
27.	Beginning or ending school or college	26
28.	Change in living conditions	25
29.	Change in personal habits	24
30.	Trouble with the boss	23
31.	Change in work hours or conditions	20
32.	Change in residence	20
33.	Change in school or college	20
34.	Change in recreation	19
35.	Change in church activities	19
36.	Change in social activities	18
37.	Moderate mortgage or loan	17
38.	Change in sleeping habits	16
39.	More or fewer family get-togethers	15
40.	Change in eating habits	15
41.	Vacation	13
42.	Christmas	12
43.	Minor violation of the law	11

RESULTS:
Add up your score.

100 and over
Your stress level has reached worrying proportions. You must change some aspect of your life to try to reduce that score.

80–100
You are over-stressed and your score is reaching the critical area. Learn to relax. See Chapter 9, "Coping with Stress" (pages 260–299), and Chapter 10, "Treatments and Therapies" (pages 300–337), for information and advice.

60–80
You are under the average amount of stress.

59 or below
You are enjoying a particularly stress-free time. Make the most of it.

TEST 3
How well are you coping with stress?

1. Do you often want to burst into tears?
2. Do you have any nervous tics/bite your nails/fidget/twiddle your hair?
3. Do you find it hard to concentrate and make decisions?
4. Do you feel you cannot talk to anyone?
5. Do you often feel irritable, snappy, and unsociable?
6. Do you eat when you are not hungry?
7. Do you feel you cannot cope?
8. Do you sometimes feel you will explode?
9. Do you often drink/smoke to calm your nerves?
10. Do you sleep badly?
11. Do you rarely laugh/feel increasingly gloomy and suspicious of others?
12. Do you drive very fast?
13. Do you feel unenthusiastic/constantly tired?
14. Have you lost interest in sex?

RESULTS:
If you answered "yes" to more than four of these questions, you need to relax more and distract yourself. Identify the problem that you think may be leading to stress and do something about it. Also try some of the following:

Listen to music—Take a break—Try meditation/yoga/relaxation—Exercise regularly—Buy a pet—Talk to a friend—Have a good time with someone you care about—Make a list of the good things in life and enjoy some of them—Make time for other people—Buy yourself something new to wear—Smile at someone—Join a club.

HOW LONG MIGHT YOU LIVE?

The charts and questions on these pages will give you an idea of how long you might expect to live. Although there are a few fixed factors, most people can take action to improve the quality of their lives. On the average, for every three people in the United States who are murdered, six die on the roads, and nearly 200 die from smoking-related diseases. You will find more information on improving life expectancy throughout this book.

TEST 1
Were you born with a long life?

ANSWER:
Your life expectancy is determined at birth by the time, the place, and your genetic make-up. In developed countries, medical care, diet, and preventive health care have improved conditions for life, so that a baby born in North America in 1988 can expect to live 20 years longer than someone born in 1888. Statistics suggest that this trend will continue.

Famine and inadequate medical care in Third World countries keep life expectancy low, yet human greed, stress, and laziness in the affluent nations still cause many premature deaths. In most countries, women live, on the average, 5 to 8 years longer than men—and the gap is widening. Whites live, on the average, 4 to 5 years longer than blacks, but the gap is beginning to narrow.

Life expectancy at birth

Kenya
India
Brazil
Portugal
Italy
Cuba
USSR
E. Germany
Greece
Belgium
W. Germany
UK
Australia
Spain
Canada
France
USA
Denmark
Sweden
Norway
Japan

Age 50 60 70 80

Men ☐ Women ☐

TEST 2
Have you inherited a long life?

ANSWER:
If your mother and father lived, or are still living, to a healthy old age, then you too stand the chance of a long life. If either of your parents died prematurely, this might affect the length of your life.

Many of the conditions and diseases that shorten life to less than the average span have a hereditary element. The most obvious of these are spina bifida, cystic fibrosis, hemophilia, and raised blood cholesterol (hyperlipidemia). Although there is no way in which a genetic pathway can be traced for the inheritance of diseases such as diabetes, breast cancer, and gallbladder disease, there is no doubt that a tendency toward these conditions does run in families. With good preventive health care, their onset can be delayed. And if they are detected early, successful treatment is often possible.

TEST 3
A matter of life and death: are you helping yourself?

1. Do you drink more than the equivalent of 4 beers or 2 shots of whiskey a day?
2. Do you have high blood pressure?
3. Do you regularly eat fried and high-fat foods?
4. Do you weigh more than the acceptable range for your height?
5. Do you smoke cigarettes?
6. Do you do little or no exercise?
7. Do you take drugs?
8. Do you work in a dangerous environment?
9. Do you live in a violent neighborhood?
10. Do you have a highly stressful lifestyle?
11. Do you drive every day?

RESULTS:
If you answered "yes" to any of the above questions then you are risking an early death. If your aim is a long life, take stock, change your lifestyle, exercise regularly, and maintain a healthy diet.

TEST 4
What are the risks of smoking?

The chart below shows how smoking reduces your life expectancy. If you have given up cigarette smoking, add a year for each five years since you stopped. The number of years lost from life expectancy through smoking is reduced as you get older because of the naturally shorter expectation of life. But the percentage of years lost through smoking increases with advancing age, so that a 65-year-old smoker stands to lose proportionally more years of those that remain than a 25-year-old. The chart on the right shows that a large proportion of men die before 65 because of their smoking habits.

The percentage of men aged 35 whose smoking habits will cause death before 65

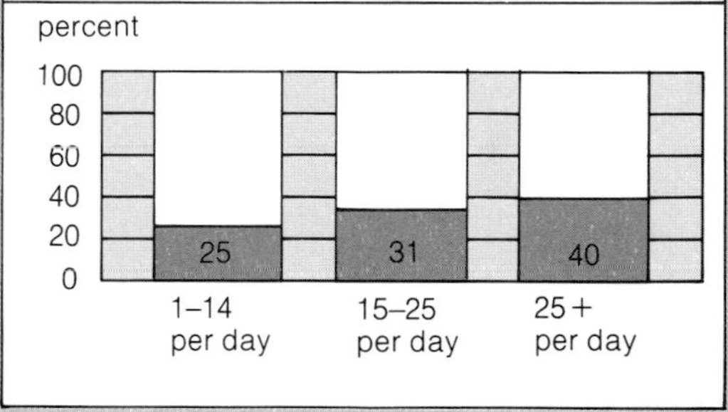
percent
100
80
60
40
20
0
25
31
40
1–14 per day
15–25 per day
25+ per day

How smoking reduces life expectancy

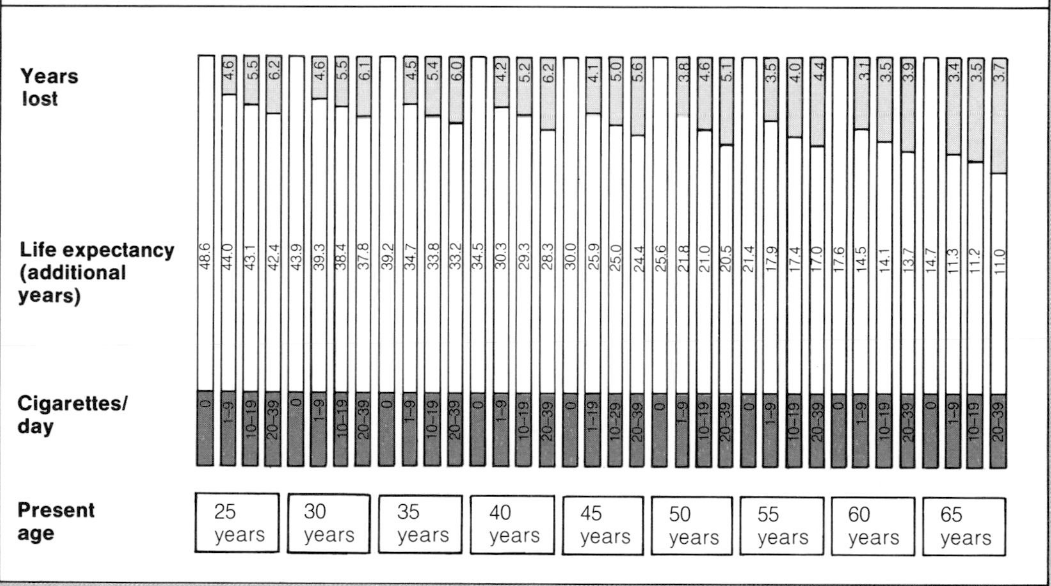
Years lost
Life expectancy (additional years)
Cigarettes/ day
Present age
25 years: 0, 1-9, 10-19, 20-39; 48.6, 44.0, 43.1, 42.4; 4.6, 5.5, 6.2
30 years: 0, 1-9, 10-19, 20-39; 43.9, 39.3, 38.4, 37.8; 4.6, 5.5, 6.1
35 years: 0, 1-9, 10-19, 20-39; 39.2, 34.7, 33.8, 33.2; 4.5, 5.4, 6.0
40 years: 0, 1-9, 10-19, 20-39; 34.5, 30.3, 29.3, 28.3; 4.2, 5.2, 6.2
45 years: 0, 1-19, 10-29, 20-39; 30.0, 25.9, 25.0, 24.4; 4.1, 5.0, 5.6
50 years: 0, 1-9, 10-19, 20-39; 25.6, 21.8, 21.0, 20.5; 3.8, 4.6, 5.1
55 years: 0, 1-9, 10-19, 20-39; 21.4, 17.9, 17.4, 17.0; 3.5, 4.0, 4.4
60 years: 0, 1-9, 10-19, 20-39; 17.6, 14.5, 14.1, 13.7; 3.1, 3.5, 3.9
65 years: 0, 1-9, 10-19, 20-39; 14.7, 11.3, 11.2, 11.0; 3.4, 3.5, 3.7

TEST 5
How will you die?

ANSWER:
The cause of your death will depend, as the chart on the right indicates, on where you live. In the developed countries (dark bands) deaths from heart disease and cancer predominate. In the developing countries (lighter bands) respiratory and infectious diseases are the more common causes of death. The differences are due to lifestyle and medical care.

Causes of death

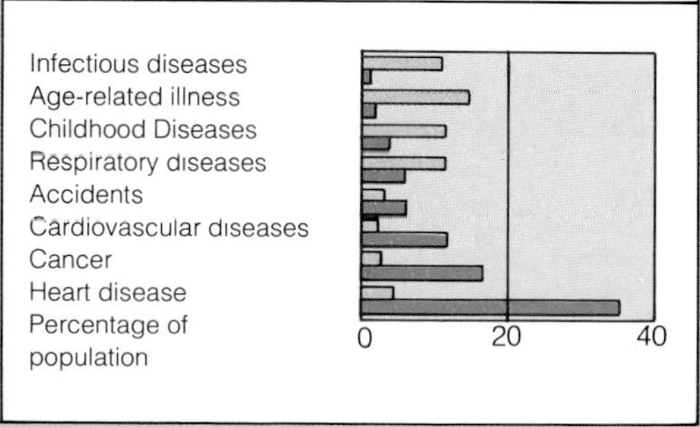
Infectious diseases
Age-related illness
Childhood Diseases
Respiratory diseases
Accidents
Cardiovascular diseases
Cancer
Heart disease
Percentage of population
0
20
40

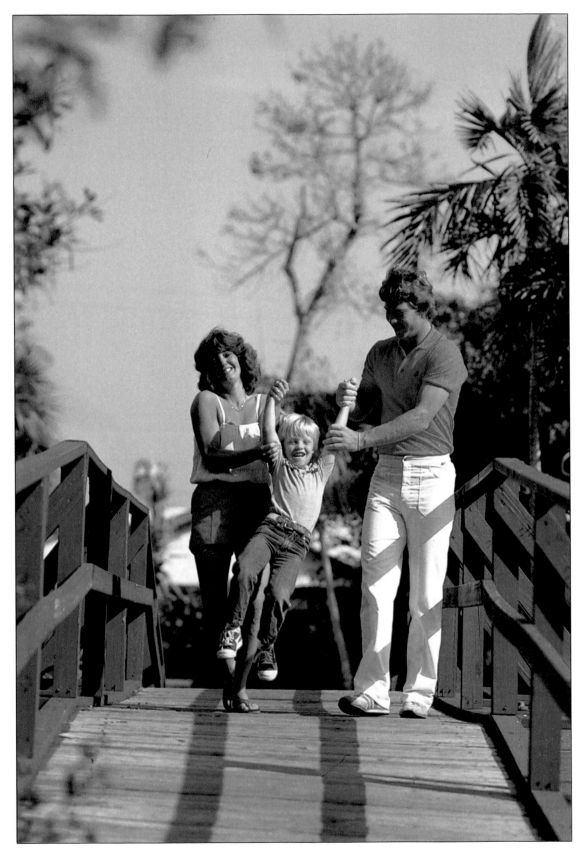

WHOLE-LIFE PROGRAMS

Whatever your age, positive thinking is one of the keys to achieving and maintaining a state of fitness and well-being. Yet even with a positive outlook, you still need to work out the individual steps that will lead you to your goal of a long and healthy life.

The whole-life programs that form this chapter are designed to help you do just that. At the same time, they will allow you, by means of cross-references, to gain access to the wealth of information in the other chapters of the book. The programs take into account the major changes that occur in your body and lifestyle as you get older, and they are grouped according to the health and fitness needs shared by people of the same age range and sex.

The whole-life programs are based on general goals that are the same for both sexes and all ages except the two youngest age groups. These goals cover the main aspects of healthy living, namely eating a balanced, healthy diet, getting sufficient exercise, learning to handle stress, not smoking, and controlling drinking. Attaining these goals is essential to achieving the central goal of every program—fitness and well-being.

Each program deals with five critical areas of your lifestyle and preventive health care: emotional and mental health, in which leisure plays a vital role; work, finance and family; fitness and body care; food and drink; and health checks.

Before you begin the program tailored to your age group and your sex, take the quizzes on pages 10–25 to find out which areas of your life are most in need of attention. Then, keeping these problem areas in mind, work your way through your whole life program, setting yourself new targets as you progress. Of course, there might be some goals that you have already achieved. That's fine, but remember that to maintain fitness and well-being you must work at them all your life.

GROWING UP

In the formative years between birth and age 13, children change from babies into young men and women on the verge of adulthood. During the childhood years living habits are formed—habits that are difficult to change later in life. Thus it is especially important that parents establish a code of behavior that will stand their

EMOTIONAL AND MENTAL HEALTH. LEISURE

● Be polite. Good manners help you to get along with other children as well as with adults.

● Be true to your word. Take time to think before you make a promise. Others will respect you for explaining that you can't do something rather than letting them down later.

● Read at least one book a week for fun. Books open up new worlds of information and imagination.

● Choose the TV programs you really want to see, and limit your viewing to one hour a day.

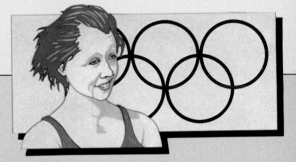

WORK, FINANCE AND FAMILY

● Help around the house. Make your own bed every day, keep your toys and books tidy, and hang up and put away your clothes every night.

● Learn to share. Let your brothers and sisters, and your friends, use your toys and books.

▲
Marjorie Gestring, American, was the youngest female ever to win an Olympic gold medal, age 13, in 1936.

FITNESS AND BODY CARE

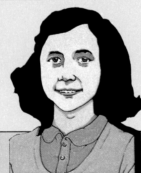

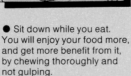

● Respect your body. Bathe every day, and wash your hair at least once a week.

◀ **Anne Frank,** Dutch, began her immortal diary while in hiding from the Nazis in 1943, age 13.

● Keep your fingernails clean, and brush your teeth after every meal.

● Learn to ride a bicycle (see pages 110–111). Once learned, this is a skill you will never lose. It is not only good exercise but also a means of independent transportation.

FOOD AND DRINK

● Sit down while you eat. You will enjoy your food more, and get more benefit from it, by chewing thoroughly and not gulping.

● Drink milk with your meals and whenever you are thirsty. It is a great thirst-quencher, and it is important to the formation of strong bones.

● Eat only small amounts of fried foods. They contain fats that are not good for your body in large quantities (see pages 52–93).

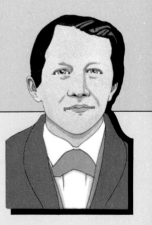

HEALTH CHECKS

● Visit the dentist every six months to have your teeth checked and cleaned. Follow instructions for proper brushing and gum care (see pages 178–179), and for wearing and caring for braces and retainers. The rewards will be healthier teeth and a beautiful smile.

Thomas Alva Edison, ▶ American, began his professional life, age 12, when he printed and published his own newspaper—the first ever to be printed on a train.

children in good stead as adult citizens. In addition, parents should encourage good health habits in their children, so that the foundations of fitness and well-being are properly laid down. It is important that children learn to eat a balanced, healthy diet, get enough sleep, and practice good hygiene.

● Understand that you are growing up emotionally. Remember that it is all right to cry when you are hurt, but learn not to use tears as a means of getting your way.
● Learn how to stand up for yourself. Don't ask or expect your parents to solve all your problems for you.

● Join a group, such as the Cubs, Brownies, or Scouts, where you can make friends and take part in a variety of activities.

Shirley Temple, ▶
American, was the youngest person to win an Oscar, in 1934, age 6.

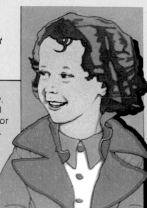

● Take a vacation away from the rest of the family occasionally. Ask your parents if you may accept an invitation to spend a weekend at a friend's house or to stay with other relatives. Go to summer camp.
● Start a hobby or activity that you have not tried before.

● Be considerate of the other members of your family. Try to understand that others might not always want to join in your activities or want you to join in theirs. Respect their privacy. Keep noise to a level that doesn't disturb others who might be studying, watching TV, or talking.

● Learn the value of money. Make your allowance last all week and try to save a little for something special you want.

● Try to do your best at schoolwork. Be prepared to ask questions when you don't understand something. Doing the best you can makes you feel good about yourself.
● Be helpful to others, particularly to younger brothers and sisters.

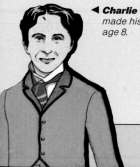

◀ **Charlie Chaplin,** *English, made his stage debut in 1897, age 8.*

● Understand how you are changing physically (see pages 186–189). As you grow, you will find some things that were difficult to do become easier.

● Regular exercise will help maintain your energy and improve your coordination.
● Try skipping rope (see pages 120–121). This simple exercise makes you fit for other sports, and can be done in a gym or outdoors or in the home.

● Learn to swim well (see pages 116–117). Swimming exercises all your muscles and improves your coordination.
● Try your hardest at sports and games. Doing the best you can is more important than being better than someone else.

● Limit the amount of salty snacks you eat. Too much salt disturbs the balance of fluids in your body (see pages 90–91).
● Candy and soft drinks are great temptations, but limit the amount you consume. Sugar is the greatest cause of tooth decay.

Franz Liszt, *the* ▶
Hungarian pianist and composer, gave his first concert in 1820, age 9.

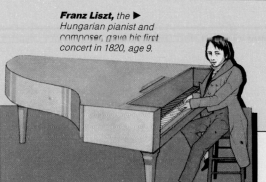

● Eat plenty of fresh fruit and vegetables. They taste good and give your body the nutrients it needs to grow (see pages 54–61).

● Have your eyesight checked once a year. Some people need to wear glasses or contact lenses to improve their vision (see pages 172–174). If you wear glasses or contact lenses, learn how to take good care of them.

● Get your height and weight checked by your family doctor once a year when you have a general check-up. Don't worry if you seem to be growing more slowly or more quickly than your friends— everyone grows at a different rate (see pages 186–187).

● Have your hearing tested regularly (see pages 175–177).

FINDING AN IDENTITY

The tempestuous teens, the years of rebellion, are those in which youngsters tend to reject—although often only temporarily—the standards of their parents and teachers. These are the years of experimentation, of striving for independence, of building self-confidence. Adolescents are adjusting to bodies that are still growing and changing, and to the awakening of sexual feelings. Under pressure from their

EMOTIONAL AND MENTAL HEALTH. LEISURE

● Recognize that you must coexist with the rest of society. Treat other people and their opinions—even if you don't agree with them—with the same courtesy and respect you want them to show you.
● Learn to make up your own mind, not just accept other people's opinions.

● Learn to cope with mistakes and failures (see pages 266–267). No one can be perfect or be a winner all the time, even if it looks that way from the outside.
● Learn how to be alone (see pages 262–265). Use the time to relax, to think, or to pursue a special interest.

WORK, FINANCE AND FAMILY

● It is easy to become very self-involved, but remember that you are part of a family. Learn how to express your interest in, and concern for, brothers and sisters, and parents and grandparents.

● Think about your future, and work hard to qualify for college entrance or a job.

▲ **Robert (Bobby) Fischer,** *American, became an International Grand Master at chess in 1957, age 14.*

FITNESS AND BODY CARE

Nadia ▶ Comaneci, *Romanian, was the first gymnast to receive a perfect score of 10 at the Olympics, in 1976, age 14.*

● Take good care of your body. Bathe or shower daily, wash your hair regularly, and brush your teeth after meals (see pages 160–183). An unkempt appearance is not attractive to anyone else.
● Go for that little extra in sports. You will enjoy the sense of achievement.

FOOD AND DRINK

● The legal age for consumption of alcohol varies from state to state. If you have reached the legal age, understand the implications of drinking (see pages 289–293). Be sure that you, not the alcohol, are in control of your mind and body.

HEALTH CHECKS

● Check your height and weight twice a year. A balanced diet and plenty of exercise should help you maintain the correct weight and body mass index (see pages 72–75). Remember that weighing too little is as unhealthy as weighing too much.

peers, many teenagers find it difficult to resist high-risk temptations such as alcohol and drugs. It is important for parents to ease young people through these problem years with sympathy and understanding, and to help them learn how to handle stress, reject cigarettes and drugs, maintain a healthy diet, and continue to get plenty of exercise.

● Understand your sexual urges (see pages 186–189).

● Develop good relationships with members of both sexes. Learn to trust, and to be trustworthy, to share your thoughts and feelings, and to be a good listener (see pages 262–263).

● Learn to organize your work time efficiently so that you can do everything you have to without needless stress. Don't put off studying until the last minute; hastily written papers and crammed-for exams do not reflect your real abilities, and can leave you feeling anxious.

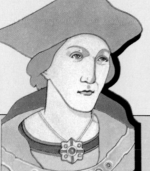

▲ **Henry VIII** *became King of England on April 22, 1509, age 17.*

● Feed your mind with new ideas. Read books, magazines, and newspapers for information and entertainment.
● Do chores around the house willingly, and lend a hand to others without being asked.

● Learn how to handle money. Make a list of all your expenditures. Decide which ones are essential—fares, lunches—and which are desirable extras. Then consider how you might earn money for these, perhaps by babysitting or walking someone's dog.

Judy Garland, American, starred in her most famous film role, Dorothy in The Wizard of Oz, *in 1939, age 17.*
▼

● Take a responsible attitude toward sexual behavior (see pages 186–189).
● Avoid drugs (see pages 280–283). They don't contribute anything positive to your life, but will harm your health and well-being even if you can't feel the effects now.

● Take up a new sport to learn new skills and meet people. Have you tried tennis or hiking?
● Be sure to get the right amount of sleep to keep your body fit and your mind alert (see pages 276–277).

▲
Louis Braille, French, invented the written language for the blind in 1824, age 15.

● Limit the amount of fast foods you eat. Fried foods, carbonated drinks, and milkshakes are high in calories and fats (see pages 52–93).
● Eat plenty of fresh fruit and vegetables. They're as fast as fast foods, but much healthier for you (see pages 52–93).

● Get the most out of your food by taking time to sit down and enjoy it. Chew thoroughly, and give your body a chance to digest before beginning your next activity. Don't watch television or argue during dinner.

● Have your eyesight checked regularly. Wear glasses or contact lenses if you need them—lenses give better all-round vision (see pages 172–174).
● Visit the dentist every six months, and practice good dental hygiene (see pages 178–179).

● See your family doctor or a dermatologist for information and advice about coping with acne.
● Girls: Check your breasts every month (see page 207). This is a vital part of your personal health care that you should continue throughout your life.

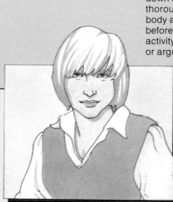

◀ *Françoise Sagan, French, published her first novel,* Bonjour Tristesse, *age 18, in 1954.*

YOUNG ADULTS

The early twenties are often years of risk-taking—traffic accidents are the greatest killers of men in this age group. These are also the years of peak physical prowess, in which the body should be worked hard.

Both career and social goals are usually uppermost in a young man's mind, although the experimental phase begun in the teens continues into the early twenties. This means that he can find it difficult to

EMOTIONAL AND MENTAL HEALTH. LEISURE

● Establish and pursue social goals, but don't be too rigid. As your self-confidence increases, you will find it easy to allow yourself to change your mind.
● Feed your imagination with books and music. Go to a museum or art gallery, see a movie or play.

◀ **F. Scott Fitzgerald,** American, published his first novel, This Side of Paradise, in 1920, age 23.

● Travel as widely as possible. Use your weekends as an opportunity to get away from your routine.

WORK, FINANCE AND FAMILY

● Make the most of your educational opportunities. Is post-graduate education or training an advantage in your chosen career?
● Learn to manage your money. Plan to make your income exceed your expenses, cutting back the latter if necessary.

● Be objective about your skills, abilities, and knowledge, and set realistic short- and long-term career goals. This is your opportunity to gain the experience you will need to progress up the career ladder.

FITNESS AND BODY CARE

● Maintain a high standard of personal hygiene (see pages 160–183), and be sure to get enough sleep (see pages 270–277).

● Balance the transition to a sedentary job by taking up another sport or new exercise. Push your body hard to get the maximum benefit from these years of peak physical ability (see pages 94–159).

● Stop smoking and keep your alcohol consumption within safe limits, particularly if you are planning to become a father. Do it for yourself, your partner, and your baby (see pages 214–215, 284–288).

FOOD AND DRINK

◀ **Rudolph Nureyev** defected from the Soviet Union when the Kirov Ballet performed in Paris in 1961, age 22.

● Control your social drinking (see pages 289–293). If you are drinking on a regular basis, you are probably drinking for the wrong reasons. Remember that alcohol can be a dangerous, debilitating drug.

HEALTH CHECKS

● Have your blood pressure checked annually, and get a complete physical check-up every two years.
● Have your vision tested in this period. If you wear glasses or contact lenses, get a check-up once a year (see pages 172–174).

keep a balance between his academic and extracurricular activities. For men who do not go on to post-graduate studies, there is the transition from student to employee, a time for testing abilities and self-confi- dence. In their jobs young men find themselves having to compete as adults in an adult world for the first time. Twenty-four is the average age for American men to marry for the first time.

● Enjoy a variety of relationships. Remember that you have plenty of time ahead of you, so don't rush into marriage.
● Learn to communicate. Make sure you express your worries, and take steps to deal with them (see pages 262–275).

● Respect your partner. Listen to her opinions and aspirations, and share yours with her. Be considerate of her need for independence and privacy (see pages 190–193).

● Take an active interest in your community, and find time to involve yourself in neighborhood activities.
● Balance work, sports, and other leisure activities, and make time to relax (see pages 272–273).

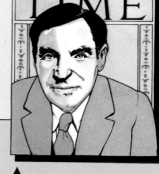

● Plan to live away from the parental home. For social and economic reasons, you might consider sharing a house or apartment with friends.
● Help to keep your home clean and tidy. Pitch in with all the chores, and be responsible for your own laundry.

● Spend time with your parents. Share your aims and achievements with them, and take an interest in their lives. Work to establish an adult-to-adult relationship.

Henry Luce, American, took the first step in building one of the biggest private publishing concerns when he co-founded Time magazine in 1923, age 25.

◀ **Charles Best,** Canadian, was the co-discoverer of insulin in 1921, age 22.

● Drive safely—your life and that of others depends on it. Don't drive at all if you are overtired, have been drinking, or have taken any medication, such as cold pills, that might make you drowsy.

● Learn about nutrition (see pages 52–93). This might motivate you to restrict your intake of junk food, and show you how easy it is to maintain a healthy diet.

● Take up cooking. It can help you to eat properly, increase your pleasure in food, and save money. It is also a pleasant and much-appreciated way in which to entertain friends.

Muhammad Ali ▶ (formerly Cassius Clay), American, won his first World Heavyweight Boxing Championship in 1964, age 22.

◀ **Charles Lindbergh,** American, made the first solo nonstop transatlantic flight in 1927, age 25.

● If you continue to take good care of your teeth, they should last you the rest of your life (see pages 178–179). Remember to visit the dentist every six months.

YOUNG ADULTS

In this group, career and social goals tend to be of equal importance. While many will be preoccupied with completing their education, 20 is the average age at which American women marry for the first time. This fact underlines the decisions that young women have to make in balancing their desires for a career and a family. Although these are the

EMOTIONAL AND MENTAL HEALTH. LEISURE

Wilma Rudolph, ▶
American, overcame the effects of polio to win 3 gold medals in track and field events in the 1960 Olympics, age 20.

● Establish and pursue social goals. Develop poise and self-confidence, and avoid being socially competitive.
● Enjoy a variety of relationships (see pages 190–193). Remember that not every romance has to lead to marriage.

WORK, FINANCE AND FAMILY

● Be objective about your abilities, and set yourself realistic short- and long-term career goals. This is your opportunity to gain the experience you will need to progress up the career ladder, and to establish a foothold if you return to work after you have children.

FITNESS AND BODY CARE

● Establish a routine of caring for your body and maintain it throughout your life (see pages 160–183).
● Find the birth control method that is best for you (see pages 196–199).

● Consider the implications of having children now (see pages 200–201).
● Stop smoking and drinking alcohol before you get pregnant (see pages 214–216, 284–293).

● Exercise to stay fit during and after pregnancy (see pages 220–227, 230–233).

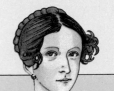

FOOD AND DRINK

● Learn about nutrition (see pages 52–93). This might motivate you to restrict your intake of junk food, and show you how easy it is to maintain a healthy diet.

● Control your social drinking (see pages 289–293). Alcohol is not a substitute for self-confidence.

Mary Shelley, ▶
English, wrote the horror classic Frankenstein in 1818, age 20.

HEALTH CHECKS

◀ **Helen Keller,** American, blind and deaf since infancy, wrote her autobiography in 1902, age 22, and graduated cum laude from Radcliffe College in 1904.

● Get a complete physical check-up every two years.
● Get a complete gynecological check-up every year. This should include a blood pressure test, a cervical smear test, and a breast examination. Review present and future methods of birth control. (See pages 196–197 and 204–207).

WOMEN 19-25

safest years for childbearing, many women choose to wait until they have achieved a position of responsibility in their career before having a child.

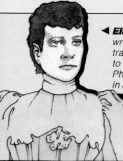

Elizabeth Seaman, *American, who wrote under the name Nellie Bly, traveled around the world in 72 days to beat the record of the fictitious Phineas Fogg, completing her journey in January 1890, age 24.*

● Feed your imagination: read books, listen to music, go to a movie, see a play.

● Travel as widely as possible. Use your weekends as an opportunity to get away from your routine. Plan and go on an exciting vacation.
● Learn to communicate. Make sure you express your worries, and take positive steps to deal with them (see pages 262–275).

● Learn to spend time alone pursuing your own special interests.
● Take an active role in your community. Look for ways of involving yourself in neighborhood activities.
● Balance work, sports, and other leisure activities, and make time to relax.

● Learn to manage your money. Plan to make your income exceed your expenses, cutting back the latter if necessary. Try to save toward a special vacation or some other treat.

● Decide whether to pursue your career after you marry (see pages 200–201).
● Plan to live away from the parental home. For social and economic reasons, consider sharing an apartment or house with friends.

● Spend time with your parents. Share your aims and achievements with them, and take an interest in their lives. Work to establish an adult-to-adult relationship.
● Help to keep your home clean and tidy. Don't let household tasks pile up until they become burdens.

● If you have just made the transition to a sedentary job, take up another sport or a new exercise to keep fit. Have you tried jogging or an aerobics class (see pages 94–159)?

● There is a great temptation during these years to "burn the candle at both ends." Make sure you get the right amount of sleep (see pages 276–277) so that you can enjoy everything you do.

Grace Bumbry, ► *American, began her distinguished operatic career as a mezzo-soprano at the age of 22 with her performance in Aida in Paris in 1959.*

● Experiment with different cuisines, and use your understanding of the principles of nutrition to prepare interesting and healthy meals for yourself, your family, and your friends.

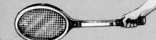

◄ Maureen "Little Mo" Connolly, *American, won the women's Grand Slam (the four major international tennis titles) in 1953, age 19.*

● Re-examine your diet if you become pregnant (see pages 220–221) and modify it to allow for the changes your body is undergoing. Don't use pregnancy as an excuse to overeat or indulge in bad eating habits.

● Check your breasts every month (see page 207). It will take only a few minutes and it could save your life.
●Visit the dentist every six months (see pages 178–179). Make a special visit if you become pregnant; some women require a calcium supplement.

● Have your vision tested in this period. If you wear glasses or contact lenses, get a check-up every year (see pages 172–174).
● Avoid crash slimming diets and excessive weight loss, which can seriously and permanently damage your health.

SETTLING DOWN

The years between 26 and 35 are a time when men begin to follow a more settled pattern of life, a fact often related to the new duties of marriage and fatherhood. In their careers, they are moving on and reaching positions of responsibility. This can be a period of increased stress and anxiety as they accept heavier workloads and new challenges in

EMOTIONAL AND MENTAL HEALTH. LEISURE

● Take all your allocated vacation time. You will be able to give more to your work and your family after you have refreshed your mind and revived your energies by taking a break.
● Analyze the effect your career is having on your social needs.

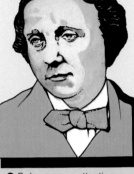

◀ **Charles Dodgson,** English, better known as Lewis Carroll, wrote Alice in Wonderland in 1863, age 33.

● Reassess your social goals in view of your achievements and altered circumstances. Keep up friendships.

WORK, FINANCE AND FAMILY

● A growing family usually makes this a period of increased expenditure. List your priorities, and actively manage your money. Understand how to use credit cards to help your cash flow, but don't let them lure you into spending unwisely.

● Balance your attention between work, home, and leisure activities. Don't let your preoccupation with your job adversely affect the other areas of your life.

● Work hard at your marriage or partnership. A good relationship is the result of nourishment and tender loving care (see pages 194–195, 200–201).
● Spend time with your parents, and foster good relations between them and your children.

FITNESS AND BODY CARE

● Push yourself physically to counteract the sedentary and stressful nature of your job (see pages 94–161). Don't use being in a hurry as an excuse to ride when you could walk, or to use the elevator instead of the stairs.

● If the sports of your earlier years no longer interest you, take up a new sport, perhaps one you can do before work or in your lunch hour (see pages 142–147).

● Play sports with your children (see pages 154–155). This not only gives you exercise, but also sets a good example for the children.
● Drive with caution, particularly if you are faced with a long journey after a tiring day at work (see pages 270–271).

FOOD AND DRINK

◀ **Edmund Hillary,** New Zealander, with Sherpa Tensing, shared the glory of being the first to reach the summit of Mount Everest age 33 on May 29, 1953.

● Avoid too many quick lunches at your desk. If pressure of work means you can't get out for a meal, vary the contents of your brown bag from day to day. Try bringing a salad and fresh fruit regularly. (See pages 52–93.)

HEALTH CHECKS

● Visit the dentist every six months. Brushing and flossing your teeth and massaging your gums will keep your mouth healthy and your breath fresh (see pages 178–179).

pursuit of promotion. This is the period in which the risk of heart and circulatory diseases begins to rise, so it is very important that you take steps to lower your risks of developing such diseases, This means, above all, paying particular attention to diet and exercise, and giving up smoking.

Alexander Graham Bell, ▶
American, invented the telephone in 1876, age 29.

● Be considerate of others at work and at home. Remember that they too have pressures and responsibilities.

● Share in the household and parenting chores, especially if your partner works outside the home too (see pages 200–201).
● Give your partner or special friend an unexpected gift that shows you care about her, and pursue an interesting activity together.

● Work hard at your job. Use your initiative and take on new responsibilities.

● Learn to recognize what makes you feel tense and irritable. What can you do to help yourself? Do you think you need professional help? (See pages 272–275, 302–337.)
● Be self-critical, and take positive action to overcome your shortcomings.

● Spend time reading to, and playing with, your children. Take an active interest in what they are doing. Be supportive of their efforts, but resist the temptation to dominate or take over their activities.

● Extend a welcome to new neighbors and new colleagues, and lay the foundations of good relationships.
● Make time in your busy schedule to have fun. Read a book, go to a concert, or see a movie.

● Discuss methods of birth control with your partner. If either of you is not satisfied with your present solution, consider alternatives (see pages 196–199).

● Reassess your appearance. Are there some areas that need special attention (see pages 142–147)? Are you taking good care of your body (see pages 160–183)?

Martin ▶
Luther King Jr,
American, won the Nobel Peace Prize in 1964, age 35.

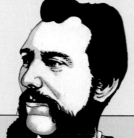

◀ *Walt Disney,* *American, created Mickey Mouse in the cartoon* Steamboat Willie *in 1928, age 27.*

● Eat and drink sensibly at business functions. Too much food and your digestion will suffer; too much drink and your job will suffer.
● Review your pattern of social drinking. Don't let drinks after work or before dinner slide into a drinking problem (see pages 289–293).

● Examine your diet and pattern of eating. Make sure you know how to control your intake of cholesterol (see pages 54–55).

John Glenn ▶
was the first American to orbit the Earth, on February 20, 1962, age 30.

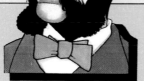

● Have your vision checked in this period. If you wear glasses or contact lenses, get a check-up every year (see pages 172–174).

● Have your blood pressure checked annually, as this is the period when the risk of heart disease begins to rise. Have a comprehensive physical check-up in this period (see pages 210–211).

SETTLING DOWN

From their mid-twenties to their mid-thirties the majority of women are concerned with completing their families. The risks associated with pregnancy gradually increase, and the risk of cancer of the breasts and cervix also increases, making regular gynecological examinations important. Women in this age group often change direction in their

EMOTIONAL AND MENTAL HEALTH. LEISURE

● Take all your allotted vacation time, and use it to get away from the normal routine at work and at home.

◄ *Valentina Tereshkova, of the Soviet Union, was the first woman to orbit the Earth, in June 1963, age 26.*

● Keep a positive outlook. If you are depressed, tense or irritable, look for the causes and take steps to deal with them (see pages 202–203, 272–275). Discuss your problems with your partner and your family. Do you think you need professional help (see pages 300–337)?

WORK, FINANCE AND FAMILY

● Work hard at your marriage or partnership (see pages 194–195, 200–201). Talk to your partner, share your daily experiences with him and take an interest in his life.

Amelia Earhart, ► *American, was the first woman to fly single-handed across the Atlantic Ocean, age 33, in May 1932.*

FITNESS AND BODY CARE

● Push yourself physically. Make time to exercise regularly. Exercise gives you the energy you need to care for your home and family; it also helps to counteract the effects of a sedentary and stressful job (see pages 94–159).

FOOD AND DRINK

● Eat sensibly (see pages 52–93). Maintain regular mealtimes, and avoid eating on the run. Make sure healthy and tasty snacks are available, particularly for the children.

● Control social drinking. Don't use drink to get rid of boredom or stress, and avoid solitary drinking (see pages 289–293).
● Eat and drink in moderation at business functions. Take these occasions into account in your overall nutritional plan.

HEALTH CHECKS

◄ *Mildred "Babe" Didrikson, American, won 17 major golf tournaments in a row in 1947, age 33.*

● Have a complete gynecological check-up every year. The chance of cancer of the breasts and cervix increases in this age group, and early detection is the best hope of successful treatment (see pages 204–207).

careers, a move commonly related to motherhood. These are the dangerous years for marriage, with divorce at its height. This is reflected in the fact that in the United States 34 is the average age at which a woman marries for the second time.

Florence Graham, ▶
Canadian, opened her first Elizabeth Arden salon in New York in 1912, age 28.

● Extend a welcome to new neighbors, and lay the foundations of good relationships.

● Reassess your career goals. Analyze how having a family will affect them (see pages 200–201), and consider if you will want to return to work after having children.
● Spend time with your parents, and foster good relations between them and your children.

● Don't get housebound. Work out a domestic routine that involves all the family in some responsibility and allows you sufficient time for your other activities.

● Get involved in the community and in the parent-teacher association. This is a good way to make new friends as well as contribute to the area in which you live.

● Learn to take a balanced view of your children. Spend time with them, and take a real interest in what they are doing. Encourage them in their steps toward independence (see pages 186–189, 264–265).

● Make time in your busy schedule to be alone. Use this opportunity to read a book, relax, or give yourself a special treat (see pages 302–311).
● Be self-critical and take positive action to overcome your shortcomings (see pages 332–337).

● A growing family usually means that this is a period of increased expenditure. Make a list of priorities and actively manage your money. Understand how to use credit cards to help your cash flow, but don't let them lure you into spending unwisely.

● Review your method of birth control with your partner. If either of you is not satisfied with it, consider an alternative (see pages 196–199).
● Stop smoking and drinking before you get pregnant (see pages 214–215, 284–293).

● Reassess the way you look. Make time to take good care of your body (see pages 160–183). Is there a particular aspect of your appearance that needs improving? If so, begin to work on it now (see pages 142–147, 232–233).

● Avoid unnecessary medications and drugs, especially during pregnancy (see pages 280–283).

Jeanette Rankin, *American,* ▶
was the first woman elected to the House of Representatives, in 1917, age 34.

Charlotte Brontë, ▼
English, published Jane Eyre *in 1847, age 31, and her sister Emily published the equally famous* Wuthering Heights *in 1848, age 30.*

● Restrict your intake of junk food, and avoid binge eating as much as crash dieting.

● If you really need to lose weight, follow a balanced program (see pages 72–83).

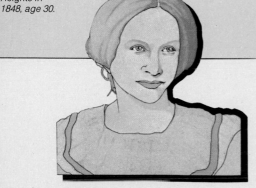

● Continue to check your breasts every month (see page 207). Consult your doctor about any changes or lumps.
● Visit the dentist every six months, and practice good dental hygiene between visits (see pages 178–179). Make a special visit if you become pregnant.

● Have your eyesight tested in this period. If you wear glasses or contact lenses, get a check-up every year (see pages 172–174).
● Have your blood pressure checked annually.

MATURE AND ESTABLISHED

The late thirties and early forties are years of anxiety for many men—years when the risk of heart disease is on the rise, years when emotional burn-out threatens. Some men at this age rush into tempestuous, and often short-lived, affairs with younger women in an effort to hold onto youth. Exercise, a healthy lifestyle, and regular medical check-ups can

EMOTIONAL AND MENTAL HEALTH. LEISURE

● Find new outlets for excess energy and ambitions: practice relaxation techniques or take up swimming (see pages 116–117, 272–273). Do something extravagant occasionally.

● Take stock of your friendships. Do you need to renew ties to old friends? Is it time to make an effort to enlarge your circle of friends?

◀ *James Joyce, Irish, published his great work* Ulysses *in February 1922, age 40.*

WORK, FINANCE AND FAMILY

● It's easy to get overloaded with responsibilities during the middle years. Work, family, and financial obligations all create mental and emotional pressure. Make a conscious effort to keep your priorities in balance (see pages 266–275).

● Find ways to spend more quality time with your family (see pages 154–155).

● If you feel you deserve a promotion, go for it.

FITNESS AND BODY CARE

◀ *Roald Amundsen of Norway became the first man to reach the South Pole, December 14, 1911, age 39.*

● Make time to exercise regularly, at least three times a week. If lack of free time is your excuse, look for new ways to increase your motivation (see pages 94–159).

FOOD AND DRINK

● Eat sensibly to help control calorie and alcohol consumption. Try new foods; don't get stuck in a rut. Many businessmen restrict the number of working lunches or parties they attend in a given week.

● Be aware that your metabolism slows, and your calorie needs decrease, as you get older. At age 45 a man needs approximately 250–300 fewer calories each day than he did at age 18.

HEALTH CHECKS

● The body performs less well as it ages; an annual physical check-up will monitor early signs of breakdown (see pages 100–101).

Jonas Salk, American, ▶ *successfully tested his polio vaccine in 1952, age 37.*

MEN 36-45

help a man cope with the underlying tension. He will feel better about himself as he enters his forties, and be likelier to stay in shape for the later years of middle age.

● Revitalize your sex life (see pages 194–195). Even if you are happily married, you and your partner can experiment sexually to keep your intimate relationship fresh.

● Take a more active role in your community. Many organizations vital to the community depend on the work of mature, experienced volunteers.
● Make sure that you take a vacation every year even if you don't have big plans.

● Read at least one good book a week, or see a movie or show.

◀ **King Edward VIII** abdicated the British throne on December 10, 1936, age 42, to marry Wallis Simpson.

● Avoid impetuous spending to keep up with friends and neighbors.

● Review your travel patterns: Are you on the road too much? Is travel wearing you out physically? If so, what can you do about it? (See pages 270–271).

◀ **John F. Kennedy** was the youngest elected American President, November 1960, age 43.

● Many men who already have children consider having a vasectomy at this time of life. Any man electing this surgery, however, should know that sterilization is usually permanent (see pages 196–199).

● Take up a new sport, perhaps something you have always wanted to try and have kept putting off—like cross-country skiing or scuba diving.

Neil Armstrong of the ▶ USA became the first man to set foot on the moon, July 20, 1969, age 38.

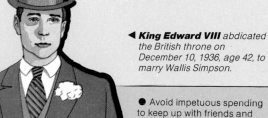

● Avoid social and unnecessary prescription drugs that provide a quick fix but no real solution to any problem (see pages 280–281).

● If you must have a drink to get through the day, you are probably developing a drinking problem. If you think you are drinking too much but cannot control it, seek help now (see pages 289–293).

◀ **Christiaan Barnard,** South African surgeon, performed the world's first heart transplant, December 3, 1967, age 45.

● Avoid eating on the run. Rushed, irregular mealtimes can lead to digestive problems and overeating (see pages 52–93).

● Have your blood cholesterol checked annually. Elevated blood cholesterol has been blamed for atherosclerosis and heart disease (see pages 53–71).

● Visit the dentist every six months. Check-ups, regular cleaning, and treatment when necessary, will help maintain healthy teeth and gums for life (see pages 178–179).

● Vision changes during these years, and most people become more far-sighted. Regular check-ups by an ophthalmologist will detect any problems (see pages 172–174).

● Get your blood pressure checked every year. High blood pressure (hypertension) is associated with kidney failure, heart disease, and stroke (see pages 95–101).

MATURE AND ESTABLISHED

A woman between 36 and 45 can exploit her vigor and experience to the full. At 36, for example, the typical woman will have sent her last child to school and will be free to reorganize her life. Many women will choose to return to work outside the home, while others will strive to advance their positions in existing careers. As women adopt lifestyles

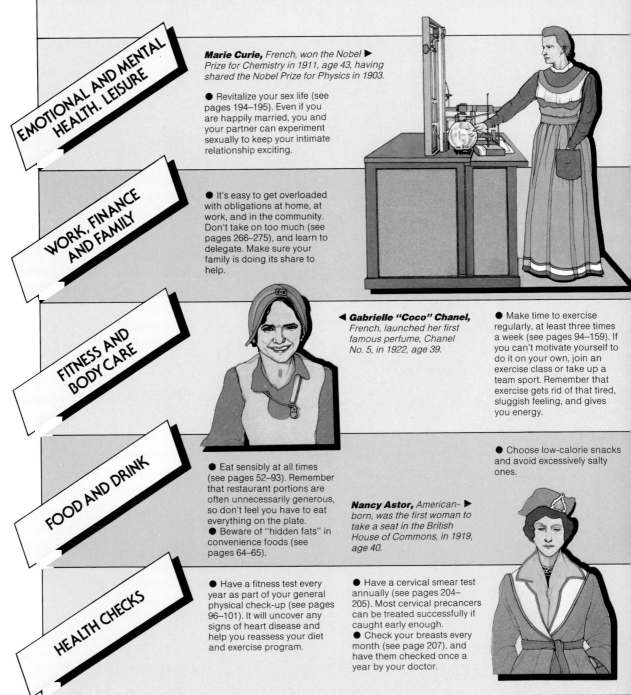

EMOTIONAL AND MENTAL HEALTH. LEISURE

Marie Curie, *French, won the Nobel* ▶ *Prize for Chemistry in 1911, age 43, having shared the Nobel Prize for Physics in 1903.*

● Revitalize your sex life (see pages 194–195). Even if you are happily married, you and your partner can experiment sexually to keep your intimate relationship exciting.

WORK, FINANCE AND FAMILY

● It's easy to get overloaded with obligations at home, at work, and in the community. Don't take on too much (see pages 266–275), and learn to delegate. Make sure your family is doing its share to help.

FITNESS AND BODY CARE

◀ **Gabrielle "Coco" Chanel,** *French, launched her first famous perfume, Chanel No. 5, in 1922, age 39.*

● Make time to exercise regularly, at least three times a week (see pages 94–159). If you can't motivate yourself to do it on your own, join an exercise class or take up a team sport. Remember that exercise gets rid of that tired, sluggish feeling, and gives you energy.

FOOD AND DRINK

● Eat sensibly at all times (see pages 52–93). Remember that restaurant portions are often unnecessarily generous, so don't feel you have to eat everything on the plate.
● Beware of "hidden fats" in convenience foods (see pages 64–65).

● Choose low-calorie snacks and avoid excessively salty ones.

Nancy Astor, *American-* ▶ *born, was the first woman to take a seat in the British House of Commons, in 1919, age 40.*

HEALTH CHECKS

● Have a fitness test every year as part of your general physical check-up (see pages 96–101). It will uncover any signs of heart disease and help you reassess your diet and exercise program.

● Have a cervical smear test annually (see pages 204–205). Most cervical precancers can be treated successfully if caught early enough.
● Check your breasts every month (see page 207), and have them checked once a year by your doctor.

similar to those of men, the danger of heart disease is increasing in this age group, in which cancer of the breast and cervix are already major risks. With this knowledge, and aware that the first blush of youth has passed, a woman should aim to remain physically and mentally fit as she approaches midlife.

● Don't become a nagger. Discuss your problems openly with your partner, and look for positive solutions (see pages 200–203).
● If all the children are now away from home, begin to think of yourself as an individual again, not just as an extension of your family.

● Learn to deal with everyday tensions, and examine ways to minimize tension-inducing aspects of your life. Make time for quiet reflection, and try new ways of relaxing (see pages 266–269, 300–311).

● Read a good book once a week, or go to a movie or show. Do something extravagant occasionally.

◀ *Dorothea Lange, American, published her deeply moving photographic record of the Depression,* An American Exodus, *in 1939, age 44.*

Emmeline Pankhurst, *English, founded the Women's Social and Political Union in 1903 to fight for women's rights, age 45.* ▼

● Take a look at your career. Can you achieve greater job satisfaction where you are? If you think you deserve a promotion, or want a change of direction, go for it (see pages 260–299).

● Reorganize your life when all the children are at school. Consider working outside the home. Look for a job that offers satisfaction, and retrain if necessary.
● Spend more time with your family in activities you can enjoy together (see pages 154–155).

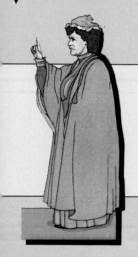

● Maintain a regular program of cleansing and moisturizing your skin, and protect it from the weather. Wear a sunscreen for protection against ultraviolet rays (see pages 162–167).

● Take a good look at yourself. Is there any aspect of the way you look that you think you should improve or change? You can do it now (see pages 260–299).

● Consider stopping the pill in favor of another method of birth control (see pages 196–199). The risk of thrombosis, which has been associated with the pill among other factors, is increased in this age group.

● If you are drinking regularly when you are alone and feeling bored, you might be developing a drinking problem. If you cannot change this pattern by yourself, seek help now (see pages 289–293).

Margaret Mitchell, ▶ *American, published* Gone with the Wind *in 1936, age 36, and won the Pulitzer Prize the next year.*

● Eat plenty of fresh fruit and vegetables; most are low in calories and in sodium/ potassium ratio (see pages 54–79), and provide fiber.

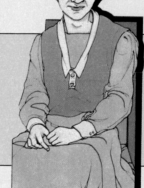

● Have your blood pressure tested annually. High blood pressure (hypertension) is associated with kidney failure, heart disease, and stroke, and indicates that a woman should stop taking the contraceptive pill.

● Most people become more farsighted as they get older (see pages 172–174). Yearly visits to the ophthalmologist will ensure that you have the right corrective lenses.
● Visit the dentist every six months, and practice good dental hygiene between visits (see pages 178–179).

INTO MIDDLE AGE

For men in the Western world heart disease is the major health risk from age 45 onward. But even in middle life it is not too late for a man to begin to take fitness and well-being seriously for the sake of his life expectancy. During the midlife transition a man might experience a deep depression or feel compelled to make sudden, frantic attempts to try

EMOTIONAL AND MENTAL HEALTH. LEISURE

● Nothing makes you old as fast and as certainly as a closed mind and a rigid attitude. Be brave enough to consider new ideas, to change your mind, and, if necessary, your behavior (see pages 236–259).

● Be hopeful of the future. You can have many more healthy years ahead of you. Look forward to, and plan for, all the things you still want to do (see pages 236–249).

Daniel Defoe, English, ▶ *published* Robinson Crusoe *in April 1719, age 59.*

WORK, FINANCE AND FAMILY

● Reappraise your working life. Is it giving you satisfaction, or are there ways you can reduce the stress (see pages 266–269)? Learn the art of delegation, and move with the times in adapting to new methods and technology.

FITNESS AND BODY CARE

◀ *Howard Carter, English, discovered the tomb of the ancient Egyptian king Tutankhamen in November 1922, age 49.*

● Make time to exercise at least three times a week. Start slowly if you have been inactive for a while (see pages 94–159, 250–255).
● Avoid unnecessary medication and drugs (see pages 280–283). Use exercise to give you energy and keep you mentally alert.

FOOD AND DRINK

● Review your drinking habits. Have you gradually increased your consumption to cope with stress at work? Remember that alcohol is ultimately a depressant, so check that you are not drinking more and feeling able to do less (see pages 289–293).

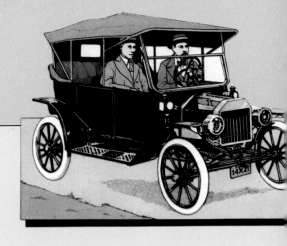

HEALTH CHECKS

Henry Ford, American, ▶ *introduced the assembly line to manufacturing in 1913, age 50.*

● Maintain regular visits to the dentist and hygienist every six months, as well as regular dental care at home (see pages 178–179).

to beat the aging process. Both of these behavioral patterns can prove fatal. However, with sensible care and attention to his physical and mental well-being, a man can reach the age of 60 with new confidence and security, ready to enjoy the next phase of his life to the full.

● Build on your experience and set yourself new goals that are a real challenge (see pages 260–263).
● Try to improve all your relationships (see pages 186–213). Spend your time with other people in a positive manner, and avoid complaining and nagging.

● Use your leisure in a creative way. Make time for constructive activity as well as for relaxation (see pages 260–299).

Marshall Field, *American,* ▶ *opened the world's first department store in 1881, age 47.*

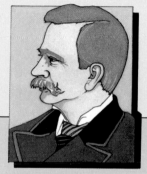

● Take pleasure in the success of younger people, and be tolerant if their perspective on life is different.
● Take all your allocated vacations. Break your routine and go somewhere new or do something different (see pages 260–299).

● Encourage your grown-up children to leave home. Continue to take an interest in their lives, but respect their independence, and build good relationships on an adult-to-adult basis.

● Begin thinking about, and planning for, retirement. Review your financial plans and attend a retirement training program (see pages 240–243).

● Consider moving when all the children have left. Discuss all the possibilities with your partner to decide what will suit you both (see pages 244–245).

● Start learning to be a good grandfather (see pages 236–239).

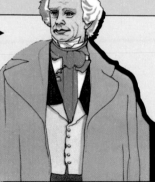

Samuel Morse, *American,* ▶ *developed the Morse Code in 1838, age 47, for use on his invention, the telegraph.*

● Take a good look in the mirror. Could you improve your appearance? Generally, men's clothing is not age-sensitive, but avoid trying to recapture youth by wearing the latest teenage fashions.

● Check your weight and body mass index (see pages 72–75), and your posture (see pages 138–141). Take positive action to get rid of any sign of a developing paunch (see pages 142–143).

● Choose foods that are low in fats and sodium to help keep your heart healthy (see pages 64–65).

Alexandre Eiffel, *French, completed his famous tower in Paris in 1889, age 56.* ▼

● Your calorie needs will have decreased if you are less active than you were just a few years ago. Make sure you adjust your eating habits (see pages 52–93).

● Eat sensibly at all times. Don't use business lunches as an excuse to pile up the calories (see pages 52–93, 338–341).

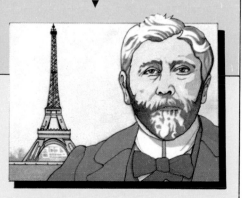

● Get your hearing tested (see pages 175–177).
● Have a thorough physical check-up every year. This should always include a blood pressure test and a prostate examination (see pages 210–211).

● Have your eyesight tested in this period. As you grow older, your vision can continue to change, and you might require corrective lenses to aid near and middle distance vision (see pages 172–174).

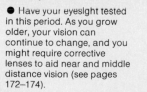

INTO MIDDLE AGE

Menopause is the greatest hurdle a woman has to leap in the years between 45 and 60— on the average it occurs at 51. Both physical and emotional problems are common in connection with the menopause, but by working for fitness of body and mind a woman can do a great deal to ease herself through this transition period. Cancer and

EMOTIONAL AND MENTAL HEALTH. LEISURE

● Be prepared to deal with an identity crisis. Now that the children are grown up and independent, your role as a mother is diminished, leaving you more time to pursue your interests (see pages 260–299).
● Set yourself new goals. Learn a new skill and a new hobby.

● Discuss your problems and concerns with your partner, look for positive solutions, and avoid nagging and complaining (see pages 200–201, 294–299).

Margaret Thatcher became ▶ the first woman British Prime Minister in May 1979, age 53.

WORK, FINANCE AND FAMILY

● Reappraise your working life. Are there ways to reduce the stress and increase the satisfaction (see pages 266–269)? Keep up with new developments and technology, and be prepared to delegate.

● Encourage your grown-up children to leave the nest and live independently. Be prepared to help them on their way, but avoid interfering. Build a good relationship on an adult-to-adult basis.

FITNESS AND BODY CARE

◀ *Rachel Carson, American, crowned a distinguished career as a marine biologist when, age 55, she published* Silent Spring, *which eventually led to the ban on the use of DDT in the US.*

● Motivate yourself to exercise. If you've been ignoring this aspect of your life, start slowly and build up to optimum fitness gradually (see pages 94–158, 250–255).
● Take positive action to combat symptoms of menopause (see pages 208–209).

FOOD AND DRINK

● Know that your calorie needs are gradually decreasing, and make minor adjustments to your normal diet (see pages 52–93).

● Avoid eating because you are bored, unhappy, or angry. Use food to nourish your body, not to pacify your emotions.

HEALTH CHECKS

● Have a thorough physical check-up every year. Make sure that this includes a complete gynecological examination, a blood pressure test, and a breast examination (see pages 204–207).

Frances Perkins ▶ became the first woman to serve in the US Cabinet when she was appointed Secretary of Labor in 1933, age 51.

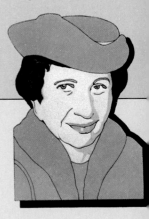

heart disease are the major killers in this age group, so regular health checks are essential. This is a time when growing children are becoming less demanding and grown-up children may already have left home. The transition can bring new freedom and enjoyment to partnerships, it's also a good time to start planning for the future.

- Keep your sex life alive and exciting, and be aware of your own and your partner's changing needs and desires (see pages 194–195).
- Take pleasure in the accomplishments of younger people, and don't be jealous of your children's youth and exuberance.

- Be hopeful about the future. You can have many more healthy and active years ahead of you, so look forward to, and start planning for, all the things you want to do (see pages 236–249).

- Avoid getting stuck in a rut that makes you feel stale and old (see pages 236–259). Be brave enough to consider new ideas.

Willa Cather, American, ▶ was the first woman to win the Pulitzer Prize, awarded for One of Ours in 1922, age 49.

- Your home might be bigger than you really need or want after the children have gone. Discuss the possibility and desirability of moving with your partner (see pages 244–245).

- Start learning to be a good grandmother (see pages 236–239).

- Start thinking about and planning for retirement. Review your financial plans and attend a retirement training program (see pages 240–243).

Mary Baker Eddy, ▶ American, founded the Christian Science Association in 1876, age 55.

- Keep abreast of new fashion developments.

- Assess your body care routine. Be sure you are making enough time to take good care of your skin, hair, nails, and particularly your feet (see pages 160–183).
- Dress well, but avoid imitating the young by donning teenage clothes.

- Make time to pursue a constructive activity as well as to relax (see pages 246–249).
- Avoid unnecessary drugs and medications (see pages 280–283). Take positive action, not pills, to overcome problems of boredom, depression, or insomnia.

- You might not be able to control what is served at social functions, but you can eat discriminatingly. Don't be embarrassed to forgo an offered dish overladen with the fats, salt, or calories you know you want to avoid.

- Be sensible about social drinking, and avoid drinking alone. Alcohol is a depressant and is high in calories (see pages 289–293).

- Women who have been through menopause are more at risk from osteoporosis, so have your bone condition checked annually (see pages 208–209).
- Continue to check your breasts every month (see page 207).

- Have your eyesight tested in this period. Choose becoming frames if changes in your vision mean you need glasses for short and middle distances (see pages 172–174).
- Get your hearing tested (see pages 175–177).

- Maintain regular visits to the dentist and hygienist every six months, as well as regular dental care at home (see pages 178–179).

▲ **Katharine Graham,** American, became sole proprietor of The Washington Post, famous for its high standard of journalism, in 1963, age 46.

ADJUSTING TO RETIREMENT

For both men and women the decade between 60 and 70 is a time of adjustment to the fact of retirement from full-time paid employment. Properly planned, these years can bring the fulfillment of all the efforts put into the previous decades of life. Positive

EMOTIONAL AND MENTAL HEALTH. LEISURE

● Put plans for retirement into action. Make sure you replace your daily working pattern with new, fulfilling activities (see pages 240–245).

● Stay young at heart and in your mind (see pages 258–259). Maintain a sharp interest in current affairs, and try to move with the times.

● Take up a new hobby, perhaps one you never had time for before (see pages 246–249), and take an active role in the community.
● Take a trip that you've always dreamed about.
● Review old friendships, and do things together, now that you have the time.

WORK, FINANCE AND FAMILY

● Be an active grandparent, and enjoy doing things with your grandchildren.
● Look into the possibility of doing volunteer work. There are often opportunities in local charity shops, in hospitals, and in community organizations (see pages 246–249).

FITNESS AND BODY CARE

● Get enough rest, but avoid sleeping too much (see pages 276–277).

▲
Boris Pasternak, *of the Soviet Union, won the Nobel Prize for Literature for his novel Dr Zhivago in 1958, age 68.*

● Exercise regularly. Remember to start slowly if you have been inactive for any length of time (see pages 250–257). Motivate yourself by joining an exercise class for your age group or club where you can participate in a sport you enjoy.

FOOD AND DRINK

◄ **Golda Meir** *became Prime Minister of Israel on March 17, 1969, age 70.*

● Make sure your diet includes at least one cooked meal a day (see pages 52–93), and avoid eating a big meal late at night.
● Eat a wide variety of foods, and maintain a balanced diet. This is just as important now as it was when you were younger (see pages 62–65).

HEALTH CHECKS

● Some loss of hearing is common in this age group. Be sure to have your hearing tested annually, and take advantage of the modern aids available to minimize this problem (see pages 175–177, 238–239).

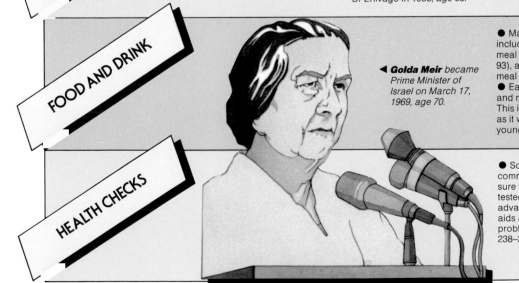

thinking and new beginnings are the keys to physical and mental fitness at this time, when a couple at last has the leisure to do things together again. But because women usually outlive men, the sixties are also the years in which widowhood often begins.

◀ **Mother Teresa of Calcutta,** Albanian, won the first Pope John XXIII Peace Prize in 1971, age 61, and the Nobel Peace Prize in 1979.

● Learn to deal with the deaths of friends and relatives, and don't be afraid to discuss your own mortality with your loved ones (see pages 258–259).
● Learn to relax, but beware of becoming apathetic (see pages 250–255, 272–275).

Eleanor Roosevelt, ▶ American, became Chairman of the United Nations Commission for Human Rights in 1946, age 61.

● Get out of the house every day if the weather allows. Visit the library, go to a museum, or just take a walk.
● Consider moving to a smaller house or apartment that will be more convenient (see pages 240–245).

● Examine your finances and know where your money is going. Avoid economizing too much, or overspending.
● Make a will or revise an existing one (see pages 258–259).

● Take good care of your body, paying special attention to problem areas such as dry skin and feet (see pages 160–183).

◀ **Noah Webster,** American, published his famous dictionary in 1828, age 69.

● Learn to accept that you might not be able to do everything as well or as easily as you used to, and be careful (see pages 256–257). Assess whether you are fit enough to continue driving.

● Avoid extremes of temperature, and always dress adequately for the weather.

● Are you as active now as you used to be? If not, reduce your calorie intake until you increase your expenditure of energy again (see pages 68–69, 338–341).

Edgar Rice Burroughs, ▶ American, became the oldest war correspondent in the South Pacific in 1942, age 66.

● Have your eyesight tested every year. If you need glasses to aid your vision, wear them (see pages 172–174, 238–239).
● As the heart ages, it becomes less efficient, so make sure you have an EKG and a blood pressure check every year (see pages 96–97).

● Women should check their breasts every month (see page 207), and have them checked by a doctor every year when they have their cervical smear test (see pages 204–206).

● Visit the dentist and hygienist every six months, and maintain good dental care at home (see pages 178–179).

OLD AND GRACEFUL

The years lived over the age of 70 should be, above all, enjoyed to the full. History shows a staggering range of achievements by men and women over 70, and there is no reason for anyone to think he or she cannot reach new heights in these decades of life. Although these are the years in which the physical aging process takes its toll, a

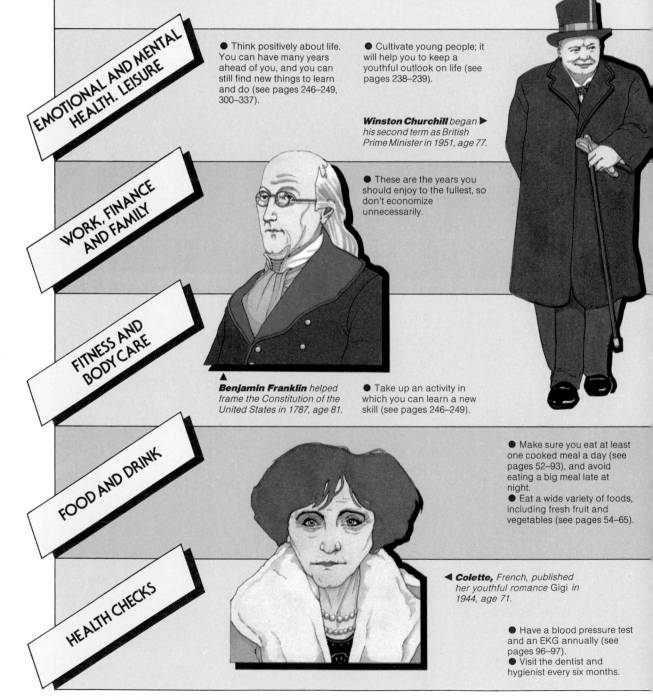

EMOTIONAL AND MENTAL HEALTH, LEISURE

● Think positively about life. You can have many years ahead of you, and you can still find new things to learn and do (see pages 246–249, 300–337).

● Cultivate young people; it will help you to keep a youthful outlook on life (see pages 238–239).

Winston Churchill began ▶ his second term as British Prime Minister in 1951, age 77.

WORK, FINANCE AND FAMILY

● These are the years you should enjoy to the fullest, so don't economize unnecessarily.

FITNESS AND BODY CARE

▲
Benjamin Franklin helped frame the Constitution of the United States in 1787, age 81.

● Take up an activity in which you can learn a new skill (see pages 246–249).

FOOD AND DRINK

● Make sure you eat at least one cooked meal a day (see pages 52–93), and avoid eating a big meal late at night.
● Eat a wide variety of foods, including fresh fruit and vegetables (see pages 54–65).

◀ *Colette, French, published her youthful romance Gigi in 1944, age 71.*

HEALTH CHECKS

● Have a blood pressure test and an EKG annually (see pages 96–97).
● Visit the dentist and hygienist every six months.

positive and youthful attitude, reflected in a willingness to learn, participate and enjoy, will pay enormous dividends in terms of the quality and length of life.

● Face up to the fact of death, and discuss it with your family (see pages 258–259, 298–299).

● Share your experience and your memories. Be prepared to help younger people; they can learn a lot from you.
● Remember to have fun. Go to the movies or a show, or just out for a meal.

◀ **Grandma Moses,** American, had her first painting exhibition in 1940, age 80.

● Make a will, or revise an existing one if necessary (see pages 258–259).

● Continue to be a good friend to your children, and a caring grand- or great-grandparent.

● Get out of the house every day if possible. Have you found some volunteer work to do? Is there an interesting series of lectures to go to at the library?

Claude Monet, French, ▶ painted his famous series of water lily pictures from 1916 to 1925, age 73 to 84.

● Most people tend to need less sleep as they get older (see pages 270–271). Avoid sleeping too much because you are bored—there are plenty of interesting things to fill your time.

● Motivate yourself to exercise, so that you maintain strength and flexibility, but don't try to do too much (see pages 250–255).

● Continue to take pride in your appearance, and maintain a routine of caring for your body (see pages 160–183).
● Take only those medications that you really need (see pages 280–283).

● Depending on your level of physical activity, you might need to adjust your calorie intake. Be sure you are eating enough to provide the energy to be active (see pages 68–69, 338–341).
● Drink plenty of fluids (see pages 90–91), especially during warm weather.

● This is the age at which you might notice a loss of hearing. There are many unobtrusive aids to help you overcome this, so have your hearing tested every year (see pages 175–177, 238–239).

● Have your eyesight tested every year (see pages 172–174).
● Women should continue to check their breasts every month (see page 207).

▲ **Barbara McClintock,** American, won the Nobel Prize for Medicine in 1983, age 81.

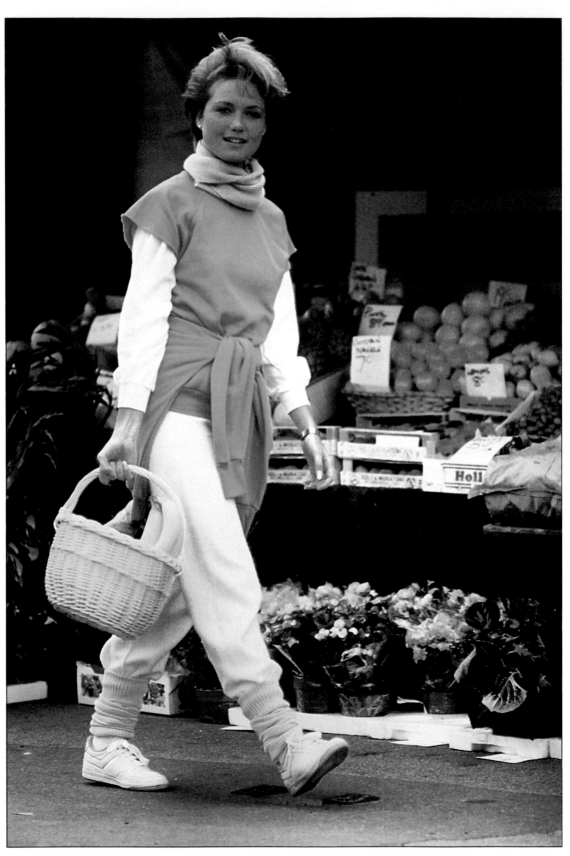

EATING FOR HEALTH

Food is the fuel that keeps the body alive, and the pleasures of the table are among the joys of life. Eating for health won't turn you into a pleasure prohibitionist. The aim is to make eating enjoyable while curbing or eliminating eating habits that work against your long-term health and well-being.

The simple guidelines in this chapter will promote fitness and health by making sure you get the nutrients you need without eating too much. They will produce good body growth and maintenance, decrease your risks of developing diet-related chronic degenerative diseases in middle age, and help to assure a good quality of life as you get older.

Although no diet guidelines come with an ironclad guarantee to protect everyone against all forms of disease, the advice given here will help you to come close to an optimal diet. In particular, it will help to make sure that you get sufficient vitamins and minerals, show you how to control the amounts of sodium and cholesterol in your diet, and make you aware of the possible causes of food allergies.

The guidelines for healthy eating apply to every member of the family, and also satisfy taste and social custom. You will find that the healthy diet is made up of foods you like. It takes the drudgery out of cooking, and helps to keep both waistlines and budgets under control. For those who need to lose weight, this chapter also contains advice for dieters.

NUTRIENTS AND FOODS

Food provides the mixture of nutrients that the body needs, not just for fitness and well-being, but for life itself. The three main classes of food are proteins, fats, and carbohydrates. They supply the body with energy and the basic building blocks needed for growth and maintenance. They are the macronutrients, the foods you must eat in considerable quantities each day in order to stay in good health.

To have a healthy diet, you must choose your macronutrients wisely. This is not always easy, since many traditional ideas about food are now being modified or changed completely as scientists continue to learn more about nutrition and how our bodies utilize food.

Until recently, for example, it was accepted that meat is an ideal source of high-quality protein, and that a perfect diet should contain substantial quantities of red meat. In many ways this is a sound notion, since protein is essential and red meat contains plenty of high-quality protein. However, the problem with eating red meat is that it is difficult to eat large amounts of it without also ingesting a lot of harmful animal fat at the same time. And nutritionists have found that there is no virtue in providing the body with more protein than it needs. The quality of protein in certain grains and legumes, which is often designated "second class," is first rate when used in the right combinations. Therefore it seems healthier to eat a more balanced mix of animal and vegetable proteins rather than emphasizing only those from animal sources.

Proteins

The human body is made of proteins: the structural parts of the body cells that stop them from collapsing are based on protein, as are the working parts of all body cells. Every protein consists of a string of building blocks called amino acids. The human body needs about 22 amino acids to make all its proteins. It can manufacture 14 of these in its cells. The others, called the essential amino acids, must be obtained from food. Much of the chemical activity of the body consists in extracting amino acids from food sources and rearranging them into new proteins. The Recommended Dietary Allowances (RDA), which are guidelines published by the National Academy of Sciences, suggest 0.8 grams of protein per kilogram of body weight.

Carbohydrates

Carbohydrates are the most underrated of the three macronutrients that the body needs. They provide the body with energy, help to control the breakdown of protein, and protect the body against toxins.

Glucose is the basic chemical that fuels the body. All the energy-producing chemical reactions of body cells are geared to using glucose, although they can use other fuels, including fats. Glucose is one of the group of carbohydrates known as monosaccharides, the simple, single-molecule sugars.

Polysaccharides, of which starch is the most important, are composed of many monosaccharide molecules and are broken down by the body into two or more sugars. Commonly referred to as complex carbohydrates, they are found in fruits, vegetables, and grains. They have a high nutritive value, providing vitamins, minerals, proteins, and fiber in addition to the sugars used for energy. Because complex carbohydrates take longer to digest than simple ones, they are more effective in staving off sensations of hunger.

Fats

Fats are an essential part of the diet, but too much of the wrong kind can be bad for your health.

All the fats you eat are composed of fatty acids, long molecules of carbon, hydrogen, and oxygen. Ounce for ounce, they produce more than twice as much energy as carbohydrates, and also carry vitamins A, D, E, and K. The body needs fats for growth and repair, and fat stored in the body tissues insulates the body, helps it to maintain a regular temperature, and cushions vital organs.

The most important feature of dietary fats is their degree of saturation, a term that refers to their molecular structure. Unsaturated fats do not produce as much blood cholesterol as saturated fats. Since a high level of cholesterol in the bloodstream is often associated with heart disease, experts recommend eating smaller quantities of saturated fats. In the average American diet today 38–40 percent of total calories are obtained from fat, about half of which is saturated fat. The American Heart Association suggests that people decrease their total fat consumption to 30 percent or less of their total calorie intake, and reduce saturated fats to about 10 percent.

All natural fats are a mixture of saturated and

unsaturated fatty acids, but generally animal fats are more highly saturated, and vegetable fats tend to be more unsaturated. There are exceptions: poultry and fish oils are high in unsaturated fatty acids, while coconut oil, a vegetable oil, is high in saturated fats.

Cholesterol

Cholesterol is a complex waxy substance that is an essential component of the walls of body cells. It is also used to make vitamin D, hormones, bile acids, and nerve tissues. It is carried around the body in the bloodstream by lipoproteins, proteins to which lipids, or fats, are attached. Some studies have shown that high levels of blood cholesterol increase the chances of having a heart attack.

Cholesterol is present in foods, but only about 15 percent of all blood cholesterol comes from the diet. Even very dramatic cuts in your consumption of cholesterol have only a slight effect on your overall blood cholesterol because most of the cholesterol in the blood is made by your body, mainly in the liver. The body continues to make some cholesterol regardless of the amount your diet contains. As a result, some of the excess dietary cholesterol may be deposited in your blood vessels; the rest is eliminated.

The best diet-related way to reduce the amount of cholesterol in your blood is to lower your intake of all kinds of fats, particularly saturated fats. A lot of saturated fat in the diet encourages the liver to pour out large amounts of cholesterol.

The type of lipoprotein on which cholesterol is carried is also an important factor influencing the risk of coronary artery disease. Most of the cholesterol in the blood is bound to low-density lipoprotein (LDL) and is called LDL cholesterol. LDL cholesterol is the major contributor to total cholesterol levels. The higher the LDL cholesterol level, the higher is the risk of coronary artery disease.

The remaining cholesterol in the blood is bound to high-density lipoprotein (HDL), and therefore is called HDL cholesterol. HDL cholesterol appears to protect against the risk of heart attacks, so the higher it is, the better.

Aim to increase your ratio of HDL to LDL cholesterol, through diet, to lower overall cholesterol levels, and exercise, which has some effect in increasing HDL cholesterol. Most Americans consume 450–500 milligrams of cholesterol a day, but the American Heart Association recommends 300 milligrams a day or less. A simple way to do this is to moderate your use of eggs and organ meats. Annual checks on blood cholesterol levels are advised, particularly for men, from midlife onward.

CHOLESTEROL AND HEART DISEASE

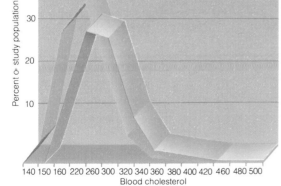

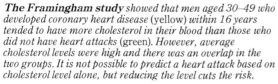

The Framingham study showed that men aged 30–49 who developed coronary heart disease (yellow) within 16 years tended to have more cholesterol in their blood than those who did not have heart attacks (green). However, average cholesterol levels were high and there was an overlap in the two groups. It is not possible to predict a heart attack based on cholesterol level alone, but reducing the level cuts the risk.

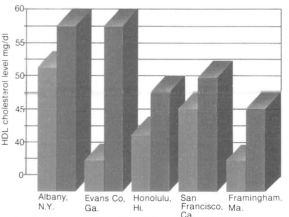

A whole range of studies of the relationship between cholesterol and coronary heart disease suggests that the higher the level of high-density lipoprotein (HDL) cholesterol, the greater the protection against such disease. The graphs show a comparison between men who developed coronary heart disease (blue) and those who did not (purple) plotted against blood HDL concentration.

FOOD GROUPS

In order to be healthy you need to obtain from your food about 40 essential nutrients—vitamins, minerals, proteins, and fats that your body cannot produce for itself or cannot produce in sufficient quantities.

It is necessary to eat many different foods to satisfy your nutrient needs. Most foods supply several nutrients, not just one or two; but no food supplies all of the essential nutrients in the type and amount you need. For example, milk provides protein, fats, sugar, calcium, phosphorus, riboflavin and other B vitamins as well as vitamins A and D, but is very low in iron and vitamin C. You cannot compensate for the lack of one nutrient by eating more of another.

A varied diet
If you eat a varied and well-balanced diet each day, you should get adequate amounts of the nutrients you need for good health. The foods you eat can be grouped according to the types and amounts of nutrients they contain. By using the information here and on pages 62–83, you can make sure that your food choices each day will give you enough protein, minerals, vitamins, and fiber while keeping your consumption of fat, sugar, and sodium within healthy limits.

Breads, cereals, and other grains
Contrary to popular opinion, the foods in this group are *not* especially fattening. It is the high-fat and high-sugar extras that you eat with them that need to be controlled. All the foods in this group supply B vitamins and iron. Whole-grain products also add fiber, magnesium, zinc, and folic acid.

Vegetables
There are three categories of vegetables: the dark green and deep yellow, the starchy, and other vegetables, such as onions, cabbage, and lettuce. Each group is important because it supplies different nutrients.

Most people should eat more vegetables, especially the dark green and deep yellow types, and dried beans or peas. They contain good quantities of folic acid, magnesium, zinc, and fiber, which are often in low supply, while adding little fat or sodium to your diet. In addition, the dark green leafy and deep yellow vegetables are especially good sources of vitamin A. The dark green types also provide the minerals iron and calcium. Cruciferous vegetables, such as cabbage and broccoli, are also thought to prevent certain kinds of cancer.

Starchy vegetables are good sources of carbohydrate, fiber, vitamins C and B_6, iron, and magnesium. Dried beans and peas are also high in protein, folic acid, and zinc. Other vegetables contribute fiber and some vitamin C.

Fruits
All fruits, especially citrus fruits, are good sources of vitamin C. They also provide folic acid, potassium, and other nutrients, and are low in calories, sodium, and fat. Those with edible seeds and skins served raw also provide dietary fiber.

Meat, fish, poultry, and eggs
These are excellent sources of protein, and good sources of phosphorus and niacin. They also add iron, zinc, vitamins B_6 and B_{12}, and trace minerals to the diet. Some items, such as the fattier cuts of red meats and processed meats are rather high in fat and calories, while other members of the group, such as poultry, are lower.

Dairy products
Milk and milk products, such as cream, yogurt, cheese, and butter, are the main sources of calcium in the diet. They also provide significant amounts of protein and vitamins A, B_2 (riboflavin), B_6, and B_{12}. Full-fat, or whole milk products are higher in fat and calories than low-fat or skim milk. Keep this in mind if you are trying to moderate your consumption of fat.

Fats, sweets, and alcohol
These foods may be fun to consume, but they supply calories and little else. The amounts you can safely eat depend on your calorie needs.

The digestive system
In order for the food you eat to be used by your body, it must go through a number of physical and chemical changes in the digestive system. The function of the digestive system is to break down complex molecules of proteins, carbohydrates, and fats into their smaller constituent molecules, to absorb those that are necessary to keep the body's biochemical systems working, and to expel the residue as feces.

It does this through a variety of mechanical and chemical processes. Chewing, for example, is a mechanical process, as are the muscular movements of the digestive tract. Hormones trigger the secretions of other chemicals—acids, enzymes, and bile—which help break down the food particles and molecules, and release the nutrients for absorption and distribution around the body.

An unhealthy diet can be a factor in causing problems ranging from tooth decay to gallstones, and possibly some cancers of the digestive tract. Stress and emotional upsets (see pages 266–269) also affect the digestive system, and can lead to disabling conditions, such as ulcers. The illustration and chart below show the relationship between diet and digestion.

DIET AND DIGESTION

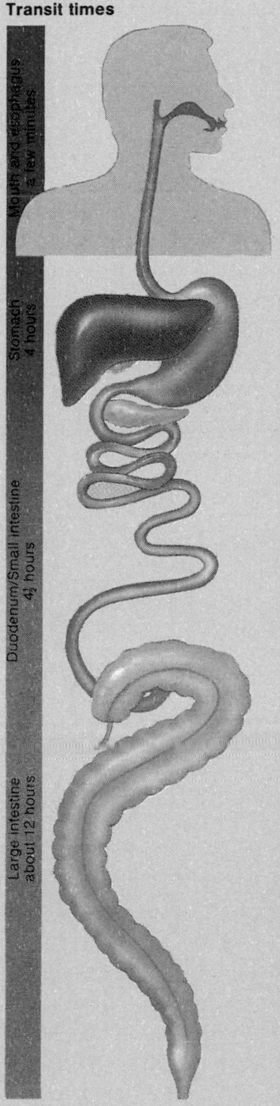

Transit times

Mouth and esophagus a few minutes

Stomach 4 hours

Duodenum/Small intestine 4½ hours

Large intestine about 12 hours

The digestive system	Problems	Prevention and remedy
Mouth and teeth Food is broken down by chewing and is moistened with saliva to start the digestive process, then swallowed as a bolus.	An infection caused by the interaction of bacteria and sugar or other carbohydrates breaks down the protective enamel and causes tooth decay.	Eating less sticky sugary foods and practicing good dental hygiene help to prevent tooth decay.
Esophagus The bolus passes to the stomach via the muscular esophagus.	Much heartburn results from the reflux of stomach acid into the esophagus.	Heartburn requires medical treatment with antacids, but eating smaller meals can help.
Gallbladder The gallbladder (*green, left*) stores bile, made by the liver, and releases it into the duodenum.	Gallstones are caused by a disturbance of fat metabolism.	A healthy diet low in animal fats seems to reduce the risk of gallstones.
Stomach A muscular sac that mixes acid fluid with food and passes it to the intestine.	Irritation, infection, or excess acid can cause pain and vomiting. Irritant foods, alcohol, and smoking can make ulcers worse.	During flare-ups avoid foods and drinks that cause problems, and try to stop smoking.
Small intestine A tube that receives strong alkaline juices from the pancreas and gallbladder, which break down fats and neutralize stomach acid. At the top end, the duodenum, the now liquid food is mixed with these digestive juices. Most absorption of food occurs in the middle and lower end.	Too much acid getting into the duodenum increases risks of dyspepsia, or indigestion, and ulcers. Duodenal ulcers are also related to alcohol, smoking, and stress. Spasms of the intestine can cause severe pain.	During flare-ups avoid foods and drinks that cause problems, and try to stop smoking.
Large intestine A tube in which food and fluid are absorbed. Food residue is formed into feces.	Constipation with the formation of small, hard feces can cause discomfort and pain.	A high-fiber diet increases fecal bulk and assists proper waste elimination.

VITAMINS

Vitamins are chemicals that your body needs to process other nutrients, help regulate the nervous system, and help form genetic material, proteins, red blood cells, and hormones. Because your body cannot manufacture its own, or enough, vitamins, you have to obtain them from your diet.

For best vitamin value, eat food in its freshest possible state, since storage, particularly in daylight, can destroy some vitamins. Careless cook-ing, such as prolonged boiling of vegetables, can also break down vitamins. The B vitamins tend to wash out of food, so use the cooking liquid as stock and in gravies rather than discard it.

Who needs supplements?

If you eat a balanced and varied diet, in most cases you will have an adequate supply of vitamins, and you will not need supplements. Vitamin pills are

ESSENTIAL VITAMINS			
Vitamin	**Best sources**	**Role**	**RDA***
Vitamin A (Retinol)	Liver, milk, eggs, butter, dark green or yellow fruits and vegetables. The body converts the pigment carotene in yellow and green fruit and vegetables to vitamin A.	Needed by body membranes, including the retina of the eye, linings of lungs and digestive system. Also needed by bones and teeth.	About 1 mg
Thiamin (Vitamin B_1)	Pork, whole grains, enriched flour and cereals, nuts, peas, beans	Ensures proper burning of carbohydrates.	1.0–1.4 mg
Riboflavin (Vitamin B_2)	Milk, cheese, eggs, liver, poultry	Needed by all cells for energy release and repair.	1.2–1.7 mg
Niacin (Nicotinic acid)	Whole grains, enriched flour and cereals, liver, poultry, lean meat	Needed by cells for proper use of fuel and oxygen.	13–19 mg
Pyridoxine (Vitamin B_6)	Liver, lean meat, whole grains, milk, eggs	Needed by red blood cells and nerves for proper functioning.	About 2 mg
Pantothenic acid	Egg yolk, meat, nuts, whole grains	Needed by all cells for energy production.	4–7 mg
Biotin	Liver, kidney, egg yolk, nuts, most fresh vegetables	Needed by skin and circulatory system.	100–200 micrograms
Vitamin B_{12}	Eggs, meat, dairy produce	Needed for red blood cell production in the bone marrow. Also needed by nervous system.	3 micrograms
Folic acid	Fresh vegetables, poultry, fish	Needed for red blood cell production.	400 micrograms
Vitamin C (Ascorbic acid)	All citrus fruits, tomatoes, raw cabbage, potatoes, strawberries	Needed by bones and teeth and by tissues for repair.	60 mg
Vitamin D	Oily fish and fish liver oils, dairy produce, eggs	Required for maintenance of blood calcium levels and thus for bone growth. Some vitamin D can be made in the skin in the presence of sunlight.	5–10 micrograms
Vitamin E (Tocopherol)	Vegetable oils and many other foods	Needed for tissue handling of fatty substances and for making cell membranes.	8–10 mg
Vitamin K	Made by intestinal bacteria; also found in leafy vegetables.	Needed for normal blood clotting.	70–140 micrograms

* *For nonpregnant, nonlactating adults*

not a substitute for a balanced diet because they do not contain energy-producing nutrients or dietary fiber. For most people, getting enough vitamins is less of a problem than moderating the amounts of calories, fat, sugar, and sodium contained in their diets.

Sometimes supplements are necessary. For example, babies need vitamin D in early infancy. Very young teenage girls who are pregnant and still growing themselves often need multiple vitamin and mineral supplements. Folic acid supplements are often given to women during pregnancy, when the need for it arises and cannot easily be supplied from food sources alone.

Total vegetarians who eat no animal food (see pages 86–89) might need supplements of vitamin B_{12} and some other nutrients, and anyone who consumes less than 1,600 calories a day for a long time might find it difficult to get the RDA for vitamins without a supplement.

Some hereditary diseases affect vitamin metabolism, and chronic intestinal diseases interfere with vitamin and mineral absorption. Other illnesses, surgery, and even some long-term medication can affect your need for specific vitamins, so that supplements are necessary. Alcoholics are often malnourished because of their unbalanced diet and disordered absorption, and use, of several vitamins and minerals, such as folic acid and some of the B vitamins. For them, a multivitamin-mineral supplement at levels close to the RDA might help to prevent malnutrition until they get their drinking under control and begin to consume regular, balanced meals.

Taking supplements sensibly

If your doctor has prescribed a supplement for you, follow his instructions; otherwise, follow these commonsense guidelines.

Before choosing a supplement, check with your doctor about safe doses, just as you would if you were taking large amounts of aspirin or allergy medicines. Vitamins and minerals can be bought in large doses without a prescription, and you are free to take as many doses as you want. However, you should not take more than the RDA, as large doses of some nutrients can have harmful effects. If a supplement contains more than 150 percent of the RDA for any nutrient, and especially when levels reach 10 to 100 times the RDA levels—a megadose—it can have harmful, druglike effects.

Infants and children, who need less of most nutrients than adults, are especially vulnerable, and can become ill if they are given megadoses of some vitamins, particularly the fat-soluble vitamins A and D, which are stored and build up easily in body tissues.

Unless your doctor has prescribed a supplement, your best choice probably is a multivitamin-multimineral product that provides no more than 100 percent of the RDA for any nutrient. You are less likely to get very high amounts by mistake with such a product, whereas single unit doses of individual nutrients often come in very large amounts.

Put your pills in a place where you will remember to take them, preferably with meals, when absorption is best. Be sure to keep them out of reach of children, who can be poisoned accidentally by eating large doses.

It has been found that "natural" vitamins, which are derived from foods, are no better than synthetic vitamins, which are manufactured to produce the same chemicals. The human body cannot tell the difference between them, but the supplements advertised as "natural" will usually cost you more. Similarly, brand-name and no-name supplements sometimes differ in the dose and the types of nutrients they contain, but are the same in other respects, except for price.

Two substances incorrectly referred to as vitamins B_{15} and B_{17} are pangamic acid, or pangamate, and laetrile. No dietary need for pangamic acid has been demonstrated and laetrile, which contains cyanide, may not be sold, or used.

Supplements in normal amounts or megadoses do not prevent or cure colds, and some can increase the risk of kidney and bladder stones, diarrhea, urinary tract irritation, and increased blood clotting. There is no scientific evidence that they help in the treatment of schizophrenia, hyperactivity, arthritis, geriatric problems, neuroses, depression, alcoholism, or mental deficiency.

Before taking supplements, check your diet. If you are not eating at least the minimum recommended number of servings of each food group (see pages 62–63), it is likely that your diet is not only deficient in some vitamins and minerals, but also too high in fat, sugar, or calories. Taking supplements is no substitute for a healthy diet.

MINERALS

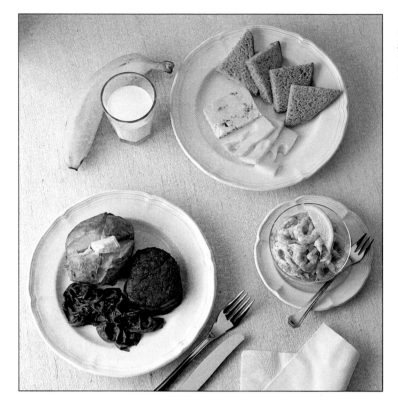

This well-balanced meal of shrimp cocktail, grilled meat, spinach, baked potato, whole-wheat bread and cheese, skim milk, and a banana is rich in the essential minerals as well as other nutrients.

Minerals are inorganic substances that your body needs for forming bones, teeth, and blood cells, for assisting in the chemical reactions of cells, and for regulating body fluids. The essential minerals—the ones the body needs to survive—are divided into two groups. The macrominerals, of which you need more than 100 milligrams a day, are calcium, chloride, magnesium, phosphorus, potassium, sodium, and sulfur. The trace minerals, of which you need a much smaller quantity each day, include cobalt, copper, fluoride, iodine, iron, manganese, molybdenum, selenium, and zinc.

How much do you need?

Your body needs only small amounts of the essential minerals, but because it cannot manufacture them, you must obtain them from your diet or from supplements. While everyone needs all the essential minerals, the amount varies according to age and other conditions, such as pregnancy. The RDA provides expert guidance as to the amount of each nutrient you need every day. Scientists have concluded that they do not know enough about some nutrients to make firm

recommendations, but they are able to advise the range of intakes that they believe are safe and adequate without being excessive. An excess of a mineral can not only be harmful in itself, but it can also interfere with the function of other minerals.

To make life easier for consumers, the Food and Drug Administration has developed a simplified standard called the USRDA. By reading the label, you can compare the statement of nutrient content of foods and supplements against this standard to find out how much of your vitamin and mineral requirements such products supply. The percentage of the USRDA on a label refers to the nutrients in a single serving or dose.

For foods that are not labeled, the information about food groups on pages 56–57 will help you to identify food sources of these nutrients.

Fortified and enriched foods

Many foods have vitamins and minerals added to those occurring in them naturally. Examples of mineral-fortified foods are iron-fortified cereals, and iron-fortified formulas for infants. Enriched foods have higher amounts of some of the nutrients that have been removed during processing added back to them. Perhaps the best known example is enriched white flour, which has iron, riboflavin, niacin, and thiamin added back to it.

Mineral supplements

Minerals are not destroyed by cooking, and if you eat a varied diet following the guidelines in this chapter, you will rarely need to take mineral supplements, but there are a few important exceptions.

Women in their childbearing years might need iron supplements because they lose iron with their menstrual periods, and must supply extra iron to the fetus when they are pregnant. Most women are prescribed iron supplements during pregnancy and for a few months afterward.

Women who cannot or prefer not to eat milk products and other foods high in calcium when they are pregnant or breast-feeding might also be given a calcium supplement, as their need for this mineral increases in order to produce a healthy fetus and milk supply.

After four to six months of age, babies might need an iron supplement in addition to iron-rich solid foods, especially if they are not eating either iron-fortified baby cereal or formulas.

You might be prescribed mineral supplements when you are ill or if you are on a very low-calorie diet, but you should avoid taking supplements if your doctor has not diagnosed a mineral deficiency. Overdoses can damage your liver, pancreas, and heart.

ESSENTIAL MINERALS			
Mineral	**Best sources**	**Role**	**RDA***
Calcium	Dairy produce, green vegetables	Essential for blood clotting and the structure of bones and teeth. Needed for working of nerves and all other electrically active body tissues.	About 800 mg in adults but more during growth
Phosphorus	Meat, dairy produce, beans and peas, cereals	Basic cell energy store, key element in cell reactions.	About 800 mg in adults but more during growth
Potassium	Avocados, bananas, apricots, potatoes and many other foods	Major mineral within body cells. Essential to fluid balance and for many cell reactions.	Not established
Magnesium	Beans and peas, nuts and cereals, leafy green vegetables	Needed by all cells. Important in electrical activity of nerves and muscles.	300–350 mg
Iodine	All seafood, iodized salt	Needed by thyroid gland.	About 0.1 mg
Iron	Liver, meat, eggs, enriched cereals	Needed in manufacture of hemoglobin, the oxygen-carrying compound in blood.	10–18 mg
Fluorine Copper Zinc	Water, fluoride toothpaste Liver, seafood, meat Seafood, meat, whole wheat, beans and peas, nuts	Helps protect teeth from decay. Needed by cells to utilize oxygen. Needed in the structure of cell enzymes.	– About 1.5 mg 15 mg
Chromium Selenium Molybdenum Manganese	Trace elements in many foods	Minor roles in body chemistry.	Minute amounts
Sodium	Most foods except fruit	Essential to fluid balance, muscle contraction, and nerve reaction.	1,100–3,300 mg

* *For nonpregnant, non-lactating adults*

Over the past two decades the dietary recommendations of experts in Western countries have moved from concentrating solely on achieving dietary adequacy (to prevent deficiency diseases), to emphasizing balance and moderation in order to decrease the risks of certain degenerative diseases. The Dietary Guidelines for Americans published by the US Department of Health and Human Services and the US Department of Agriculture recommend that everyone should eat a variety of foods that will provide sufficient amounts of the essential nutrients and energy to maintain a desirable weight. They suggest you eat foods with adequate starch and fiber; avoid too much fat, cholesterol, sugar, and sodium; and drink alcoholic beverages in moderation, if at all.

How does the American diet compare to these guidelines? The information available shows that, like that of most highly industrialized Western countries, it is higher in fat, sodium, cholesterol, sugar, and alcohol, and lower in dietary fiber and starchy carbohydrates than is thought to be best for health. What could be more typical than a hamburger, french fries, a thick milk shake, and a big slice of pie? It is all right to eat such a meal occasionally, but as regular daily fare it poses risks of potentially dangerous excesses in calories, saturated fats, salt, and sugar, as well as a deficiency in fiber.

The healthy diet is a distillation of all the discoveries and advances in nutritional thinking that have taken place since World War II. Its aim is to promote growth, health, fitness, and vitality, to maximize enjoyment, and to reduce the risks of diet-related diseases.

Healthy adults can get all the nutrition and energy they need by eating the right number of servings from each of the main food groups (see pages 56–57) every day, as shown in the table below, and by following the key principles of variety, balance, and moderation.

Variety
The more variety there is in your diet, the less likely you are to develop either a deficiency or an excess of any single nutrient. And because

GUIDE TO A HEALTHY DIET		
Food group	**Daily servings**	**1-serving equivalents**
Breads, cereals and other grains	6–11	1 slice of bread, or 1 small roll or muffin, or $\frac{1}{2}$–$\frac{3}{4}$ cup hot cereal, or 1 oz ready-to-eat cereal, or $\frac{1}{2}$ cup pasta or rice. A hamburger bun or whole English muffin is 2 servings.
Vegetables Dark green and deep yellow Starchy Others	3–5 At least 1 At least 1 At least 1	A small salad, or $\frac{1}{2}$ cup of cooked vegetables
Fruits Citrus Melons, berries Others	2–4 At least 1 At least 1	1 medium whole fruit, or 1 cup sliced or wedged fruit, or 4–6 oz juice
Meats, fish, poultry, and eggs	At least 2	A serving is 2–3 oz. You can count 1 egg as 1 oz meat. Other alternatives are: 1 cup cooked dried beans = 2 oz lean meat, poultry, or fish plus 2 slices of enriched or whole-grain bread.
Dairy products	At least 2/ 3 for teens, pregnant and nursing women	8 fl oz milk, or 1–2 oz cheese, or 6–8 oz yogurt
Fats, sweets, and alcohol	Moderation	

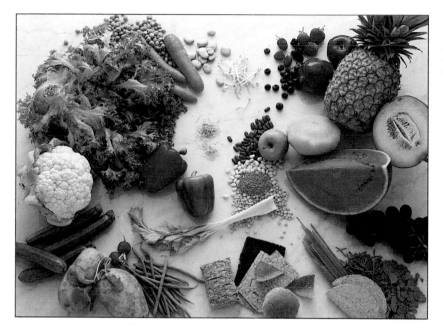

Dietary fiber is found in such a wide range of tasty fruits, vegetables, whole grains, and whole-grain products that it should be easy to increase the amount in your diet to the recommended level.

variety also keeps eating interesting and pleasurable, the less likely you are to become bored and careless about your diet.

Balance

It is important to balance your food consumption with your energy production in order to achieve and maintain a desirable weight. The Dietary Guidelines for Americans point out that it is equally important to achieve a balance among the types of energy-producing nutrients—fats, carbohydrates, and proteins—that you eat. They recommend diets that are low in fats, especially saturated fats, and high in complex carbohydrates and fiber.

Moderation

It is not always true that if a little is good for you, more is better. The Dietary Guidelines for Americans, The American Dietetic Association, the American Heart Association, the American Diabetes Association, and the American Cancer Society all recommend moderation in the diet. It has been noted that most people would benefit from reducing their intake of calories, fat, cholesterol, sugar, and salt. It is also true that there is no health advantage in eating, say, more protein than you need—it doesn't make your muscles bigger or improve athletic performance. But whereas an excess of protein is not thought to be harmful, excesses of some minerals and vitamins can be.

Fiber

Grandma used to call it roughage, and most people need to eat more of it to achieve better dietary balance. Fiber promotes a healthy digestive tract, helps to prevent constipation, and reduces the risk of hemorrhoids. Scientists are studying the possible role played by fiber in preventing certain digestive diseases and cancers.

Dietary fiber is material from plant foods that cannot be digested by the human stomach, and can be only partly digested in the human intestinal tract. There are several different types of fiber, and you need to eat a variety of foods to make sure you benefit from them all. Most of the fiber you eat comes from whole-grain products, and fruits and vegetables, particularly their skins.

Most Americans eat about 10–20 grams of dietary fiber daily. The National Cancer Institute recommends that you should eat about twice that, bringing total consumption to 25–35 grams a day, depending on the size of the individual. The best way to increase your intake of fiber is to eat several servings of fiber-rich foods every day. High-fiber supplements have no special advantages, and you should avoid them unless they are prescribed by your doctor.

The medical experts all agree that to have a healthy diet most Americans need to eat less sugar, less sodium, and less fat.

Less sugar

Most Americans eat too much sugar. The average individual uses 130 pounds of sugar and other calorie-laden sweeteners a year, or about a third of a pound a day. Most of this is sucrose, the kind of sugar that is in the sugar bowl, but it also includes "hidden" sugars and sweeteners in a wide variety of foods. Food manufacturers know that most people like the sweet taste, and so processed and prepared foods tend to have a high sugar content. This includes not only very obvious foods such as jams and jellies, cookies and candy, ice cream and cake, honey and syrups, soft drinks and breakfast cereals, but also canned fruits and vegetables, soups, sauces, and juices.

You do not actually need to eat sugar to be healthy, for the body's nutritional need for glucose can be supplied by many other carbohydrates. Moreover, most foods high in added sugars, such as candy and other sweets, are a highly concentrated source of calories but contain little or no vitamins and minerals, whereas foods

SODIUM

Sodium is essential to fluid balance, muscle contractions, and nerve reactions. Most of us eat far more than the RDA of 1,100–3,300 mg, mainly in the form of table salt. Sodium occurs naturally in most foods, except fruit. The salt content rises dramatically when food is processed or cured, as the figures show. You can reduce your consumption of sodium by using less salt at the table and in cooking, eating fewer processed and convenience foods, and choosing foods with a low sodium/potassium ratio. These include most fresh fruits and vegetables.

Average daily consumption of salt

Most people eat about 0.33 oz of salt a day. This list shows what percentage of that total is contributed by some common foods.

Table salt	32
Cereal products	27
Meat, eggs, milk	19
Cheese, cream, ice cream, fats	15
Root vegetables	2
Other vegetables	3
Fish	1
Fruit and sugar	trace
Beverages	trace
Total	100

Sodium/potassium content of some common foods

Food	Sodium mg/100g (3.5 oz)	Ratio sodium 1mg potassium
Bread, whole-wheat	560	3.5
Cheese, Cheddar	610	5.08
Butter, salted	870	58
Margarine	800	160
Bacon, unsmoked, raw	1,470	6.39
Haddock, fresh	120	0.40
Haddock, smoked	1,220	4.2
Potato, boiled	4	0.01
Potato, chips	550	0.46
Peas, fresh	1	0.002
Peas, canned	230	1.77
Peas, frozen	2	0.02
Tomato ketchup	1,120	1.90

Eating less fat

Here are some easy ways to reduce the amount of fat, particularly saturated fat, in your diet.

- Broil, bake, or boil your food rather than fry it.

- Cook stews and casseroles in advance; cool and remove the fat before reheating and serving.

- Drain fat from the pan before serving.

- Substitute broth for some of the fat you would normally use in cooking.

- Choose lean meat, fish, poultry, and dried beans and peas as your sources of protein.

- Trim excess fat off meats, and remove skin from poultry.

- Cut down on the amount of sauces and salad dressing you add to foods in cooking and at the table.

- Switch from whole milk to skim or low-fat milk.

- Choose low-fat soft cheeses and medium-fat hard cheeses.

- Limit your consumption of butter, cream, hydrogenated margarines, shortenings, coconut oil, and foods made with these products.

- Read food packaging labels carefully to find out both the amount and types of fat contained in processed foods.

- Choose food products marked "low fat."

---

that are naturally high in sugar are more likely also to contain other nutrients. Sweets, particularly sticky ones, stay in the mouth longer and increase the risks of tooth decay.

Less sodium

The Recommended Dietary Allowances state that a safe and adequate level of sodium consumption is 1,100–3,300 milligrams a day, yet many people eat as much as 7,000 milligrams. There is no evidence that eating this much does you any good, and increasing evidence that it might do you harm if you suffer from, or have a predisposition to, high blood pressure. Medical experts estimate that about 20 percent of the American population is genetically predisposed to a form of high blood pressure that is sensitive to sodium in the diet. Since there is no simple test that can predict who will develop high blood pressure, it makes sense for everyone to reduce sodium consumption.

Salt and sodium are not the same. Table salt is sodium chloride, and is about 40 percent sodium by weight. Sodium is found naturally in many foods, and is added to many foods and beverages during processing. A number of over-the-counter medications, such as aspirins, antacids, and some laxatives, are also high in sodium. About one-third of the sodium you eat comes from salt added to food at the table or during cooking; as much as one-half comes from processed foods; and the remainder comes from natural foods. Therefore, the easiest way to reduce the amount of sodium in your diet is to cut down on the amount of salt and the quantity of processed foods you eat.

When it comes to saltiness, humans are creatures of habit. The tendency is to think a food is salty when it has more salt than you are used to, however high or low that level may be. Thus, what is salty to one person can be bland to another. Luckily, it takes only a short while to get used to lower levels of saltiness.

Less fat

The American Heart Association, the American Cancer Society, and the National Cancer Institute all suggest that diets should not exceed 30 percent of calories from fat. If you eat 2,500 calories a day, this is about 83 grams, or the equivalent of about seven tablespoons of butter. If you eat 2,000 calories a day, it is about 67 grams of fat; and if you eat only 1,500 calories, it is about 50 grams, or about the amount in 2 ounces of butter.

You do not have to change what you eat to reduce the fat in your diet, but you do have to change how often or how much of it you eat. The menus on pages 80–85 all contain 30 percent or less fat.

As you decrease your fat consumption, you should increase the amount of calories you get from complex carbohydrates, such as whole-grain products, fruits and vegetables, cereals, and other starchy foods. These will give your body the energy it needs as well as other nutrients and dietary fiber.

EATING HABITS

Obesity afflicts at least 28 percent of adult women and 19 percent of adult men in America. Many others consider themselves more than pleasingly plump. In spite of all the diet books and diet foods, obesity doesn't seem to be declining.

Appetite control

Why do some people have such difficulty controlling their appetites? Actually, over the long term, most people do quite well and remain at approximately the same weight for considerable lengths of time. Although there does seem to be some rather imprecise control over appetite, it does not appear to be sufficiently finely tuned to keep many people at their desired weights.

When scientists first studied hunger and appetite, they assumed that eating was largely, if not entirely, regulated by the body's need for food, which was expressed through a strong hunger drive originating in the hypothalamus in the brain. But the hypothalamus isn't the only control—it acts like a telephone exchange, processing and distributing information arising from, or destined to go, elsewhere in the brain or the body.

Snacking can be healthy if you choose your food sensibly, but avoid eating on the move.

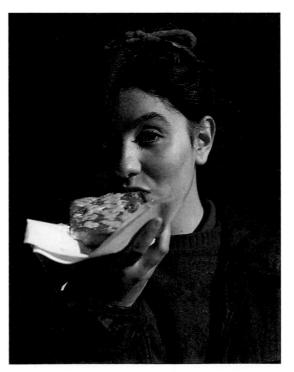

Gradually scientists have become aware that in affluent societies, where people very seldom go without food for more than a few hours or, at most, a day at a time, appetites are influenced more by social, environmental, and emotional pressures than by internal physiological cues or signals. This is good news since it suggests that not all fat people are predestined to be so. However, it is also bad news since it means that many external factors encourage overeating.

The enormous variety of tempting foods available, especially those high in fat, sugar, and calories, but low in bulk, make it easy to overeat. Seductive food advertising, television commercials, and the prevalence of high-calorie menus in cafeterias and restaurants also make it hard to watch the waistline. Other people, especially those you live with and are fondest of, might also encourage you to eat more than you otherwise would. And some people react to stress or depression by eating even when they aren't hungry.

Fast foods and convenience foods

Americans today eat at least a third of their meals away from home. At home, you may rely on prepared and packaged foods to save time in cooking. Always check that convenience foods do not violate the principles of variety, balance, and moderation. Choose items that help to fill gaps in the food groups. Many fast-food places now have salad bars, and if you take only a little dressing, salads are low in fat, sodium, and calories, and, of course, add dietary fiber. When choosing convenience foods for home use, read the nutritional labels carefully to make sure the products fit in with your eating plan.

Snacking

Snacking—eating between meals or instead of them—is a fact of life for most people. As far as the human body is concerned, it doesn't make a bit of difference whether you eat foods at mealtimes or space them out through the day. The problem is that some people tend to choose snack foods, that are high in fats, sugar, and calories, but don't carry their share of the protective nutrients, and fail to eat a balanced diet. This has given snacking a bad name, which it doesn't really deserve. If you eat healthy snacks, and pay attention to the guiding principles of moderation, balance, and variety you don't have to give up snacking entirely.

Good choices of snack foods are fruits, vegetables, low-fat milk products, and small servings of any of the other foods in the basic food groups. Many foods are not inherently bad for you, but you need to be careful with high-fat and high-calorie items because it is easy to eat large amounts without feeling you have eaten very much. Similarly, you should eat high-salt snacks only in moderation. Sticky, sugary snacks are particularly bad for dental health.

CHOOSING HEALTHY SNACKS		
Food group	**Good**	**Less desirable**
Milk products	Low fat milk, cheeses, and plain yogurt	Chocolate milk, ice cream, milk shakes, fruited yogurt
Breads, cereals	Popcorn, soda crackers, plain toast, hard rolls, pretzels, pizza, corn chips	Cake, pie, sweet rolls, frosted desserts, cookies
Meat, fish, poultry, eggs	Egg salad, chicken, ham, hamburgers, hot dogs, luncheon meats	
Fruit and nuts	Fresh or water-packed fruits, nuts, peanut butter alone, unsweetened juices, diluted juices	Syrup-packed canned fruits, jams, jellies, preserves, sweetened fruit drinks and sodas
Vegetables	Fresh, frozen, or canned vegetables, potato chips	Candied or glazed sweet potatoes
Other foods	Sugarless soft drinks, gums, black tea and coffee	Added sugar drinks, candy, honey, sugar, syrups, carbonated sugary sodas

ENERGY AND CALORIES

The energy values of foods are commonly described in terms of "calories." In fact, what most people call a calorie is actually a kilocalorie, or 1,000 calories. A kilocalorie is the scientific term for the amount of heat needed to raise the temperature of a liter (slightly more than a quart) of water by one degree Centigrade (1.8 degrees Fahrenheit). You might sometimes see the energy values of foods referred to in kilojoules (kJ) or megajoules (MJ), as this country increasingly adopts metric units of work energy. One calorie equals about 4.2 kJ or 0.0042 MJ.

Calories in foods

Although we eat thousands of foods prepared in many different ways, all food can be thought of in terms of the amount of energy it liberates when it is finally used for energy by the body's cells. Foods vary in their energy value, and thus in their caloric value, depending on the amount of energy-yielding substances—fat, carbohydrate, protein, and alcohol—they contain. Fat produces the most calories for its weight: 9 calories per gram. Carbohydrates, such as sugar and starch, and protein produce about half as much: 4 calories per gram. Alcohol produces about 7 calories per gram. Water, dietary fiber, vitamins, minerals, and other constituents of food such as flavors, colors, and preservatives do not affect the caloric value of a food.

Some foods are said to be high in caloric density. This means that they are high in calories for their weight. Foods such as butter, alcohol, and chocolate are high in caloric density. Foods such as carrots and lettuce, which are high in water, are low in caloric density.

Calories and weight

Day to day, you have to keep your energy intake and output in balance to keep your weight constant. If you eat more energy than you burn, your body will store the excess as fat. For every 3,500 calories that you accumulate, you will gain roughly one pound of fat. Similarly, if you burn more energy than you eat, your body will use the energy-yielding nutrients its cells are made of—especially fat from the fat cells—and you will lose weight. The number of calories that you need to keep your weight steady depends on your age, size, lifestyle (especially the amount of exercise you get), body composition, and heredity.

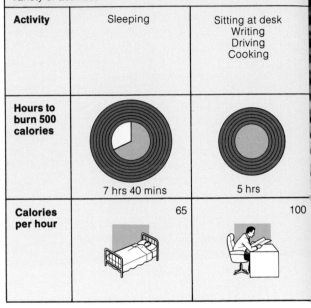

HOW YOU USE ENERGY
The amount of energy you burn in a day depends on the amount and type of exercise you do. The chart is a guide to the number of calories burned per hour in a variety of activities.

Activity	Sleeping	Sitting at desk Writing Driving Cooking
Hours to burn 500 calories	7 hrs 40 mins	5 hrs
Calories per hour	65	100

Comparing foods according to the calories they contain reveals the high energy content of fatty and sugary foods. An average-size slice of a 9-inch pecan pie, for example, is the caloric equivalent of a whole plateful of fruit. Each contains approximately 500 calories, or roughly one-quarter of the recommended daily caloric requirement of a sedentary woman.

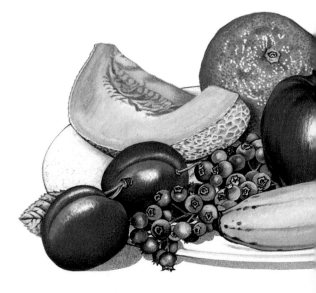

Walking (2 – 3 miles per hour) Dancing Badminton	Brisk walking (3 – 5 miles per hour) Tennis Skating Bicycle riding Gentle jogging	Slow running Soccer Climbing	Sawing wood Swimming Skiing	Running Squash Competitive swimming Water polo Weight-lifting
2 hrs	1 hr 40 mins	1 hr 15 mins	1 hr	45 mins
250	300	400	500	650

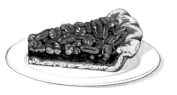

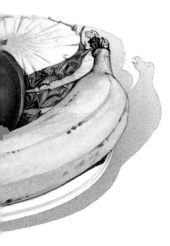

DAILY CALORIE NEEDS
The chart shows recommended average daily energy allowances for various age groups. If you are much taller or more muscular than average, or are extremely active, you should adjust your caloric intake upward. If you have a small frame and do little exercise, your caloric consumption should be lower than average.

Category	Age years	Weight pounds	Height inches	Energy needs (with range) (calories)	
Infants	to 6mo	13	24	675	(560 – 860)
	6 – 12mo	20	28	950	(725 – 1,225)
Children	1 – 3	29	05	1,300	(900 – 1,800)
	4 – 6	44	44	1,700	(1,300 – 2,300)
	7 – 10	62	52	2,400	(1,650 – 3,300)
Males	11 – 14	99	62	2,700	(2,000 – 3,700)
	15 – 18	145	69	2,800	(2,100 – 3,900)
	19 – 22	154	70	2,900	(2,500 – 3,300)
	23 – 50	154	70	2,700	(2,300 – 3,100)
	51 – 75	154	70	2,400	(2,000 – 2,800)
	76 +	154	70	2,050	(1,650 – 2,450)
Females	11 – 14	101	62	2,200	(1,500 – 3,000)
	15 – 18	120	64	2,100	(1,200 – 3,000)
	19 – 22	120	64	2,100	(1,700 – 2,500)
	23 – 50	120	64	2,000	(1,600 – 2,400)
	51 – 75	120	64	1,800	(1,400 – 2,200)
	76 +	120	64	1,600	(1,200 – 2,000)
Pregnant				+ 300	
Nursing				+ 500	

THE MEANING OF METABOLISM

Metabolism is simply the sum of all the chemical activities of the body's cells. In order to carry out these activities, the cells need food energy. The food you eat is broken down in the digestive system (see page 57), absorbed into the bloodstream, and then distributed around the body for use or, in the case of some surpluses, storage. The cells trap food energy in the chemical adenosine triphosphate, or ATP. When the cells split the high-energy bonds of ATP, they can then harness the energy and liberate it either as heat, or, in some specialized cells such as muscle cells, as mechanical work, like walking or skiing.

The basic fuel
Glucose is the basic chemical fuel that cells use most easily. The carbohydrate food you eat is converted to glucose in the liver. It is then delivered to the blood, which carries it to the cells. Here each glucose molecule is altered chemically, then enters an extraordinary series of reactions within a kind of self-perpetuating circle, known as the Krebs cycle. During the course of the cycle, oxygen is used up—that is, the cycle is aerobic— and a good deal of energy is liberated as heat. In fact, as your cells carry out their normal activities, they produce more than enough heat to keep you warm. You don't need to exert energy to stay warm unless you are in a very cold place.

The other fuels
If glucose is in short supply, the cells can use the breakdown products of other carbohydrates, protein, fats, and alcohol. When you go on a reducing diet, fats are used in excess, especially if the diet is very low in carbohydrates. When fats are burned in this way, they produce small chemical leftovers called ketones, which many cells cannot use. People who are starving produce many ketones, since they too are burning a lot of fat. Some diabetics are unable to use glucose efficiently and also burn more fat than their cells can handle, and so produce ketones if they are not given insulin. Ketones smell like nail polish remover and leave a bad taste in the mouth. They can be a telltale sign that someone is trying to lose weight too quickly.

When glucose is lacking, many body proteins are also used as fuel. If there is also very little fat available, as sometimes happens in people who are extremely underweight, proteins can be burned very quickly. Because your cells are

THE KREBS CYCLE
The Krebs cyclē is the body's energy cycle. Energy from glucose and, when glucose is not available, from other carbohydrates, fats, and proteins is converted into a chemical form capable of rebonding phosphates and re-forming molecules of adenosine triphosphate, or ATP (*right*). These are needed for all body activities. As a result of the chemical reactions of the cycle, the waste products carbon dioxide and water are formed and then eliminated from the body.

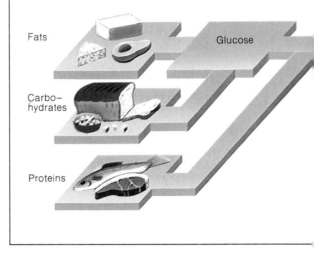

Fats

Glucose

Carbo-hydrates

Proteins

structured from protein, the use of body protein for energy means that the body is destroying itself. This is the last resort of human metabolism, and can be a very dangerous result of starvation, fasting, or illness.

Storing food energy: glycogen loading
Energy production over the long run depends on a chemical fuel, such as glucose, and oxygen being available. Carbohydrates are the most readily available source of food energy, and with fats are the major source of energy for muscle contraction. You need enough carbohydrate in your diet to take care of your immediate energy needs, and a little extra to be converted to glycogen and stored in the liver and muscles.

Glycogen is the form of starch your body makes to supply its quick-energy needs. Glycogen is essential for repeated muscle contractions, but it is a short-term form of storage. Only a limited amount of it can be held in the body at any given time and this amount does not vary according to how fat or thin you are. Excess food energy cannot be eliminated from the body, and so is stored as fat under the skin and around the

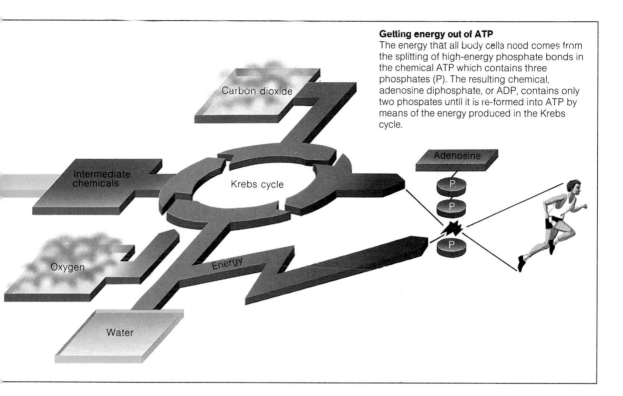

Getting energy out of ATP
The energy that all body cells need comes from the splitting of high-energy phosphate bonds in the chemical ATP which contains three phosphates (P). The resulting chemical, adenosine diphosphate, or ADP, contains only two phospates until it is re-formed into ATP by means of the energy produced in the Krebs cycle.

organs. When the glycogen is exhausted, even though the fat is broken down to provide a sizable amount of energy, the muscle fibers will fail to contract properly and weakness will result.

Glycogen, or carbohydrate, loading is the process of manipulating the diet and amount of exercise to increase glycogen stores in muscles, and thereby, it is hoped, increase the capacity for continuous, exhausting, and prolonged—over 90 minutes—exercise. The usual glycogen content of the body is only about one pound, or roughly 3,500 calories. If you follow several days of carbohydrate deprivation with several meals of very high carbohydrate content while continuing to exercise all the time, you can increase your muscle glycogen content a good deal above these levels. Glycogen loading does not affect your performance in short-term activities, for which the body's normal stores are more than ample. However, it can be advantageous in endurance activities, such as long-distance running.

Exercise and exhaustion
Vigorous physical activity requires a lot of energy. Sometimes the cells are worked so hard

that not enough oxygen reaches them. The cells can continue to liberate energy, but the body can sustain anaerobic activity—activity without oxygen—only for a limited period of time. In muscles, for example, anaerobic activity leads to the build-up of lactic acid, which makes the muscles sore and signals that they need to rest.

Resting metabolism
While some people are apparently able to eat a lot but never gain a pound, others who seem never to eat very much gain weight anyway. One factor that helps to explain this paradox is the resting metabolism, the rate at which the body uses up energy while at rest. When it is tested under very special conditions, it is called the basal metabolic rate, or BMR.

Resting metabolism varies widely with age, sex, body size, and shape. BMR is closely related to the amount of lean tissue a person has, and so tends to be higher in men than in women. It rises with exercise and decreases with age as the body loses lean tissue. For many Americans, at least half of their total energy needs are used by their resting metabolism.

A significant report issued by the National Institutes of Health in 1985 concluded that obesity has many negative implications for health. It creates psychological burdens, increases the risks or severity of many illnesses, and decreases longevity. A national study by the American Cancer Society found that obese men had a higher rate of death from cancers of the colon, rectum, and prostate, and obese women had a higher rate of death from cancers of the uterus, ovaries, breast (after menopause), gallbladder, and bile ducts than those who were within the normal weight range. People who are too fat are also more likely to suffer from high blood pressure, high blood cholesterol, and stroke. Maturity onset diabetes is also more common among the obese. While diabetes is inherited, weight reduction may control it.

Who is obese?

The graphs of mortality figures for men and women (opposite) show the risks associated with obesity. Because people have different shapes and sizes, the graphs use the body mass index (BMI) as a measure of obesity. To obtain the index, which is an international scientific standard, the weight of the person in pounds is divided by his or her height in inches squared, and the resulting figure is multiplied by 725, as shown in the example on page 73.

There is no threshold, or single point, of fatness at which being obese increases the health risks. However, in the United States obesity is considered clearly present and treatment is strongly advised at a body mass index greater than 27.8 for men, and 27.3 for women, which is about 20 percent above the desirable weight. People who are extremely obese—that is, 100 pounds over their desirable weight—have enormously greater health risks than people with normal weights.

Not everyone who is obese is greatly overweight. A National Health and Nutrition Examination Survey showed that about eight million Americans were obese but not particularly heavy. This occurs when people are physically inactive. Since they rarely use their large muscles, they have lower amounts of lean tissue and higher amounts of fat. These balance out on the scales, but not in their shapes, which look rather flabby. You can tell if you fall into this category by doing the "pinch" test (see page 14); if you can pick up

more than about one inch, you might be overfat.

Some people, such as athletes in the contact sports, have very heavy builds, heavy bones, and very large muscles. Their weights might be above the desirable range even though they are not really fat. However, usually they are less than 20 percent overweight. Being an athlete or an ex-athlete is no insurance that you fall into this category, and it is particularly unlikely if you are now very sedentary. Overweight and overfatness *usually* go together, and more than 20 million Americans are both overweight and obese.

Smoking: an added risk

The health risks of being fat are increased among those people who smoke. The graphs opposite show the death rates for nonsmokers and those who smoked more than 20 cigarettes a day. They demonstrate that there is no point in worrying about a minor degree of obesity if you have a separate major risk to health such as smoking. A nonsmoker has to be enormously obese to have the same risk of death as a smoker of an acceptable weight. Suppose, for example, that you are a nonsmoking woman with a body mass index of 29, which is clearly obese. Your risk of death is exactly the average for the whole population. It would be less if you were thinner, but not a lot. However, if you smoke, your risks are higher at all degrees of overweight. Although it has not been proven, it is possible that, even if you smoke, the risk of death might be less if you eat a healthy diet and are physically fit, even if you remain at exactly the same weight. Clearly, however, the best thing you can do for your health and longevity is to stop smoking (see pages 284–288).

Reducing the risks

Almost everybody who is 20 percent or more overweight will reap health benefits from losing weight. Weight reduction often saves the lives of extremely fat people who develop heart and breathing problems because of their obesity. If you have high blood pressure or high blood cholesterol or triglyceride levels, you will benefit from losing weight. If you suffer from coronary heart disease, gout, or conditions that are worsened by weight, such as emphysema and arthritis of the weight-bearing joints, you could probably get some relief by losing even a relatively small amount of weight.

BODY WEIGHT: THE RISKS OF OBESITY AND SMOKING

The graphs show the risk of death for men and women in relation to weight and to smoking 20 cigarettes a day. Weights are calculated in terms of body mass index (see chart below). The risk to life is calculated in relation to average mortality. A risk factor of less than 1.0 means that you are likely to live longer than the average.

The risks of smoking can be seen to be much greater than those of overweight. If you are obese *and* a smoker you are putting your life doubly at risk. For further explanations see text.

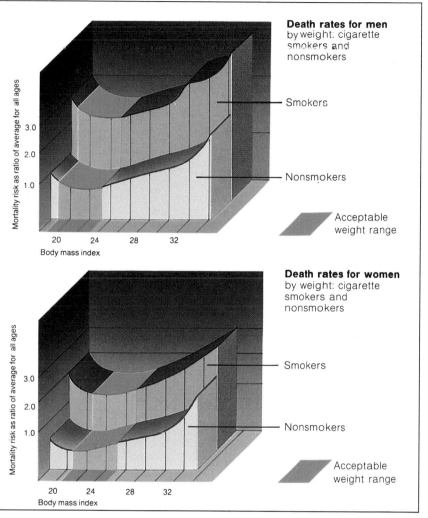

Death rates for men by weight: cigarette smokers and nonsmokers

Smokers

Nonsmokers

Acceptable weight range

Death rates for women by weight: cigarette smokers and nonsmokers

Smokers

Nonsmokers

Acceptable weight range

BODY MASS INDEX

Work out your own body mass index with the help of the example given here. Then calculate, if necessary, a target range within the acceptable range indicated in the graphs above. If you start a reducing diet you should aim to lose no more than 2 lb of weight a week.

The body mass index (BMI) is a useful measure of obesity (or the lack of it). Both BMI and target weight can be easily worked out with the help of a calculator.

$$BMI = \frac{\text{weight in pounds}}{(\text{height in inches})^2} \times 725$$

(The "conversion factor" of 725 is necessary because BMI is an international measure usually calculated using metric measurements.)
Take the example of a woman who weighs 168 lb and is 5 ft 5 in (65 in) tall.

$$BMI = \frac{168}{65 \times 65} \times 725 = \frac{168}{4,225} \times 725 = 0.04 \times 725 = 29$$

This BMI is well over the upper limit of the acceptable range, so this woman would be advised to lose weight.

To calculate a target weight corresponding to a BMI of your choice, use this formula:

$$\text{Target} = \frac{BMI \times Ht^2}{725}$$

So, if the chosen BMI of the woman in the example was 23, her target weight would be:

$$\frac{23 \times (65)^2}{725}$$

$$= 134 \text{ lb}$$

This means a weight loss of 34 lb.

You can get a rough idea of whether you are too fat, or too thin, by using the tables of weight for height and frame opposite. It is difficult to judge your frame size simply by guessing, so use the instructions and table at the top of page 75 to calculate it. Next, measure your height barefoot, and weigh yourself without any clothes—the most accurate reading will be in the morning before breakfast. Then read across from your height to the appropriate frame size and compare your weight to that given in the table.

The range of weights given in the tables is based on the lowest mortality rates among large numbers of insured people. The newest weight-for-height tables were issued in 1983, and show desirable weights to be slightly higher than in previous tables. If you have a health risk factor such as high blood pressure, high serum cholesterol, or high blood sugar, you should check with your doctor since it is possible that a lower weight than the range shown on these tables might be best for you.

Overweight children

The weight-for-height tables given here are not suitable for children or young adults under the age of 21. You should discuss the proper weights for your children with a physician. Do not put any child on a weight reduction diet without consulting a doctor because growth and maturation as well as eating behavior and the relationship between the child and its parents can be adversely affected by the wrong kind of diet.

You should not ignore obesity in a child. It is not a healthy condition, and children can suffer in their relations with other children because of their appearance and inability to keep pace in physical activities. Although being overweight in childhood does not necessarily lead to obesity in adulthood, it does increase that risk. Adults who eat a healthy diet, lead a physically active life, and keep their weight under control are good role models. Avoiding the use of food as a reward, encouraging more physical activity, and limiting snacks to fruits, crackers, and other low-calorie items are good habits to form in childhood.

The elderly

The desirable weights in the tables opposite were calculated for young and middle-aged adults, and can be different for the elderly. If you are over 60,

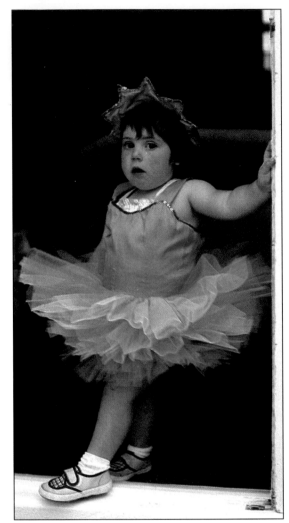

Being overweight is unhealthy at any age. The unhealthy eating practices that lead to obesity often start in childhood. It is easier to change to a healthy way of eating at an early age than to try to change bad eating habits years later.

use the tables as a rough guide, but you should consult your doctor about your optimum weight. At any age, but especially among older adults, any weight loss of five to 10 pounds or more that is not intentional, should be discussed with a doctor. Such loss might signal the existence of an unsuspected medical condition that needs investigation.

FIND YOUR FRAME SIZE

1. Bend your forearm so that it is at a 90-degree angle to your shoulder.
2. Turn your wrist in toward your body.
3. Place the thumb and index finger of your other hand on the most prominent bones on each side of your elbow, or have someone else do it.
4. Measure the space between your fingers with a ruler or tape measure. (Don't measure the distance around your elbow, but across your elbow in a straight line.)
5. Find the correct height for your sex on the table opposite.
6. If your elbow breadth falls in the range given on the table, you have a medium frame. If it is smaller, you have a small frame. If it is larger, you have a large frame.

	Height without shoes	Elbow breadth for medium frame
Men	5'1" – 5'2" 5'3" – 5'6" 5'7" – 5'10" 5'11" – 6'2" 6'3" up	$2\frac{1}{2}$" – $2\frac{7}{8}$" $2\frac{5}{8}$" – $2\frac{7}{8}$" $2\frac{3}{4}$" – 3" $2\frac{3}{4}$" – $3\frac{1}{8}$" $2\frac{7}{8}$" – $3\frac{1}{4}$"
Women	4'9" – 4'10" 4'11" – 5'2" 5'3" – 5'6" 5'7" – 5'10" 5'11" up	$2\frac{1}{4}$" – $2\frac{1}{2}$" $2\frac{1}{4}$" – $2\frac{1}{2}$" $2\frac{3}{8}$" – $2\frac{5}{8}$" $2\frac{3}{8}$" – $2\frac{5}{8}$" $2\frac{1}{2}$" – $2\frac{3}{4}$"

DESIRABLE WEIGHTS FOR HEIGHT BY FRAME

	Height (without shoes)		Weight in pounds (without clothes)		
	Feet	Inches	Small frame	Medium frame	Large frame
Men	5	1	123–129	126–136	133–145
	5	2	125–131	128–138	135–148
	5	3	127–133	130–140	137–151
	5	4	129–135	132–143	139–155
	5	5	131–137	134–146	141–159
	5	6	133–140	137–149	144–163
	5	7	135–143	140–152	147–167
	5	8	137–146	143–150	150–171
	5	9	139–149	146–158	153–175
	5	10	141–152	149–161	156–179
	5	11	144–155	152–165	159–183
	6	0	147–159	155–169	163–187
	6	1	150–163	159–173	167–192
	6	2	153–167	162–177	171–197
	6	3	157–171	166–182	176–202
Women	4	9	99–108	106–118	115–128
	4	10	100–110	108–120	117–131
	4	11	101–112	110–123	119–134
	5	0	103–115	112–126	122–137
	5	1	105–118	115–129	125–141
	5	2	108–121	118–132	128–144
	5	3	111–124	121–135	131–148
	5	4	114–127	124–138	134–152
	5	5	117–130	127–141	137–156
	5	6	120–133	130–144	140–160
	5	7	123–136	133–147	143–164
	5	8	126–139	136–150	146–167
	5	9	129–142	139–153	149–170
	5	10	132–145	142–156	152–173
	5	11	135–148	145–159	155–176

The old saying that an ounce of prevention is worth a pound of cure is the best advice for keeping your weight in line. Once you become fat, it is difficult to slim down and stay that way.

The principles for getting back down to a healthier weight are straightforward. Your body is like a bank account. If you put in more calories than you draw out, the surplus builds up as fat. If you use up more calories than are in the account, you have to cover the deficit from another source, which is body tissue. Most of the body tissue that is used for this purpose is fat, which is good if you are trying to slim down. But some lean tissue, which is needed for bodily work, is also used up, and that is undesirable. The way you try to lose weight influences the proportions of fat and lean tissue that will be burned for fuel, how well your needs for protein, vitamins, and minerals are met, and what your fluid balance will be—all elements of nutritional health. For most people, the best way to lose weight is a combination of a modest decrease of 500 to 1,000 calories a day, and an increase in physical, particularly aerobic, activity.

Can you do it yourself?

It is a good idea to have a medical check-up before embarking on a weight-reducing program, but you are probably safe going on a diet by yourself *if* you have only 10 to 15 pounds to lose, and follow the guidelines given here. Use the checklist at right to see if you need to consult a doctor.

Choosing a diet

An enormous number of reducing diets are published in books and magazines every year. It is important to choose one that will help you to lose weight in a nutritionally healthy way, and encourage you to adopt a healthy pattern of eating for the rest of your life.

If your diet is not medically supervised, be sure it includes at least 1,200 calories a day; below that you risk nutritional and metabolic deficiencies. Your usual calorie level minus the calorie level of the diet will determine how quickly you lose fat. Two people on the same diet will lose weight at different rates if their usual calorie intakes differ.

Make sure your diet is balanced and contains the Recommended Dietary Allowances for vitamins, minerals, and proteins (see pages 54–61). On reducing diets, protein is not used quite as efficiently as normally. Too little protein at this

---

Medically supervised dieting

You need to consult a doctor before you begin a weight-reducing diet if any of the following points apply to you.

● You are more than 15 pounds over normal weight.

● You have been heavy for most or all of your life. You need special support to help you overcome longstanding habits.

● You are pregnant; dieting can endanger your unborn child.

● You are a child or adolescent; growing bodies need special help to put on lean tissue while losing fat.

● You have a health problem such as high blood pressure, diabetes, high blood cholesterol; the doctor might suggest additional measures.

● You are determined to follow a crash diet of less than 800 calories a day.

● You are considering the use of appetite suppressants or drugs; these are best prescribed by a doctor.

● You suffer from emotional illness; dieting might cause added stress with which you might not be able to cope.

● You develop symptoms of physical problems while on a diet, including sudden chest pains, nausea, fainting spells, or depression.

If you do need medical help, select a physician who is interested in you and your weight problems, and can refer you to a registered dietitian for assistance in meal planning.

---

time needlessly increases the breakdown of body protein to keep other cells working properly. Too much protein does not seem to have any side effects, but such a diet can be expensive.

Your diet should also contain at least 100 grams (about three ounces) of carbohydrate, so that lean tissue doesn't have to be broken down to keep blood sugar up. When your daily diet supplies less than this amount of carbohydrate, or less than a total of 800 calories, ketones build up and your body tends to lose a great deal of water in the urine. Unlike the loss of fat weight, water weight loss is temporary, and weight reappears as soon as you are off the diet. Diets very high in carbohydrates are often also very high in dietary fiber; such diets may be more satisfying to some people, and thus more effective, for this reason.

Surprisingly, you also need to eat some fat on a reducing diet. One-half to one ounce of fat per day is absolutely necessary to provide the essential fatty acids and to carry the fat-soluble vitamins A, D, E, and K. Considerably more fat than this (at least one to two ounces) is usually necessary to make menus most Americans would find palatable. High-fat diets are not recommended, since they might increase blood fat levels. They might appear to work because they are so low in carbohydrates that they cause you to lose a few pounds of water weight temporarily.

Weight loss products

It is impossible to keep all the bad and ineffective weight loss diets and devices out of the marketplace. As a consumer, you should try to determine if the advertising and marketing practices that are employed are honest. For example, avoid diets that use pyramid marketing schemes, in which everyone who goes on the diet becomes a salesperson who tries to sell it to other people. You can also be sure that any diet that claims 100 percent success or a revolutionary breakthrough is not telling the whole truth; even experts have failures among their patients. And products that are sold door to door by silver-tongued salespeople are also best avoided until you check them out with your state Public Health Department, your county cooperative extension agent, or your doctor.

Be suspicious of any plan whose sponsors complain that it has been suppressed by the medical profession. There are few secrets or conspiracies in science. For example, there are diet doctors who claim to have special diet pills and hormone shots that the rest of the medical profession does not possess. Many studies have been made of diet pills. Some of the appetite suppressants do provide a boost to dieters at first, helping them to control their appetites and stick to the diet in the first few months. However, by the end of the diet there are usually few differences in weight loss between those who took appetite suppressants and those who did not. Hormone shots and other types of pills have not been found to be effective in speeding weight loss, and some have risks of their own. For these reasons medical experts do not recommend them.

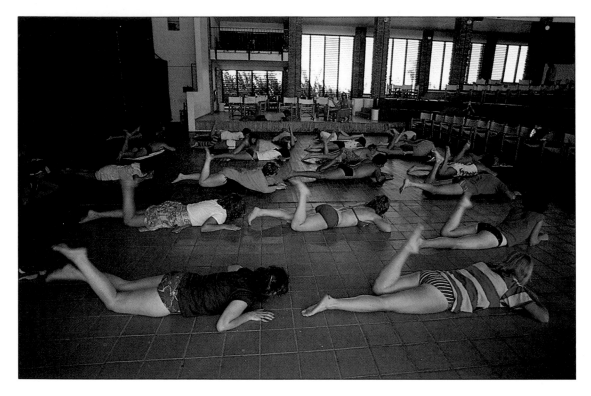

You are more likely to succeed in losing weight if you increase the amount of exercise you do while decreasing the number of calories you eat. You will benefit from the extra fitness and trimmer looks, and from the fact that you need a less rigid diet when your energy output increases. Increased activity does not make you eat more. In fact, it helps you to burn up excess calories while you are doing it, and helps to keep your resting metabolism from decreasing.

The physical activity you choose doesn't have to be vigorous to help you. If you have been sedentary until now, include more walking, stair climbing, and lifting in your daily routine. Do a little more each day. Then add vigorous aerobic exercise, which takes you to your maximum level of endurance, several times a week. This can burn off significant amounts of calories.

Choose the activity that you like the most because then you're more likely to keep it up. If you are embarrassed about your shape and weight, you might prefer to exercise by yourself or with someone close to you. If you find that you are more successful with group support, you might make your scheduled exercise program a

Many organized weight-reducing groups make physical exercise a major feature of their program. Participants meet regularly, and at each session may be given advice about their diets, and then weighed, before exercising.

social occasion with friends or join an exercise class. See "Getting Fit, Staying Fit" (pages 94–159) for help in devising an exercise program.

More help

Commercial weight loss firms are very popular. They offer the advantages of group support, a diet plan, and a program of physical activity. Those that use diets over 800 calories and have reasonable charges are best; avoid those that insist you pay a large sum in advance.

Health farms, spas, or other live-in facilities have the advantage of controlling the total environment of the dieter and thus keeping food temptations to a minimum. They usually offer high-quality accommodation, a diet plan, exercise, massage, saunas, and other beauty treatments. They can be a useful way to get started, but are helpful in the long term only if they teach you new eating habits. Avoid establishments that insist on rigid crash diets.

At a health farm the emphasis is on low-calorie diets served in luxurious surroundings. The problem is that visitors stay for only a short time. This inevitably means that there is an element of crash dieting involved in the weight loss. Despite this, many people who treat themselves to a vacation at a health farm find it valuable in terms of well-being, even if they do not achieve a permanent weight loss.

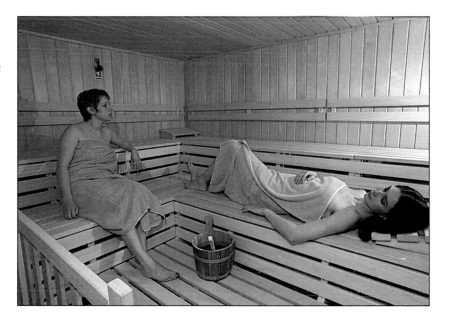

The weekly weigh-in is an essential part of the Weight Watchers approach to dieting. At meetings members are encouraged to talk openly about their weight and are given help to handle the emotional problems with which overeating and overweight are often associated. Advice is given on choosing an appropriate eating program with the aim of educating members into recognizing and accepting a lower energy input.

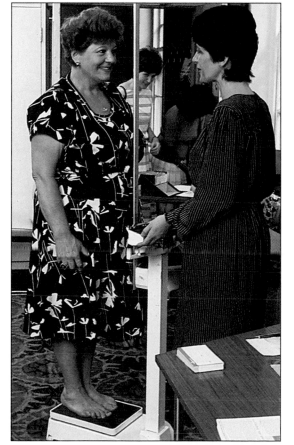

Chart your progress

Even if you do not attend a group weighing session, you can use similar methods at home to chart your progress.

● Write a list of numbers, say 1 to 20, representing your target weight loss in pounds. Cross off each pound as you lose it.

● Make a graph of your weight against time. Fill in points on the graph each week as you weigh yourself.

REDUCING DIETS

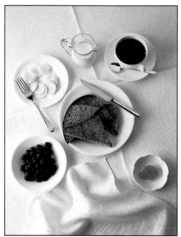

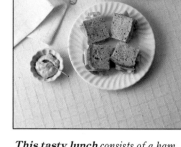

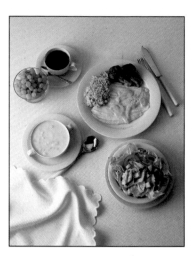

An appetizing and well-balanced breakfast *of fresh blueberries, whole-wheat toast and marmalade, a hard-boiled egg, skim milk, and black coffee (see 1,200-calorie menu, Day 3).*

This tasty lunch *consists of a ham and cheese sandwich on rye bread, tossed salad with blue cheese dressing, an orange, and low-fat milk (see 1,800-calorie menu, Day 3).*

A hearty meal *of vegetable chowder, followed by baked flounder, broccoli, brown rice, and salad with French dressing, with grapes for dessert (see 2,400-calorie menu, Day 3).*

The menus shown in the table opposite provide a moderately low-calorie reducing diet that is relatively low in fat, and adequate in protein, vitamins, and minerals for short-term use (a week or two). If you wish to follow this diet for a longer period of time, you would be wise to include a multivitamin-mineral supplement, as it is difficult for a diet with such a low calorie level to meet the Recommended Dietary Allowances for certain nutrients, even with careful planning.

Making choices
These menus illustrate several points you need to keep in mind when evaluating other weight-reducing diets.

First, this reducing diet is only moderately low in calories. You should check with your doctor if you are considering a diet below this calorie level. Very restrictive diets make it difficult to include all the protein, vitamins, and minerals that you need to lose weight safely, and since they also cause changes in body fluids and metabolism, they need to be medically supervised.

Second, a good reducing diet does not wholly eliminate any group of foods, and any diet that does is likely to be nutritionally inadequate.

Third, although you don't have to give up any food completely, you do have to control portions. You will note that the menus shown here indicate small portions, and that very high-calorie items

are used relatively rarely.

Many people don't realize how big a difference small changes in their diet can make. For example, if these menus included whole milk instead of skim, vegetables with added cooking fat, pie or cake instead of fruit, and fatter cuts of meat, they would have included several hundred more calories each day.

Fourth, how you prepare your food is as important as how much you eat on a low-calorie diet. Select lean cuts of meat and trim off the visible fat. Choose lower-fat fish, and eat poultry without the skin. Roasting, broiling, boiling, steaming, and poaching are low-calorie cooking methods; avoid frying and sautéing. Get used to drinking tea and coffee black and unsweetened; milk, cream, and sugar are high in calories. The menus on pages 81–83 allow for a cup of unsweetened black tea or coffee after meals.

A diet to live with
Look at the menus here and you will see that with a few additions and larger portions they can easily be used for maintaining weight. In the long run the only way to keep obesity under control is to control calorie consumption and lead a physically active life. For this reason, reducing diets have to be adaptable not just for a week or a month, but for a lifetime.

This reducing diet is suitable for nonpregnant adults. The amount of weight you will lose depends on the difference between your previous calorie intake and the diet. For example, if your weight is steady on 2,400 calories, you will have a calorie deficit of 1,200 calories a day, or 8,400 calories by the end of a week, and you should lose 2.4 pounds of fat.

1,200-CALORIE MENUS				
Day	Breakfast	Lunch	Dinner	Snacks
1.	½ cup fresh orange juice 1 shredded wheat biscuit with ½ sliced banana 1 cup skim milk	Tuna salad: ¼ cup tuna fish (water-packed), 2 tsp mayonnaise, 1 tbsp celery, 1 tbsp bean sprouts, 2 small lettuce leaves 1 small pita bread 1 cup tomato juice 1 small apple	4 oz broiled center slice ham ¼ cup mashed yams ½ cup black-eyed peas ½ cup spinach 4 radishes ½ cup fruit cocktail (water-packed) 1 cup skim milk	1 small peach 1 cup diet soda
2.	½ fresh grapefruit 1 tsp sugar ⅓ cup All Bran cereal 1 cup skim milk	Turkey sandwich: 2 oz sliced turkey, 1 tsp mustard, 1 tsp soft margarine, 2 lettuce leaves, 2 slices tomato, on 2 slices whole-wheat bread 1 small fresh nectarine 1 cup skim milk	3 oz lean round steak braised in beef bouillon and herbs 1 medium boiled potato 1 tsp soft margarine ½ cup cooked carrots ½ cup cooked Brussels sprouts ½ cup tossed green salad with tomato 1 tbsp low-calorie Italian dressing ¼ medium cantaloupe	2 graham crackers 1 small pear Herbal tea
3.	½ cup fresh blueberries 1 small hard-boiled egg 1 slice whole-wheat toast 2 tsp orange marmalade 1 cup skim milk	1 cup yogurt made from skim milk ½ cup fresh sliced strawberries 4 small rye crispbreads 1 tsp soft margarine 1 cup tomato juice	4 oz trimmed braised veal cutlet ½ cup spaghetti 1 tsp soft margarine ½ cup Italian-style green beans ½ cup cauliflower with 1 tbsp red pepper 1 small slice angel food cake 1 tbsp frozen raspberries in own juice	½ cup carrot and celery sticks 1 pear
4.	¾ cup strawberries with 2 tsp sugar 1 slice oatmeal toast 2 tsp strawberry jam 1 cup skim milk	Greek salad: ½ cup spinach, ½ cup lettuce, 1 oz feta cheese, 1 oz anchovies, ½ cup tomato slices, 2 Greek olives, 1 tbsp low-calorie Greek salad dressing 4 bread sticks 1 orange ½ cup iced milk	Fresh celery sticks and radishes 1 serving baked haddock with tomato and basil sauce, with 1 tsp margarine ½ cup brown rice ½ cup cooked broccoli ½ cup cooked carrot slices ½ cup fresh pineapple chunks	2 graham crackers 1 cup diet ginger ale
5.	½ cup bran flakes 1 fresh sliced peach 1 blueberry muffin 1 cup skim milk	½ cup low-fat cottage cheese ¼ fresh cantaloupe 1 slice raisin bread	Carrot and celery sticks 3 oz baked turkey, no skin ½ cup mashed potato with 1 tsp butter 2 tbsp cranberry sauce ½ cup cooked green beans ½ small butternut squash with brown sugar ½ cup fruit soup	¼ cup fruit ice 1 cup skim milk
6.	½ grapefruit with 1 tsp sugar 1 slice whole-wheat toast 2 tsp grape jelly	1 cup low-fat yogurt 1 large apple 3 small rye crackers 1 cup tomato juice	4 oz flank steak 1 large baked potato 1 tsp soft margarine ½ cup cooked broccoli spears 1 cup tossed salad ½ cup fresh orange ambrosia	1 cup skim milk 2 small plums
7.	1 cup orange juice 1 cup oatmeal with 1 tbsp brown sugar 1 slice cinnamon toast 1 tsp soft margarine 1 cup skim milk	½ cup low-fat cottage cheese 1 serving molded gelatin fruit salad on leaf lettuce 2 pineapple rings (water-packed) 1 cup iced tea	4 oz lean ground beef hamburger with soy extender, on French bread with 2 tsp catsup, 2 tsp mayonnaise, ½ green pepper sliced, pickle slices, onion 1 cup cucumber and tomato salad 1 cup skim milk ½ cup peach slices (water-packed)	Peanut butter sandwich: whole-wheat bread with 1½ tsp peanut butter, 1 tsp jelly 1 cup diet soft drink

SAMPLE MENUS/1,800 CALORIES

The menus shown here are suitable for many mature women. Each day's menus illustrate four principles of low-fat eating.

- Select lower-fat milk products.
- Select lean, lower-fat meats: remove skin from poultry and trim excess fat from meat.
- Use low-fat food preparation methods.
- Reduce the amount of fats added at the table.

These menus allow for a cup of unsweetened black coffee or tea after meals, if desired.

1,800-CALORIE MENUS

Day	Breakfast	Lunch	Dinner	Snacks
1.	$\frac{3}{4}$ cup fresh grapefruit juice 1 scrambled egg 2 slices banana-nut bread	Chicken salad sandwich: 2 oz chicken, 1 tbsp celery, 1 tsp onion, 2 tsp mayonnaise, 2 slices pumpernickel bread 1 orange 1 cup skim milk	4 oz lean-only chuck pot roast $\frac{3}{4}$ cup mashed potato $\frac{1}{2}$ cup green beans 1 cup spinach salad 1 tbsp Italian dressing 1 slice enriched Italian bread 1 tsp soft margarine $\frac{1}{2}$ cup orange-pineapple fruit cup	1 cup raw vegetable sticks: carrots, celery, green pepper $\frac{1}{4}$ cup bean dip or yogurt dip
2.	$\frac{1}{3}$ cup fresh sliced peaches $\frac{1}{3}$ cup bran with $\frac{1}{2}$ cup 1% fat milk 1 slice raisin toast 1 tbsp marmalade	2 oz hamburger with 1 oz American cheese and hamburger bun $\frac{1}{2}$ cup coleslaw with mayonnaise-type salad dressing Small bag potato chips 1 cup 1% fat milk	1 serving chicken cacciatore $\frac{1}{2}$ cup enriched spaghetti $\frac{1}{2}$ cup Italian green beans $1\frac{1}{2}$ cups mixed green salad 1 tbsp Italian dressing 1 slice Italian bread 1 tsp soft margarine $\frac{1}{2}$ cup seedless grapes	1 cup orange juice 1 medium pear 2 small squares unsalted soda crackers
3.	$\frac{1}{4}$ medium honeydew melon 1 toasted enriched English muffin 1 tbsp orange marmalade 1 hard-boiled egg 1 cup 1% fat milk	Ham and cheese sandwich: 1 oz lean ham, 1 oz Swiss cheese, 2 slices rye bread, 2 tsp mayonnaise-type salad dressing, 1 tsp mustard $1\frac{1}{4}$ cups tossed mixed salad 1 tbsp blue cheese dressing 1 medium orange 1 cup 1% fat milk	1 serving flounder Florentine 1 medium baked potato 2 tbsp sour cream $\frac{1}{2}$ cup green peas 1 small whole-wheat roll 1 tsp soft margarine $\frac{1}{2}$ cup fresh strawberries	1 medium corn muffin 1 tsp margarine $\frac{1}{2}$ cup low-fat blueberry yogurt
4.	$\frac{1}{2}$ cup fresh orange juice 2 slices pumpernickel toast 1 tbsp jam 1 cup fortified skim milk	Turkey salad: 2 oz sliced turkey, 1 cup Boston lettuce, $\frac{1}{2}$ cup spinach, $\frac{1}{2}$ tomato, $\frac{1}{4}$ cup sliced green pepper 3 tbsp green goddess dressing 1 small slice sourdough bread 1 tsp soft margarine 1 fresh apple 1 cup skim milk	1 serving bean salad 1 serving baked fish with spicy sauce $\frac{1}{2}$ cup Brussels sprouts $\frac{1}{2}$ cup brown rice 2 Parker House rolls 2 tsp margarine 1 pear	1 slice gingerbread
5.	$\frac{1}{2}$ medium fresh grapefruit 2 slices whole-wheat toast 1 tbsp strawberry jam 1 cup fortified skim milk	$\frac{3}{4}$ cup canned vegetable juice $1\frac{1}{2}$ cups green salad with $1\frac{1}{2}$ oz Swiss cheese 1 tbsp French dressing 2 bran muffins 2 tsp soft margarine 1 small nectarine 1 cup fortified skim milk	1 large carrot, cut into sticks 4 oz lean broiled ground beef $\frac{1}{2}$ cup mashed potatoes with 1 tsp soft margarine $\frac{1}{2}$ cup green beans 1 baked apple with 2 tsp brown sugar	3 graham crackers 1 cup orange juice
6.	$\frac{3}{4}$ cup grapefruit juice 2 buckwheat pancakes 1 tbsp maple syrup 1 tsp soft margarine 1 cup fortified skim milk	Pouch sandwich on Syrian bread: 2 oz lean beef, 1 tbsp onion, 1 tbsp Cheddar cheese, 1 tbsp lettuce, 1 tbsp tomato $\frac{3}{4}$ cup fresh fruit cup: oranges, apples, bananas 1 cup skim milk	4 oz lean-only baked ham 1 small baked sweet potato $\frac{1}{2}$ cup cooked spinach 1 cup tossed mixed salad 1 tbsp Italian salad dressing 1 small corn muffin 1 tsp margarine $\frac{1}{2}$ cup canned pineapple with $\frac{1}{2}$ cup lemon sherbet	24 goldfish crackers 1 cup light beer 1 fresh apple
7.	1 small orange, $\frac{1}{2}$ cup oatmeal with 1 tsp brown sugar $\frac{1}{2}$ cup low-fat fortified milk	1 cup split pea soup Chicken salad sandwich: 2 oz chicken, 1 tbsp celery, 1 tsp onion, 2 tsp mayonnaise, lettuce, 2 slices rye bread 1 small peach 1 cup skim milk	1 serving beef with Chinese-style vegetables $\frac{1}{2}$ cup enriched white rice 2 coconut bars	$\frac{1}{2}$ cup pineapple chunks in own juice 2 slices banana-nut bread 1 cup skim milk

SAMPLE MENUS/2,400 CALORIES

The week's menus shown here are suitable for many mature, relatively sedentary adult men. Younger and more active men and teenage boys usually need more calories than this. They can eat larger portions or add extra foods.

The menus for each day include foods from all the food groups to provide all essential nutrients. They include minimal amounts of fats, sweets, and alcoholic beverages. An unsweetened cup of black tea or coffee is permissible after meals, if desired.

2,400-CALORIE MENUS

Day	Breakfast	Lunch	Dinner	Snacks
1.	¾ cup fresh orange juice 1 large soft-cooked egg 2 slices banana-nut bread	Tuna salad sandwich: 2 oz tuna (water-packed), 1 tbsp celery, 1 tsp onion, 2 tsp mayonnaise, 2 slices whole-wheat bread 1 fresh pear	4 oz lean-only chuck pot roast ¾ cup mashed potato ½ cup cooked green beans 1 cup spinach salad 1 tbsp Italian dressing 1 tsp soft margarine 1 cup orange-pineapple fruit cup	1 cup assorted raw vegetable sticks ½ cup bean dip 6 whole-wheat crackers 1½ cups grapefruit juice
2.	½ cup fresh strawberries 2 shredded wheat biscuits with ½ sliced banana 1 tbsp sugar	3 oz hamburger with 1 oz melted cheese 1 hamburger bun 1 tsp catsup 2 slices pickle 1 large serving french fries 1 cup lemonade	1 serving chicken cacciatore 1 cup enriched spaghetti ½ cup cooked zucchini squash 1½ cups mixed green salad 1 tbsp Italian dressing 2 slices enriched Italian bread 2 tsp soft margarine 1 medium peach ½ cup Chianti wine	2 graham crackers
3.	¾ cup fresh orange juice 1 large scrambled egg 1 bagel 2 tbsp cream cheese 1 tbsp raspberry jam	2 chicken sandwiches; 3 oz sliced chicken, 2 leaves lettuce, 3 tsp salad dressing, 4 slices whole-wheat bread 1 serving three-bean salad 1 medium, fresh apple	1 serving vegetable chowder 1½ servings baked flounder ½ cup cooked broccoli spears ½ cup brown rice 1½ cups mixed green salad with tomato 1 tbsp French dressing 1 cup seedless grapes	1 slice gingerbread 1 medium, fresh pear
4.	¼ medium cantaloupe 2 medium corn muffins 2 tsp soft margarine 2 tsp grape jelly 1 cup whole milk	1 large lean-only pork chop ½ cup black-eyed peas ½ cup enriched rice 1 large enriched hard roll 1 tsp soft margarine ½ cup sliced peaches (water-packed) ¾ cup apple cider	1 serving flounder Florentine 1 medium baked potato 2 tbsp sour cream ½ cup cooked frozen green peas 1 small whole-wheat roll 1 tsp soft margarine 1 cup vanilla yogurt with ½ cup fresh strawberries	1 whole enriched English muffin 2 tsp soft margarine 1 tbsp marmalade
5.	½ medium grapefruit 2 slices whole-wheat toast 1 tsp soft margarine 1 tbsp apple jelly	¾ cup canned tomato juice Chef's Salad: 2 oz turkey, 1 oz ham, 1½ oz Swiss cheese, 1½ cups mixed greens 1½ tbsp French dressing 2 small peaches	4 oz broiled lean ground beef 2 ears corn on the cob 3 tsp soft margarine 2 rye rolls 1 baked apple with 2 tsp brown sugar	Peanut butter sandwich: whole-wheat bread, 1 tbsp peanut butter, 2 tsp grape jelly 1 cup fresh orange juice
6.	¾ cup fresh orange juice 3 whole-wheat pancakes 2 tsp soft margarine 1 serving blueberry syrup	2 beef tacos ¾ cup fresh fruit cup: oranges, apples, bananas	4 oz lean-only roast loin of pork 1 medium sweet potato ½ cup fresh collard greens 1¼ cups tossed salad 1 tbsp Italian dressing 2 enriched biscuits 1 tbsp honey	4 graham crackers 1 fresh apple 1½ cups fresh orange juice
7.	¾ cup pineapple chunks (water-packed) 1 cup oatmeal with cinnamon and 3 tbsp raisins 2 tsp brown sugar	1 cup split pea soup Stuffed tomato: 1 medium tomato, 2 oz cooked chicken, 1 tbsp celery, 1 tsp onion, 2 tsp mayonnaise 6 rye crackers 2 tsp soft margarine ¾ cup lemon sherbet	1½ servings beef with Chinese-style vegetables ¾ cup enriched white rice 1 serving apple crisp	

A HIGH-FIBER DIET

These menus provide about 30 grams or more of dietary fiber a day, which is at least twice as much as most Americans usually eat. They illustrate several points that you need to keep in mind in following a high-fiber diet.

It is important to include whole-grain products, which contain nearly the entire edible portion of the grain.

Be sure to eat plenty of fresh fruits and vegetables each day, preferably with their skins.

Concentrate on eating several servings of fiber-rich foods throughout the day. These menus include at least one high-fiber food at each meal, and allow for after-dinner tea or coffee, if desired.

To benefit from all the kinds of dietary fiber it is important to eat a variety of plant foods.

HIGH-FIBER DIET MENUS

Day	Breakfast	Lunch	Dinner	Snacks
1.	Skim milk Bran buds cereal 1 fresh peach Whole-wheat toast Soft margarine Coffee	Lettuce and tomato salad with lemon dill dressing and tabbouleh (cracked bulgur wheat) Sliced chicken on pumpernickel bread with mayonnaise Skim milk Orange	Broiled haddock with lobster and shrimp stuffing Broccoli Brown rice Green pepper, endive, escarole, and lettuce salad with French dressing Fresh pineapple chunks	Rye Krisp Apple Chocolate milk
2.	Grapefruit broiled with brown sugar All Bran and skim milk Bran muffin with margarine Skim milk Coffee	Cucumber, lettuce, and tomato salad with bean sprouts and low-fat yogurt dressing Tuna salad sandwich on whole-wheat bread Pear Skim milk Oatmeal cookies	Three-bean salad with vinaigrette dressing Lemon-baked chicken with orange sauce Baked potatoes with mock sour cream made from low-fat yogurt and chives Green beans Carrots Strawberry shortcake with fresh strawberries and homemade biscuits	Peanut butter sandwich on whole-wheat bread Skim milk Apple
3.	100% bran cereal with skim milk Blackberries Apricot nectar Corn muffin Coffee	Bean soup Ham and Swiss cheese sandwich on rye bread Celery and carrot sticks Skim milk Nectarine Coconut macaroon	Flounder in green tomato sauce Brown rice Green beans Whole-wheat roll and soft margarine Carrot salad Skim milk Sliced peaches and peach sherbet	Bran muffin with marmalade Orange and grapefruit sections Skim milk
4.	Raisin bran with skim milk Oatmeal toast with raspberry jam Orange Skim milk Coffee	Chicken tacos with Mexican hot sauce Tortillas Mexican flag salad: white beans, red pepper, and green beans Skim milk Tea Pear	Finger vegetables with low-fat yogurt dip Roast loin of pork (lean meat only) Baked winter squash Broad green beans with sesame seeds Brown rice with pan gravy Fresh fruit cup	Graham crackers Cantaloupe Skim milk
5.	All Bran with skim milk Nectarine Blueberry and bran muffin with blueberry jam Coffee Skim milk	Fresh fruit salad with low-fat cottage cheese, and sweet dressing Rye Krisp Lemonade	Finger vegetables Boston baked beans Peas Brown bread Tossed green salad Ambrosia of oranges and shredded coconut	Fresh strawberries Popcorn Skim milk
6.	Oatmeal with wheat germ Skim milk Prunes and apricots Whole-wheat raisin English muffins with peanut butter Coffee	Lentil soup Tuna salad sandwich on dark bread with lettuce Skim milk Nectarine	Mixed green salad with French dressing Baked fish in spicy sauce Cooked fresh zucchini squash Cooked fresh carrot rounds Steamed bulgur wheat with soft margarine added at table Concord grapes	Bran buds and skim milk Apple
7.	Shredded wheat with peach slices, milk and sugar Orange juice Whole-wheat muffin with peach jam Coffee Skim milk	Egg salad sandwich on dark rye bread with lettuce and tomato on the side, celery and carrot sticks Skim milk Apple	Whole-wheat spaghetti with low-fat meat balls and tomato sauce Whole-wheat rolls and soft margarine Italian broad green bean, cauliflower, and pepper vegetable medley Tossed salad with Italian dressing Skim milk Cantaloupe	Carrot sticks Bran muffin with raspberry jam Apples

This diet will provide about 1,000–1,500 milligrams, or about half a teaspoon, of sodium a day. It is suitable for people who wish to reduce the amount of sodium they eat, as well as those who have been told by their doctor to follow a low-sodium diet because of illness. If you are in the latter category, check with your doctor that this diet is suitable for you, since there are many different levels of sodium restriction. The menus include optional tea or coffee after dinner.

When eating out, ask for your order to be unsalted and choose main dishes that are broiled, as salt can then be easily omitted. Choose side items that are not usually salted, such as baked potatoes. With salads, ask for oil and vinegar on the side so you can make your own dressing.

LOW-SODIUM DIET

Day	Breakfast	Lunch	Dinner	Snacks
1.	Orange juice Low-sodium muffin with low-sodium margarine Soft cooked egg Skim milk Coffee	Small portion broiled fresh flounder Low-sodium bread with low-sodium margarine Fresh broccoli, unsalted Low-fat milk Peaches	Roast beef Green beans Carrot coins Boiled rice Green salad with low-sodium dressing Whole-wheat rolls and low-sodium margarine Bananas and strawberries	Baked apple with sugar Apple Unsalted crackers
2.	Shredded wheat with banana and milk Pineapple chunks Low-sodium muffin with strawberry jam Skim milk Coffee	Tomato stuffed with chicken tarragon Tossed salad with low-sodium dressing Low-sodium bread with low-sodium margarine Tea Pears	Beef with Chinese stir-fried vegetables (no salt or MSG added) Boiled rice Green salad with low-sodium dressing Fortune cookies and pineapple chunks	Banana-nut bread Orange Low-fat milk
3.	½ grapefruit Low-sodium toast with low-sodium margarine and jam Low-fat milk Puffed rice with milk Coffee	Tomato juice Chef's salad with low-sodium cheese, turkey, mixed greens, and low-sodium French dressing Low-sodium corn bread and low-sodium margarine Peach	Broiled lean ground beef Ear of corn with low-sodium margarine Fresh cooked green beans Sliced beefsteak tomatoes with parsley, peppers, and low-sodium vinaigrette dressing Baked apple with brown sugar	Plums Graham crackers Skim milk
4.	Orange sections Low-sodium muffin with low-sodium corn oil margarine and blueberry jam Low-fat yogurt Coffee	Gazpacho (cold vegetable soup) Chicken sandwich with mayonnaise and bean sprouts on whole-wheat bread Lettuce with celery seed dressing Pears Skim milk	Veal scallopini Noodles cooked without salt Asparagus spears cooked without salt Whole-wheat dinner rolls with low-sodium margarine Lemon sherbet with sliced strawberries	Oatmeal cookies Apple Orange juice
5.	Cantaloupe Low-sodium whole-wheat pancakes with blueberry sauce Low-fat milk Coffee	Pasta salad with low-sodium dressing Low-sodium bread with low-sodium corn oil margarine Fresh fruit cup with oranges, apples, and bananas Iced tea	Roast loin of pork (lean meat only) Baked sweet potato Fresh cooked spinach Tossed salad with low-sodium dressing Biscuits with honey and low-sodium margarine Angel food cake with strawberries	Grapefruit juice Low-sodium crackers Seedless grapes Skim milk
6.	Orange juice Scrambled egg Low-sodium toast with jam Skim milk Coffee	Sliced chicken sandwich with lettuce and mayonnaise on whole-wheat bread Bean salad with oil and vinegar dressing Apple Skim milk	Finger vegetables Baked codfish with green pepper and onion dressing Baked potato with yogurt and chives Low-sodium bread with low-sodium corn oil margarine Broccoli Tossed salad with low-sodium dressing Fruit cup	Pear English muffin and jam Skim milk
7.	Fresh strawberries Shredded wheat with sliced banana and sugar Low-fat milk Coffee	Tuna salad sandwich with celery, onion, mayonnaise, and no salt, on whole-wheat bread Pear Apple juice	Pot roast, lean-only chuck steak cooked with herbs and no extra salt Mashed potatoes, with no salt added and low-sodium corn oil margarine Green beans boiled with no salt added Spinach and tomato salad with low-sodium dressing Whole-wheat dinner rolls with low-sodium corn oil margarine Orange pineapple fruit cup	Apple Graham crackers Low-fat yogurt with fruit

Several types of diets eaten in America today are loosely described as vegetarian. The most common is actually a semivegetarian diet in which no red meat is eaten, although poultry, fish, milk, and eggs are consumed. Next comes the lacto-ovo vegetarian diet, in which no animal flesh is consumed, but milk products and eggs are allowed. The strictest and least common is the vegan diet, in which no animal flesh or animal products are eaten. These distinctions are important from the nutritional standpoint because the nutrient consumption and deficiencies of vegans are quite different from those of lacto-ovo and semivegetarians.

In addition to these limitations, many vegetarians often use only organically grown, natural whole foods or health foods, and avoid highly processed, fortified and enriched foods, as well as vitamin-mineral supplements.

Is vegetarian better?

Some vegetarians choose their diet because of religious beliefs, or because they feel that animals should not be killed for food. Some think that besides being healthier, vegetarian diets provide spiritual advantages beyond the boundaries of nutrition. However, many omnivorous people are now turning to the vegetarian style of eating, believing it is better for their health.

From the health standpoint, vegetarian diets do have a lot of good points. Compared to the usual American diet, they generally contain less fat, fewer calories, less sugar, and, because of the emphasis on fruits, vegetables, and grains, less sodium and more dietary fiber—in fact, just what medical experts and nutritionists everywhere now recommend. However, vegetarians are neither more nor less healthy than someone who follows the healthy diet outlined earlier in this chapter (see pages 62–65).

Since the whole or partial elimination of animal and/or dairy products clearly restricts your nutrient sources, all vegetarian diets require careful planning to minimize health risks and maximize health benefits. Dietary difficulties among vegetarians are usually related to an insufficiency, rather than an excess, of calories and nutrients. This can be an even greater problem for people who have especially high nutrient needs, such as expectant and nursing mothers and children.

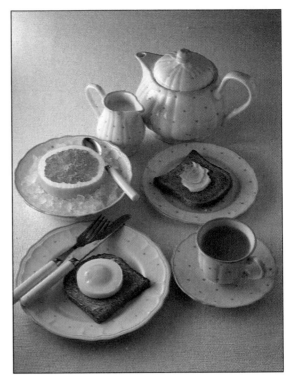

A vegetarian breakfast suggestion: half a grapefruit, poached egg, whole-wheat toast with polyunsaturated margarine, tea with skim milk.

Problems of a vegan diet

The risks of deficiency diseases are greatest on a vegan diet, particularly when combined with a self-imposed restriction to eating whole foods. In addition, children and adults with small appetites may find it difficult to eat the large quantity of vegetable foods necessary to provide enough protein and/or carbohydrate.

A study of growth in a large number of vegetarian children under six years of age, carried out at Tufts University in Boston, suggested that the growth of vegan children was somewhat diminished. The main cause seemed to be the lower level of energy rather than a protein deficiency. In part, this is because there is little fat in a vegan diet. Some of the children also had high risks of deficiencies of vitamins D and B_{12}, which can also limit growth.

Do not put a child on a vegan diet until you have consulted a physician to make sure that the particular diet meets all the child's nutrient needs.

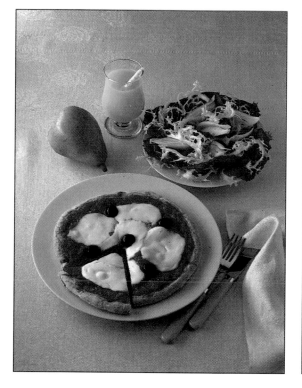

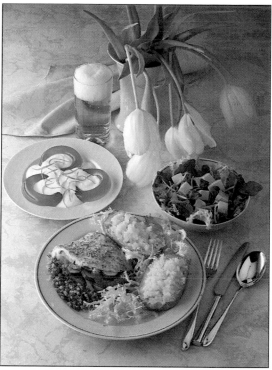

A meat-free lunch: *whole-wheat pizza, mixed salad, a pear, pure orange juice.*

An alternative dinner: *buckwheat and vegetable casserole with yogurt topping, baked potato, tofu salad, orange gelatin with yogurt, beer.*

Switching to a vegetarian diet

If you are thinking of switching to a vegetarian diet, it is usually best to do so gradually, in order to avoid any temporary digestive disturbances. Try giving up red meats first, followed by white meats, such as pork and veal, then poultry, and finally, fish and seafood. At each stage, replace the protein-rich meats with plant proteins from legumes (dried peas and beans), seeds and nuts, as well as vegetables, dairy products, and eggs.

Aim to get as much variety as possible, and follow the diet suggestions on pages 88–89 to avoid the possibility of nutrient deficiencies. Since some nutrients are in a lower concentration, absent or in a less available form in plant than in animal foods, you need to understand the contributions of all the food groups in order to make the correct choices. This is particularly important if you plan to adopt a vegan diet. Lacto-ovo vegetarians, who can obtain iron from eggs, and can find in fortified milk products certain minerals and vitamins that are in short supply in vegetables, have a distinct advantage in this regard. Consuming milk and eggs does not mean, however, that you should reduce the quantity or range of plant foods you eat, since each plant group provides different nutrients.

Growing children, pregnant or nursing women, or anyone recovering from a serious illness, may need to supplement a vegetarian diet by taking vitamin-mineral tablets.

Vegans have to be particularly careful about their choice of foods if they are to avoid serious deficiencies, particularly of vitamin B_{12}, which is found only in foods of animal origin. The effects of vitamin B_{12} deficiency may not be apparent for many years, but may ultimately lead to serious damage to the nervous system.

Vegan diets are considered in more detail on page 88. Since switching to this type of diet clearly involves extensive changes, you will almost certainly find it helpful to consult a doctor or dietitian before you do so.

VEGETARIAN DIETS/2

The meals suggested on page 89 are an example of a day's balanced eating for a lacto-ovo vegetarian. The calorie level, based on a single serving of each item, just meets the needs of an average woman, and the fat level is 34 percent. Use the calorie tables on pages 338–341 as a guide if you want to increase or decrease the calorie level of the menus. As in all healthy diets, there is a good deal of emphasis on fresh fruits, vegetables, and whole-grain products. The dishes show that even though vegetarians do not eat meat, they do have a wide and varied menu.

Reduce all the "empty-calorie" foods you eat, that is, those high-calorie, low-nutrient density foods like cakes, pies, alcoholic beverages, and soft drinks. Replace them with natural and unrefined foods, which supply a more balanced mix of proteins, vitamins, and minerals as well as calories. This has been done in most of the menus shown opposite; for example, instead of high-calorie, rich desserts and soft drinks, the emphasis is on fruits, juices, and whole-grain products.

Building protein

For most Americans, a big concern in following a vegetarian diet is to ensure that they are getting enough protein-rich foods. Contrary to popular opinion, you do not have to eat meat to be healthy. The human body does not specifically require animal protein, but it does need certain amino acids and the nitrogen found in protein.

These needs can be met by either animal or plant sources. However, the concentration of the essential amino acids in plants is lower, and the essential amino acid patterns are not as well balanced as they are in animal sources. Therefore it is important to include a mixture of proteins from whole grains, legumes, seeds, nuts, and vegetables high in protein so that the different amino acids in each can supplement and complement each other. These complementaries must be combined in the same meal, although not necessarily in the same dish, to be effective.

The lacto-ovo vegetarian menus here assure that a proper balance is achieved by combining at each meal several different protein-rich plant foods and acceptable foods from animal sources, such as milk and eggs. Together these provide all the essential amino acids. When planning other meals, be sure you include one of the following combinations:

- Legumes with grains
- Legumes with seeds and nuts
- Dairy products or eggs with any vegetable protein.

On a lacto-ovo vegetarian diet it is often a good idea to use low-fat or skim milk products since they supply large amounts of high-quality animal protein inexpensively and without a lot of fat or calories. Eggs are also a good source of animal protein that can be included in moderation. At the same time, legumes, seeds, and nuts deserve special emphasis because they are good sources of particularly high-quality plant protein.

Most lacto-ovo vegetarians also find it helpful to increase their intake of whole-grain breads and cereals because, in addition to supplying protein and other protective nutrients, they provide needed energy.

It is important to eat a variety of fruits and vegetables. The iron in vegetarian diets tends to be less available to the body than the iron in diets that are high in red meat and other animal products. It is a good idea to include citrus and other fruits high in vitamin C with meals because vitamin C enhances iron absorption.

Some vegetarians use meat analogs, which are commercially produced plant protein products that look like meat, to add variety to their meals and for convenience. For people who are in the process of changing to a vegetarian diet these foods might make the transition easier. However, they are not essential for maintaining a well-balanced vegetarian diet.

Vegan diets

Vegan, or total vegetarian, diets involve the near total avoidance of animal foods of any type. It is much more difficult to make sure that your nutrient needs are met on these diets since there is no practical source of vitamin B_{12} or vitamin D in plant foods. There are few plant sources rich in calcium or riboflavin and, as has been noted, the iron in plant-only diets is more difficult for the body to absorb. In addition, zinc, magnesium and iodine, protein and caloric intakes, might also be too low. Because of these potential shortfalls, it is helpful to consult a registered dietitian or a physician who is knowledgeable in clinical nutrition for assistance in planning diets. This is especially important for infants, young children, growing teenagers or pregnant or nursing women on a vegan diet.

In addition to the dietary recommendations for lacto-ovo vegetarians, vegan-vegetarians are usually advised to use a fortified soybean milk drink, or a nutrient supplement that provides vitamin B_{12}. Nutritional yeasts (not brewer's yeast, baker's yeast, or live yeast) are special types of yeast grown on vitamin B_{12}-enriched media to provide that vitamin. Commercially prepared soy and sesame seed drinks are usually fortified with calcium and vitamins A, D, and B_{12}, and can help to increase intakes of nutrients that might otherwise be low in the vegan's diet.

Vegans need to be especially careful to use a variety of protein-rich legumes and whole grains, and to include some seed or nut products in their meals every day to make sure that the mixture of proteins they get is of high quality. Good examples are beans with corn or rice, whole-grain cereals with legumes and green leafy vegetables, and peanuts with wheat or rice.

By increasing their consumption of dark green leafy vegetables, legumes, nuts, and dried fruits, they also ensure that their iron intakes are sufficient. Vitamin D supplements or liberal exposure of the skin to sunlight each day will fulfill requirements for this vitamin.

VEGETARIAN DIET

Day	Breakfast	Lunch	Dinner	Snacks
1.	Oatmeal with sliced peach and sunflower seeds Whole-wheat toast with peanut butter Skim milk Herbal tea	Vegetarian vegetable soup Bean spread and lettuce sandwich on pumpernickel bread Buttermilk Fresh fruit cup	Tortillas Green salad with French dressing Tamale pie Broccoli Stewed tomatoes Skim milk Fresh pineapple slices	Apple crisp Apple juice Yogurt
2.	Hot whole-wheat cereal with low-fat milk and raisins Homemade whole-wheat bread with marmalade Fresh orange juice Low-fat milk	Low-fat cottage cheese with fresh fruit salad of plums, blueberries, seedless grapes, pineapple, and strawberries on a bed of lettuce Raisin bread and apple butter Lemon-grass tea	Finger vegetables Boston baked beans Boston brown bread and cream cheese Mixed salad with French dressing Broccoli Low-fat milk Angel food cake with peaches	Cranberry juice Graham crackers with peanut butter Low-fat milk
3.	Blueberry buckwheat pancakes with maple syrup $\frac{1}{2}$ grapefruit Yogurt Herbal tea	Corn chowder Soyburger sandwich with lettuce on whole-wheat bread with catsup Buttermilk Peach	Tahini with pita bread appetizer and finger vegetables Eggplant stew with tomato and cheese topping Winter squash Spinach salad with Greek dressing Baklava	Cheese pizza Low-fat milk Orange
4.	Orange Stewed prunes Toasted English muffins with scrambled tofu Skim milk	Bean soup Corn muffins with honey Small tossed salad with Italian dressing Low-fat milk Dates and apricot halves	Macaroni and cheese Broccoli Baked squash with brown sugar Whole-wheat bread with soft margarine Tomato juice Cantaloupe	Skim milk Trail mix Sesame seed crackers with jelly
5.	Bran cereal with low-fat milk Bran muffin with marmalade Fresh sliced oranges Low-fat milk	Split pea soup Stuffed peach salad with cottage cheese and sunflower seeds Raisin bread Low-fat milk Apple	Vegetable juice cocktail Vegetarian antipasto Lasagne Fresh broccoli with lemon Garlic French bread Chef's salad with Italian dressing	Peanut butter and jelly on whole-wheat bread Low-fat milk Pear
6.	Scrambled eggs Pumpernickel toast with soft margarine Orange juice Low-fat milk Herbal tea	Chili bean soup Swiss cheese sandwich on rye with lettuce, tomato, bean sprouts, and mustard Fruit salad Low-fat milk	Lentil nut loaf with mushroom gravy Carrots and cauliflower with parsley Lettuce, endive, escarole, and tomato salad with Caesar salad dressing Pumpernickel bread with margarine Strawberries	Cornbread with soft margarine and honey Apple
7.	Wheatena with milk Prune-grapefruit juice Bran muffins with peanut butter Low-fat milk	Cheese enchiladas Tacos and guacamole Sliced tomatoes with vinaigrette dressing Low-fat milk Papaya with lemon	Tomato juice Nutburgers in vegetarian gravy Baked potato with sour cream Green peas and carrots Fresh garden vegetable salad and buttermilk dressing Pineapple	Yogurt with honey Orange juice Concord grapes Graham crackers

FLUIDS

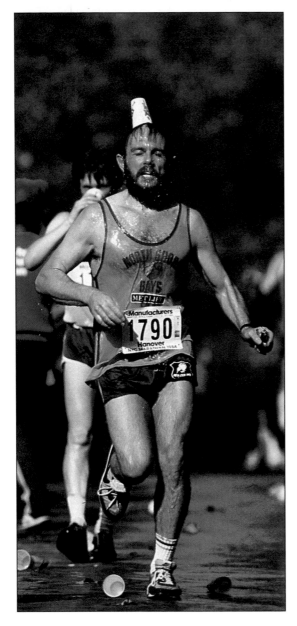

A marathon runner loses 10 to 12 pints of water during a race, which makes it important to replace lost fluid at feeding stations along the course. Runners are usually offered a choice between pure water and water with added glucose and vitamins; pure water is the better choice.

Water is one of the essentials of the diet. All bodily functions use it, and it helps to keep the body cool. About 60 percent of the body is composed of water; the exact proportion varies, depending chiefly on body fatness. Fatter people have a lower percentage of water because fat cells contain very little of it.

To stay in good health, your water consumption and output need to balance, and the water within your body needs to stay in the right place. Most of this happens automatically. Your hunger and thirst regulate your intake of water and minerals, and your kidneys control output. The sophisticated physical and chemical mechanisms that keep you alive also automatically ensure that all the body water, and the minerals dissolved in it, remain in the right compartments in the body—most of the sodium outside the cells, and most of the potassium inside.

Diet and fluid balance

You get the water you need in food as well as drink. Most food contains a high percentage of water—fruit and vegetables are about 80 percent water, cooked rice and pasta are about 70 percent, and bread is about 35 percent. Generally, about 7–10 eight-ounce glasses of fluid a day in addition to the food you eat is as much as you need.

Getting too little water is rarely a problem. Athletes and others who sweat a great deal lose sodium, potassium, and chloride as well as water during vigorous exercise. Most people get enough water and minerals in their normal diet to meet even these needs. The kidneys are able to regulate water, sodium, and potassium levels in the urine when there are alterations in water and salt intakes, or losses through sweat and moist air exhaled through the lungs. You do not need to take salt tablets or special "sports" beverages, powders, or foods. In fact, if such products are sweet and quench the thirst, they might discourage you from drinking enough, and thus do more harm than good.

You don't need to worry about drinking too much water. You won't become waterlogged, since the kidneys will quickly adjust the amount of fluid in your body; and you won't rapidly gain weight, since pure water provides no calories. Remember, however, many other fluids, particularly soft drinks, alcohol, fruit-ades, juices, and milk shakes, are high in calories.

All body cells *are bathed in a watery fluid similar in composition to the sea water in which life evolved. Of all the fluid in the body, 37.5% is made up of this extracellular fluid. Some 55% is inside the cells; the remaining 7% is in circulation in the bloodstream. The diagram shows average daily water intake and loss for an adult man living in a temperate climate. In hotter climates, water drunk and sweat produced increase markedly. Metabolic water is that made by body cells as a result of their functioning.*

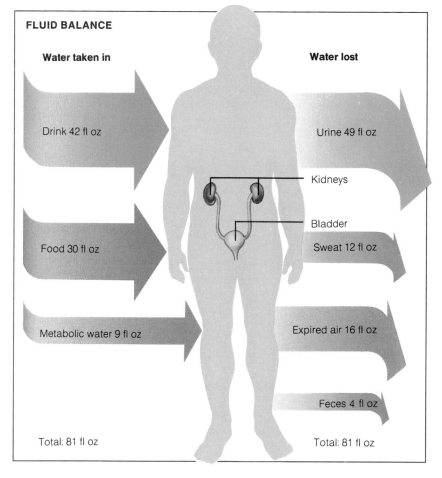

FLUID BALANCE

Water taken in

Drink 42 fl oz

Food 30 fl oz

Metabolic water 9 fl oz

Total: 81 fl oz

Water lost

Urine 49 fl oz

Kidneys

Bladder

Sweat 12 fl oz

Expired air 16 fl oz

Feces 4 fl oz

Total: 81 fl oz

Your diet can temporarily affect your fluid balance. Crash diets can lead to a loss of a few pounds of body water, but they soon return (see pages 76–77). Drinks containing alcohol and caffeine, including coffee, tea, and some colas, act as weak diuretics, increasing the amount of fluid expelled by the kidneys. Taken in excess, they can cause dehydration, which stresses the heart and blood vessels, and makes it more difficult for the body to rid itself of excess heat. Severe dehydration, when water losses are more than about two percent of body weight, can increase the pulse rate and body temperature, resulting in fatigue, apathy, and decreased performance.

Special situations
Although the body usually keeps its fluid needs in balance, in certain circumstances you need to consciously increase your fluid intake. When you have a high fever, you need to remember to drink plenty of fluids to replace the water you lose by evaporation. If you go to a hotter climate, or the weather becomes hot and dry, it takes your body some time to acclimatize, and you will lose a good deal of water as sweat. You should make a conscious effort to drink plenty of water for about a week after you first encounter such conditions.

If you undertake unusually heavy exercise, weigh yourself (preferably nude) before and afterward. If you lose more than two percent of your body weight, you need to drink more before and during the activity to compensate for losses in sweat and evaporation. Keep fluids, preferably chilled water, nearby and remember to drink periodically even if you don't feel thirsty. If you monitor how well you are replacing your water losses, eventually you will learn to drink enough automatically.

FOOD ALLERGIES AND PROBLEMS

Certain foods do not agree with some people, and might even make them ill. The symptoms of food-related problems are variable, and may arise as a result of any of four basic causes.

The simplest is a food dislike. An individual might sometimes or always find the appearance or taste of a food unpleasant or disgusting. The problem is easily solved by avoiding that food.

Intolerances to a food or a substance in food are more complicated. A food problem is considered psychological if an individual does not have a food allergy, which can be determined through immunological tests, but always develops a variety of physical and behavioral symptoms when he is aware that he has eaten the offending substance. Symptoms do not develop when he is unaware of eating the substance.

If a person always develops signs and symptoms whether or not he is aware of the presence of the substance—and his immunological tests are normal—he is said to have a physiological food problem, or a food intolerance. This means that his symptoms are caused by his body's inability to digest or absorb the substance.

Finally, if a person always has adverse reactions when he eats the offending substance, and his immunological tests are abnormal, his problem is a food allergy. The symptoms are caused by the reactions of his immune system to the food in question.

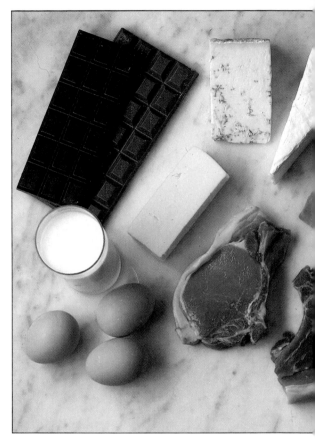

Detecting food problems

Fortunately, most food-related problems cause only temporary discomfort (although some can be lethal), but they all need to be dealt with. Because treatments differ, it is important to distinguish, with the help of a reputable doctor, which kind of problem a person suffers from.

The usual procedure is to put the individual on a very simple elimination diet, which consists of a few basic foods that are almost never associated with food allergies or intolerances. Symptoms are monitored for several weeks, and foods are gradually added back to the diet. If symptoms then occur, more sophisticated tests are used to determine which kind of problem is present.

In one such test, known as the double blind challenge, or provocation test, opaque capsules containing the suspected substance are alternated randomly with a nonactive substance, and eaten with the elimination diet. If the person always responds to the presence of the substance,

even when he is unaware of it, with asthma, eczema, allergic rhinitis ("stuffy nose"), hives, or other physical reactions, the possibility of his having a true allergy or physiological intolerance is strengthened. Further tests to establish tolerance and immune response to certain substances, such as lactose, fat, and gluten, might then be undertaken.

Allergists sometimes inject a suspected allergen (allergy-causing substance) under the skin. If the person has an allergy, a skin irritation will develop at the location of the injection. Another test, the cytotoxic test, in which the suspected food is placed with white blood cells from the patient, is not used by reputable specialists.

If a person taking the double blind challenge does not always respond, or develops only less clear-cut symptoms, such as nausea, headache, behavioral problems and general discomfort, psychological causes of intolerance will be suspected. These need to be explored.

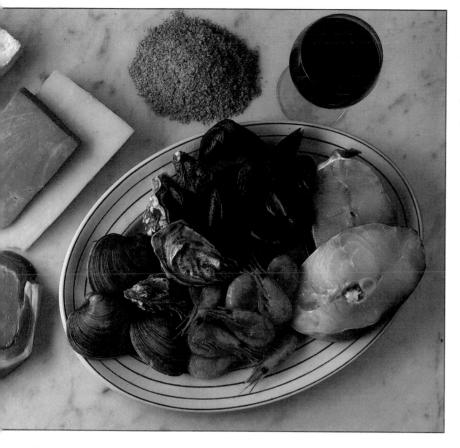

Almost every sort of food has been blamed at some time for causing problems ranging from rashes to migraine headaches. These may be the results of psychological or physiological intolerances as well as allergies. Some of the foods that are often associated with adverse reactions are illustrated here.

Common offenders

Although medical experts agree that there are true food allergies and intolerances, it is not clear how prevalent or widespread they are. When double blind food challenges are used to establish their presence, only 10–15 percent of suspected food allergies are actually confirmed and found to have a physiological cause.

True food allergies and intolerances are much more common in children than in adults. The most common intolerance is to lactose, milk sugar. The most common allergies are to the proteins in milk, eggs, wheat, and peanuts. Because these problems can affect growth and health, they need to be identified early. Breast-feeding and the gradual introduction of solid foods, with common offenders introduced later in infancy, and only gradually, can help to prevent some of these problems. However, it is unwise to put infants or children on special diets until a doctor diagnoses the problem and recommends a diet that includes all the necessary nutrients.

Food allergies and intolerances also occur in adults, although food might not always be the cause. Some drugs, for example, can cause headaches when people taking them eat certain foods. And there is evidence that in some people who suffer from migraine headaches, certain foods trigger the attacks, although no single food appears to be the cause. People who suffer from migraine headaches should take double blind food tests administered by an allergist to determine if foods are involved.

Cause for controversy

There are widely conflicting opinions about whether allergic reactions to food additives and colorings are the triggers of hyperactivity, hyperkinesis, fatigue or depression in either children or adults. The evidence is inconclusive, but if you suspect food to be the cause of a problem, you should be checked for allergy.

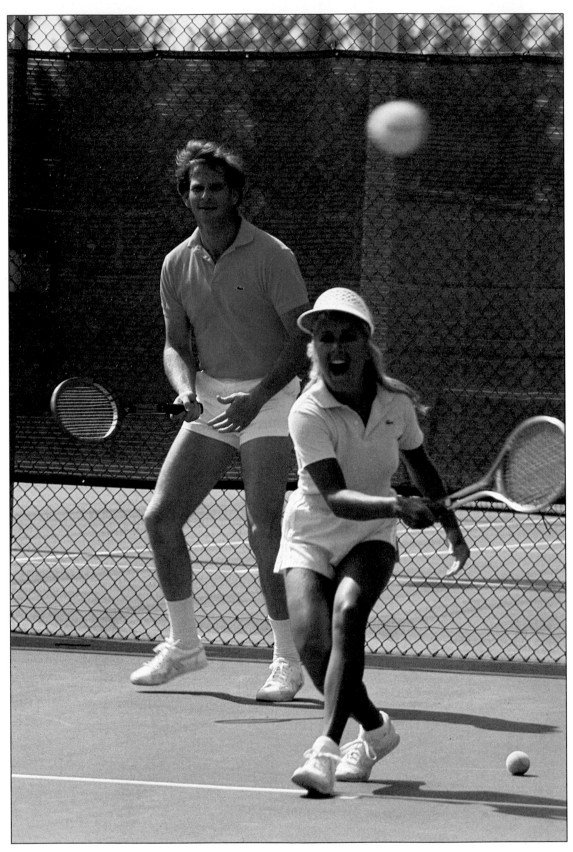

GETTING FIT, STAYING FIT

Health, vitality, and long life are desirable goals for everyone, but they are not achieved without effort. Because many of the habits of modern life do more to diminish health than to increase it, fitness has to be worked at. If you are resolved to take a positive attitude toward your health and well-being, and to prevent problems rather than simply treating them as and when they occur, then physical fitness must be an essential part of your life.

Being fit has many advantages, from helping you to control your weight to giving you a better night's sleep. There is impressive evidence that people who exercise frequently, and in the correct way, are less prone to heart attacks, strokes and other life-threatening conditions, and live longer than people whose existence is sedentary. You cannot, however, build up a store of fitness that will last for life. You need to exercise regularly all your life, and should exercise more, not less, as you get older.

The type of exercise that is most effective in improving fitness is aerobic exercise. The word aerobic means "with oxygen," and all aerobic exercise uses oxygen. The oxygen reaches the body by being breathed in through the lungs and distributed to working muscles via the blood, which is pumped around the circulation by the heart. Aerobic exercise usually involves vigorous exercise sustained over a period of several minutes, and its effect is to increase the efficiency of the lungs, heart, and blood circulation, which are known collectively as the aerobic system. Short, sharp bursts of activity, which rely on the body's reserves of oxygen and are described as anaerobic, do not produce a similar improvement.

This chapter gives you many examples of aerobic activities, as well as specific programs to follow. Everyone should be able to find an activity, or a mixture of activities, that will be enjoyable and help aerobic fitness. In addition, there are exercises that will help improve your strength and mobility, and aid relaxation and stress management.

Exercise helps you look and feel your best. Few adults who have taken the trouble to get fit will ever allow themselves to become inactive again. Having the support and encouragement of those around you will make getting and staying fit easier and more enjoyable, and involving others in fitness will help you, and them, to achieve a healthier and more productive lifestyle.

WHAT IS FITNESS?

THE HEART

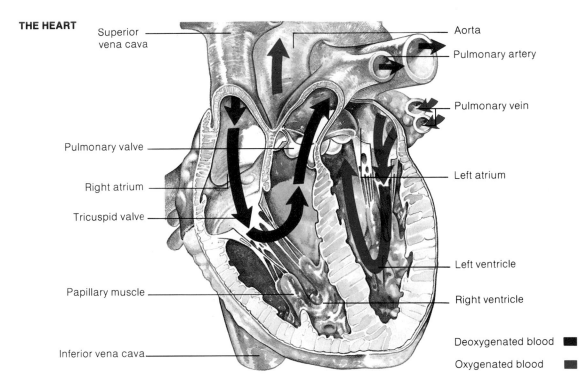

Superior vena cava

Aorta

Pulmonary artery

Pulmonary vein

Pulmonary valve

Right atrium

Tricuspid valve

Left atrium

Left ventricle

Papillary muscle

Right ventricle

Deoxygenated blood ■

Oxygenated blood ■

Inferior vena cava

The heart consists of two pairs of pumping chambers, the right and left atria and ventricles. Deoxygenated blood delivered from the venae cavae enters the right atrium, then the right ventricle, which pumps blood to the lungs for reoxygenation. Oxygenated blood returns to the left atrium, then the left ventricle. This is the thickest-walled, highest-pressure chamber.

During a single heartbeat, the two atria contract, filling the ventricles. Then the two ventricles contract, sending blood back into circulation. As you get fit, the amount of blood pumped out at each stroke is increased. In endurance training, there is a modest increase in heart wall thickness. Strength training increases wall thickness more. This is not as desirable, since it might impair function.

Most people consider themselves basically healthy as long as they do not suffer from any disease or infirmity. But fitness is more than that. Fitness means having efficient circulation, muscular strength and stamina, and good balance; it means being agile and well-coordinated. Being physically fit makes you look good and feel well, enables you to live energetically and enjoy life more, and improves your mental efficiency.

The most important muscle

The first measurement of your fitness is the performance of your heart. The heart is a muscular organ, whose contractions pump blood around the body. Like any other muscle, the heart depends on a constant supply of oxygen to sustain activity, and so its fitness is inextricably linked with the lungs (see pages 98–99). The difference between the heart and other body muscles is that the heart must keep working all

the time to sustain life.

Diseases of the heart and arteries are responsible for the majority of deaths in the Western world. The key process in causing these diseases is the formation in the artery walls of a waxy, cheeselike substance called atheroma, which contains large quantities of cholesterol. The arteries are the vessels that carry the blood on its outward journey from the heart. If an artery becomes blocked with atheroma, the tissues downstream from the blockage become starved of oxygen, and will suffer.

Nowhere is the formation of atheroma more serious than in the coronary arteries—the arteries that supply blood to the heart itself. Blockage of these arteries leads to heart attacks and causes angina pectoris, which is experienced as a severe cramplike pain.

The combination of a healthy diet (see pages 53–93) and aerobic training (see pages 98–99) provides the best means of reducing the risk of atheroma—unless you smoke cigarettes. Smoking cigarettes lowers the efficiency of the aerobic system (the lungs, heart, and circulation) and greatly increases the tendency toward atheroma formation. If you do smoke, then stopping is the most beneficial thing you can do for your health (see pages 284–288).

Training for a fit heart

As you start to exercise, your heart suddenly needs to pump much more blood. Fitness training improves your heart's performance and ability to do this. The easiest way of monitoring the improvement in heart function is by the pulse rate (see pages 12–13). A typical nonsmoker has a pulse rate of about 65–70 beats a minute (in a smoker it is, on the average, 5 to 10 beats higher). As aerobic fitness increases, the resting pulse rate, which is best taken in the morning on awakening, falls to about 60 beats a minute or even lower.

Not only does the resting pulse rate fall with increased fitness, but the rate to which it increases during exercise also falls. Thus an unfit person may have a pulse rate of, say, 120 while climbing stairs, whereas a fit colleague might have a rate of only 80 or 90 beats a minute.

The total amount of blood the heart pumps in a minute is its cardiac output. At rest, this is nearly 11 pints, and it is little changed by increased fitness. However, since a fit heart beats less often per minute to produce this same output, the amount of blood it pumps at each stroke—its stroke volume—must be greater.

The heart's stroke volume increases dramatically with aerobic training. Furthermore, the fit heart responds to an increase in load by a much greater increase in stroke volume than the unfit heart, which merely tries to compensate by beating faster. Getting fit also means that your heart has a lot less work to do. If your resting pulse falls by 10 beats a minute, it would, for example, beat 600 fewer times an hour, and 14,400 fewer times a day.

Aerobic training also produces a fall in blood pressure, a measure of the resistance to blood flow in the vessels and, indirectly, of the efficiency of the circulation. Since high blood pressure is often associated with heart disease, a fall in the pressure shows progress to a healthier heart.

THE ELECTRO-CARDIOGRAM

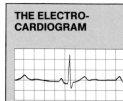

The electrocardiogram (EKG) records the heart's electrical activity. The largest deflections in the tracing represent the contractions of the ventricles. An EKG taken during exercise helps to detect heart disease. It also reflects the changes that occur in the heart rate with increased fitness.

BLOOD PRESSURE

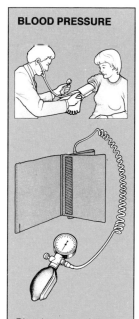

Blood pressure is normally taken in the main artery of the arm. A cuff is wrapped around the upper arm and inflated to a pressure that stops blood flow down the artery. As the cuff is slowly deflated, the return of flow can be detected either by feeling for the pulse or by listening over the artery with a stethoscope. The pressure reading at this point indicates the peak, or systolic, pressure in the system. As the cuff is deflated further, it is possible to detect the lowest, or diastolic, pressure that is reached in the system in the pause between heartbeats.

If your systolic pressure is below 140 millimeters (mm) of mercury and your diastolic pressure is below 90 mm, then, as a rule, all is well, although there is a great deal of individual variation.

AEROBICS

Every minute of your life, your body is burning up fuel with oxygen to produce energy. When you are doing something that demands that working muscles be supplied with extra oxygen, this type of activity is described as aerobic. It should make you breathe harder and more deeply. It should not mean, however, that you are so out of breath that you are forced to stop the activity altogether.

Obtaining oxygen

The aerobic system is responsible for carrying oxygen from the air into the muscle fibers. The lungs are the organs that provide the link between the body and the outside world. Air is moved in and out of the lungs through the airways. They are arranged like a tree, with air entering through the main trunk, the trachea, then passing down the two main bronchi that lead into the lungs. The airways then split into smaller and smaller branches until the air finally reaches the minute sacs, called alveoli.

Oxygen is extracted from the air at the level of the alveoli. Each alveolus is surrounded by a rich network of capillaries—tiny blood vessels—and oxygen crosses the alveolar walls into the blood in this network. This process of oxygen absorption is accompanied by an exchange in the reverse direction, with the waste product carbon dioxide being released from the blood back into the air along with unwanted water vapor.

Once the process of gas exchange has taken place, oxygen is carried onward in the bloodstream bound to hemoglobin, the red pigment in red blood cells. The heart and circulation (collectively called the cardiovascular system) are responsible for carrying the blood to the muscle cells, where oxygen is exchanged for carbon dioxide and used for energy production.

Blood also transports fuel—mainly glucose—for combustion and energy release. The muscles contain their own store of glucose in the form of the chemical glycogen, but can also use energy obtained from the body's fat stores.

Aerobic training

The purpose of aerobic training is to improve, at all levels, the efficiency of the oxygen delivery system and the efficiency with which the muscles produce energy. In health terms, the benefits to be gained from aerobic exercise are enormous and include weight loss, increased life expectancy, and an enhanced feeling of well-being. In contrast, an improvement in your ability to exercise anaerobically (defined in the chart below) offers much less benefit, since it tends to foster mere muscle development.

The aerobic system is best trained by exercising continuously a little below your maximum capacity (see pages 102–103). If you are running, for example, it is best to do so at a speed at which you can hold a conversation.

In order to achieve a significant improvement in your level of aerobic fitness you should gradually exercise for longer periods of time and maintain a steady increase in the intensity of exercise. The best way to make exercise more intense is to cover a given distance over a shorter period of time or to "handicap" yourself by wearing wrist or ankle weights while you perform the exercise.

FITNESS VOCABULARY

The vocabulary of fitness contains many terms that are often used incorrectly or which cause confusion. These include:

Anaerobic exertion
This is exercise of high intensity and usually brief duration, as in sprinting. In this type of exercise, the energy needs of the muscle cells cannot be met rapidly enough by the aerobic system. In anaerobic exercise, energy is produced quickly, without the use of oxygen—hence its name.

Isometric exertion
In this activity, muscles are made to work against a static resistance, so that they expend energy but do not produce movement. An example is pressing your hands palm-to-palm. While this builds up muscle strength, it has no useful effect on aerobic fitness and might increase blood pressure to dangerous levels.

Isotonic exertion
Working muscles in a particular part of the body contract at varying speeds against a constant resistance. Lifting weights and sit-ups are both examples of this.

Isokinetic exertion
Exercise in which muscles contract at a constant speed against varying degrees of resistance. Variable resistance equipment (see pages 134–135) is designed to produce isokinetic muscle activity.

THE OXYGEN CYCLE

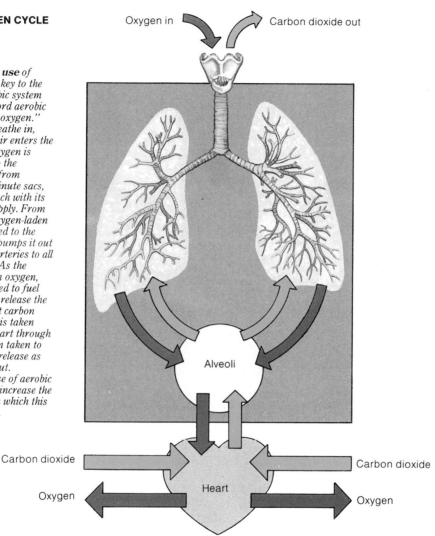

Oxygen in

Carbon dioxide out

Alveoli

Carbon dioxide

Oxygen

Heart

Carbon dioxide

Oxygen

The body's use of oxygen is the key to the way the aerobic system works; the word aerobic means "with oxygen." When you breathe in, oxygen-rich air enters the lungs. The oxygen is absorbed into the bloodstream from millions of minute sacs, the alveoli, each with its own blood supply. From the alveoli, oxygen-laden blood is carried to the heart, which pumps it out through the arteries to all body tissues. As the tissues take in oxygen, which is needed to fuel the cells, they release the waste product carbon dioxide. This is taken back to the heart through the veins, then taken to the lungs for release as you breathe out.

The purpose of aerobic training is to increase the efficiency with which this system works.

Calisthenics
Involves rhythmic exercises, usually in place, but is not fully aerobic. The amount of exertion necessary to increase the heartbeat rate up to levels that produce a significant increase in aerobic fitness is much more strenuous than a 15- to 30-minute run, swim, or bicycle ride. In conjunction with aerobic exercise, calisthenics is useful for building strength and endurance.

Interval training
Short bursts of high-level exertion interspersed with periods of rest or low-level activity. As the period of intense activity is increased, the greater the aerobic training effect.

Long, slow distance
A form of training that can be applied to any aerobic activity. It involves exercising over long distances at a low level of energy output. This form of training has a preferential effect on slow-twitch muscle fibers (see pages 102–103), and may also make muscles more likely to burn up fat reserves.

Tempo training
This means running middle or longer distances at racing pace.

Fartlek
A type of interval training that involves repeated variations of pace. Fartlek training should also take place over varied terrain and gradients, and is an excellent form of training for distance running. The word means "speed play."

FITNESS TESTING

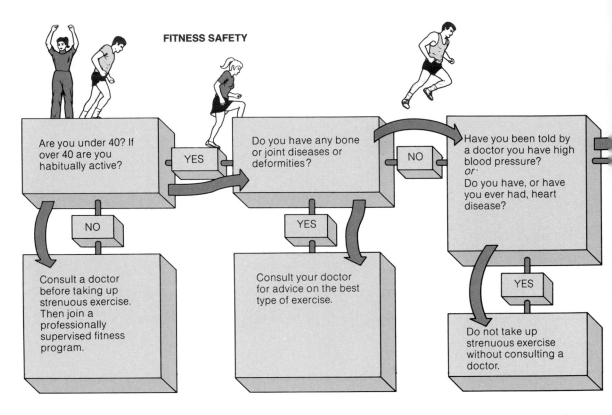

FITNESS SAFETY

Are you under 40? If over 40 are you habitually active?

YES

Do you have any bone or joint diseases or deformities?

NO

Have you been told by a doctor you have high blood pressure?
or
Do you have, or have you ever had, heart disease?

NO

YES

YES

Consult a doctor before taking up strenuous exercise. Then join a professionally supervised fitness program.

Consult your doctor for advice on the best type of exercise.

Do not take up strenuous exercise without consulting a doctor.

Fitness testing is useful on two counts. It can determine whether you are at risk—particularly from heart attack—if you take up exercise. It can also measure your levels of muscle performance and of heart-lung, or aerobic, fitness. As a result of this type of testing, your need for increased aerobic activity can be assessed.

A full fitness test includes a physical examination, and measurements of height, weight, and percentage of body fat. Your blood and urine will be analyzed to detect signs of disease. The blood analysis includes a measure of its cholesterol content, since cholesterol levels are related to the risk of heart disease.

The electrical activity of your heart is measured as an electrocardiogram (EKG), both when you are resting and when you are exercising. This dual measurement is important in the detection of heart problems that might make exercise risky, since the signs of heart trouble do not necessarily show up on the record made while you are sitting or lying quietly at rest. Your heart rate is also a useful guide to fitness, indicating the improvements that might be expected with increased aerobic exercise.

Your blood pressure measurements are also taken at rest and during exercise, again with the aim of detecting cardiovascular problems that could be improved by a more health-conscious lifestyle. The exercise part of the fitness assessment is usually performed on a treadmill or an exercise bicycle.

A doctor will analyze the results of your tests and advise you about your fitness and the steps you should take to improve it. He or she might suggest that you lose weight and recommend a healthy reducing diet combined with regular aerobic exercise. Your heart and lung function tests might also indicate that you need to increase your aerobic activity as well as give up smoking and reduce your consumption of alcohol.

If the tests reveal that you have heart disease, the advice you are given will depend on the extent of the problem and on your doctor's attitude toward treatment. But whatever your state of fitness, and whatever recommendations are made, you will be advised about the need for, and frequency of, follow-up fitness tests to assess your progress. (See "Whole-life Programs," pages 26–51.)

Follow the pathways *shown on the chart to discover whether or not it is safe for you to exercise. As a general rule, it is wise to make sure that you see a doctor before you start an exercise program. Remember that the EKG, taken while you are exercising, is probably the best test to have.*

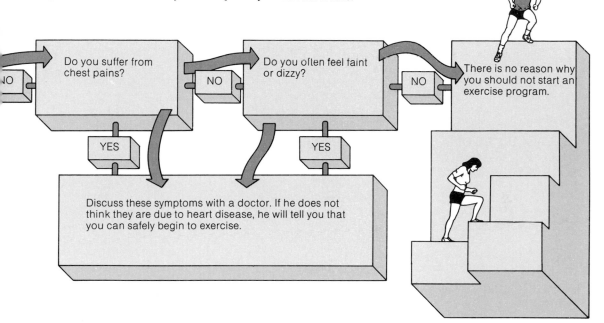

NO

Do you suffer from chest pains?

NO

Do you often feel faint or dizzy?

NO

There is no reason why you should not start an exercise program.

YES

YES

Discuss these symptoms with a doctor. If he does not think they are due to heart disease, he will tell you that you can safely begin to exercise.

THE TREADMILL

The treadmill is a piece of equipment central to fitness testing. The person being tested is "wired up" for EKG recordings and breathes into a mouthpiece connected to a computerized air analyzer. (In noncomputerized systems, air is collected in huge bags for laboratory analysis.) At the start of the test, the belt of the treadmill moves so that the person is moving at a walking pace. As the test progresses, the speed can be increased so that the person breaks into a run, or the treadmill can be made to rise into an incline. In both instances this means that the person's aerobic system is having to work harder.

The test continues until the doctor supervising it considers (from the subject's age, the degree of distress, and from the readings on the recording apparatus) that it is no longer safe to continue. Analysis of the results is followed up with advice about future activity.

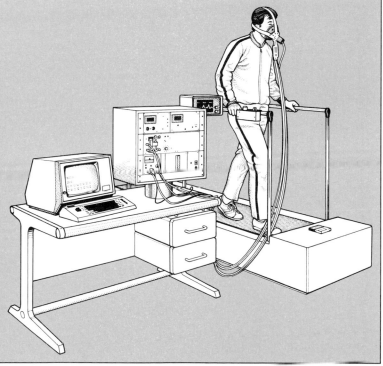

FITNESS GOALS

Even if your immediate goal is to improve just one aspect of yourself, perhaps to lose weight or feel more energetic, you will benefit from exercise in many more ways as your respiratory and cardiovascular systems become more efficient and your muscles get stronger (see opposite page).

Using oxygen

Measurements of the amount of oxygen you are using while exerting yourself as hard as possible reflect the function of the aerobic system as a whole. The lungs have to be working hard to get oxygen into the bloodstream and the heart has to be pumping well to push the blood out to the muscles. Similarly, the muscles have to be operating at full stretch to take up oxygen from the blood, and use it to produce the energy needed for mechanical work.

Oxygen usage can be measured accurately using the type of sophisticated equipment illustrated on page 101; it is expressed as the maximum amount of oxygen a person can consume per pound of his body weight. This amount of oxygen is called the VO_2 (max). As a general rule,

the larger your VO_2 (max), the fitter you are. In most people, VO_2 (max) increases with fitness and with the efficiency of the respiratory and cardiovascular systems.

Your VO_2 (max) begins to increase as soon as you begin a program of aerobic training. VO_2 (max) cannot be increased indefinitely—its upper limit is genetically determined. But most people are working well below their potential. Improvement in VO_2 (max) means an increase in your capacity to exercise.

Muscles and performance

The muscles upon which physical activity depend are made up of fibers. Each muscle works by contracting its individual fibers; this shortens the muscle and moves the joint on which it acts.

Muscles are made up of two types of fiber, known as fast- and slow-twitch fibers because

Many companies *and corporations are now realizing that they have much to gain by promoting the pursuit of fitness. Not only are sickness rates lowered, but fitter staff usually perform more efficiently.*

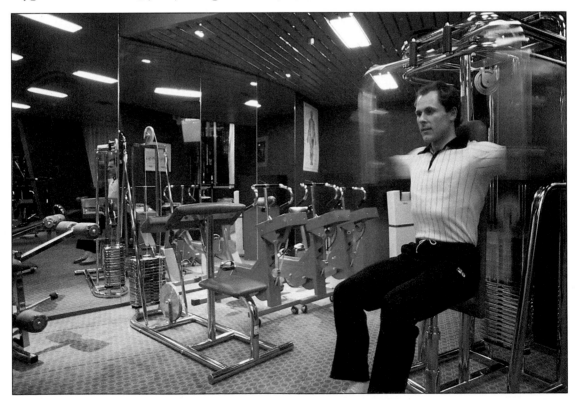

IMPROVEMENT IN VO₂ (MAX)

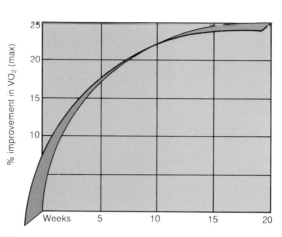

When a sedentary person *begins an aerobic exercise program, his or her VO_2 (max)—a measure of aerobic fitness—rises fast, as the graph shows. After 15 weeks, there is usually an improvement of more than 20%. The purpose of aerobic training is to use as great a percentage of your improved VO_2 (max) as possible during sustained exercise and to maintain that improvement.*

they twitch either fast or relatively slowly when electrically stimulated under experimental conditions. As a rule, the more fast-twitch fibers you have, the better your ability for explosive bursts of activity, and the more slow-twitch fibers you have, the better your capacity for endurance exercise. Unfortunately, there is no way of telling which type predominates without removing a piece of muscle tissue (a biopsy) and examining it under laboratory conditions.

When you exercise aerobically for a long period of time, your muscles will be burning glucose (made from glycogen stores in the muscles themselves and in the liver) and some fatty acids. After about two to two and a half hours, the glycogen runs out, which is what happens when marathon runners "hit the wall." However, with improved endurance training, the relative contribution of fatty acid "burning" improves so that the glycogen stores last longer.

If you can get your muscles switched on to fat burning during each exercise session, exercise will be of considerable help in keeping you slim. The best way of promoting fat burning is long, slow distance (see page 99), in which you exercise for long periods at 30 to 40 percent of your maximum effort.

RATING A HEALTH CLUB

Along with the enthusiasm for health and fitness has come a new industry; health clubs have been around for many years, but they are no longer only the body-building emporiums they used to be. Exercising in a facility designed for that purpose can have real benefits. For many people, motivation increases and is more easily sustained in the company of others with similar goals. A good health club or gym can offer a great deal in terms of equipment, facilities, and expert supervision and instruction. Not the least of these benefits is the opportunity to establish a structured routine for your workouts.

If you are considering joining a health club, be certain you make an informed decision based on a number of factors. In order to be a viable part of your fitness program, the club must be convenient to either your home or workplace. Proximity is of the utmost importance in adhering to a schedule.

Before you make a financial commitment, define your fitness goals and be sure that the club can meet them. Make a list of the activities that interest you and visit the club to see the facilities. As the fitness industry has expanded, many different companies have begun to manufacture equipment. Ask the staff person who shows you the club to explain the specific benefits of the machines that are available, and see if they meet your needs. If you are a jogger who prefers to run indoors, you'll want a club that has many treadmills available. These machines, as well as rowing machines and exercise bicycles, are generally used for longer periods of time than the circuit weight equipment: you won't want to stand around waiting because there are not enough machines for the number of people. Check also that equipment is maintained in good working order.

Some clubs that advertise a swimming pool have one that is scarcely larger than your bathtub at home. If lap swimming is your choice of activity, be sure the pool is large enough so that you can do a proper workout and don't get dizzy doing turns.

If you are interested in aerobic exercise, check that the floor is sprung wood—not carpeted tile or cement—to protect you from injury. Ask to see the shower and locker room facilities to check for cleanliness, and enquire about the availability of towels and other services.

The general atmosphere of the club is an important factor. Most health clubs play music to work out by. If you dislike rock and roll, for example, and that's all they play, either choose another club or bring your own headphones. The club might offer additional services at an extra cost, including nutrition counseling, lectures on topics such as stress management and stopping smoking, massage therapies, and beauty services. Investigate the credentials and experience of those who offer the services to be sure they are qualified.

On your tour notice the attitude of the staff: are instructors talking to each other or paying careful attention to club members? How do the staff respond to your questions? Try to visit each facility you consider at least twice; once during peak hours to check class size, traffic flow, and equipment availability. Shop around for seasonal and promotional prices, and ask about off-hour memberships—they are often a bargain.

A reputable club will require certain information from members, which should include some tests as well as a medical history. Ask if there is fitness testing available and how it will help you to measure your progress. Most important, check out your physical and personal safety as a club member. Use the checklist below to help you make an informed decision.

Health club checklist

● Is the club close enough to home or work?
● What qualification or degrees do instructors have?
● Is there always someone on the premises who knows how to perform cardiopulmonary resuscitation (CPR)?
● Does the club have emergency medical equipment, such as oxygen, on hand?
● Is there adequate supervision at all times?
● Is the pool area clean and well maintained?
● Is the membership fee within your realistic budget?
● Are the other members people you would like to know?
● Do the facilities meet your needs in terms of fitness goals?
● Are class times convenient?
● Will there be room for you when you want to go?
● Are the instructors friendly and supportive?
● What is the cancellation/freezing policy in case you move or travel for your job?
● Does the club have affiliation with others in different cities, states, or countries that you might visit regularly?

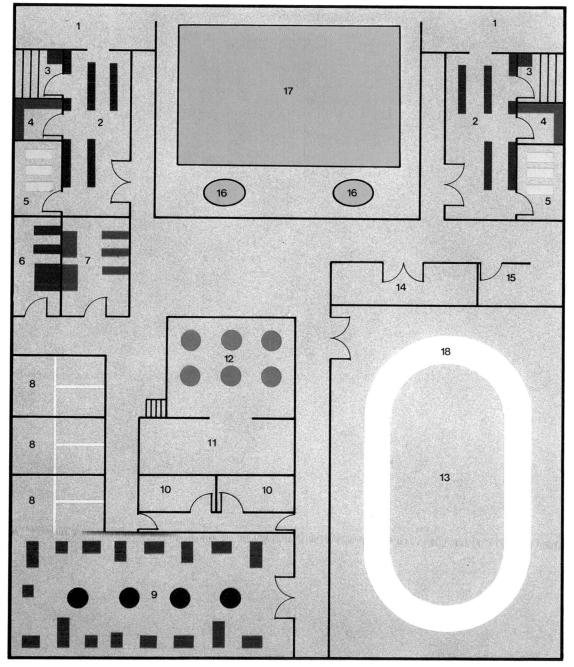

A typical health club has the facilities shown in this plan. The key indicates the major area allocations.

Key

1 Showers
2 Locker room
3 Sauna
4 Steam room
5 Sundeck
6 Massage room
7 Beauty treatment room
8 Racket ball court
9 Weight-training room
10 Offices
11 Snack bar
12 Relaxation area
13 Gym
14 Shop
15 Reception desk
16 Whirlpool bath
17 Swimming pool
18 Running track

WARM UP, COOL DOWN

Warming up and cooling down should be an integral part of any type of exercise or sport, particularly aerobics, for it is dangerous and inefficient to leap immediately from rest to maximum activity. When you are at rest, your blood circulates more or less evenly through your body, facilitating the healthy functioning of all vital organs. When a specific part of the body is called into action, a greater blood supply carrying oxygen is sent to the working part. Warm up is essential to signal to your body that a certain group of muscles will be in need of an increased oxygen supply. A few minutes of slow swimming,

jogging, or bicycling before you start to work a little harder is usually satisfactory. Pay attention to any pain or stiffness you might feel and add extra stretching for that area.

Use the exercises shown here to warm up and cool down your joints instead of, or in addition to, swimming, jogging, etc. Joints are vulnerable because muscles, tendons, and ligaments attach there. Along with the slow warm-up movements, add movements that will ease and lubricate the joints into action.

It is especially important to warm up before a race or competition, for cold muscles are much

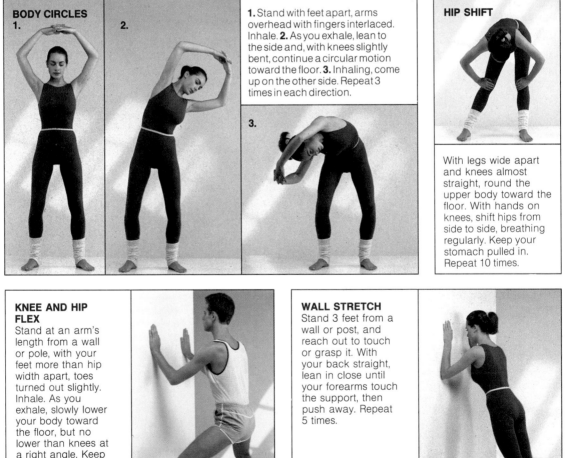

BODY CIRCLES

1. Stand with feet apart, arms overhead with fingers interlaced. Inhale. **2.** As you exhale, lean to the side and, with knees slightly bent, continue a circular motion toward the floor. **3.** Inhaling, come up on the other side. Repeat 3 times in each direction.

HIP SHIFT

With legs wide apart and knees almost straight, round the upper body toward the floor. With hands on knees, shift hips from side to side, breathing regularly. Keep your stomach pulled in. Repeat 10 times.

KNEE AND HIP FLEX

Stand at an arm's length from a wall or pole, with your feet more than hip width apart, toes turned out slightly. Inhale. As you exhale, slowly lower your body toward the floor, but no lower than knees at a right angle. Keep your knees bent over your toes and your back straight. Inhale on the way up. Repeat 5 times.

WALL STRETCH

Stand 3 feet from a wall or post, and reach out to touch or grasp it. With your back straight, lean in close until your forearms touch the support, then push away. Repeat 5 times.

more likely to be injured, and the extra stimulus of competition tempts many people to drive too hard before the full blood flow through their muscles is established. It is important to recognize that these exercises are an adjunct to aerobics and should not exhaust you before you begin to cover any ground.

Runners particularly benefit from warm-up exercises, as running incorporates only a limited range of movements. To warm up, use the swing through, body twists, body circles, and wall stretch, which put the big muscle groups through a variety of motions. Gradually increase the

duration of each exercise so that you give each muscle a stretch lasting 30 seconds or more.

The period after exercise is even more important. If you stop exercising suddenly, the body can suffer from shock, and the muscles tend to shorten, with subsequent stiffness and loss of flexibility. First, reduce the exercise you are doing to a slow pace, then use the knee and hip flex, hip shift, knee hugs, and ankle circles. They give the important muscle groups a mild stretch before you shower and rest. As with the warm-up exercises, gradually increase the duration of each cool-down exercise.

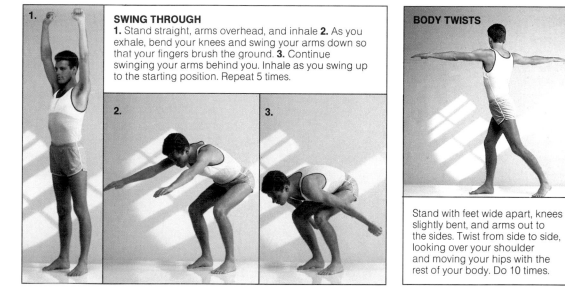

SWING THROUGH
1. Stand straight, arms overhead, and inhale **2.** As you exhale, bend your knees and swing your arms down so that your fingers brush the ground. **3.** Continue swinging your arms behind you. Inhale as you swing up to the starting position. Repeat 5 times.

BODY TWISTS

Stand with feet wide apart, knees slightly bent, and arms out to the sides. Twist from side to side, looking over your shoulder and moving your hips with the rest of your body. Do 10 times.

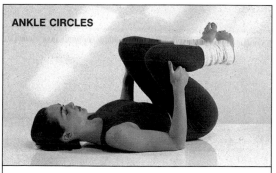

ANKLE CIRCLES

Lie on your back, with your knees into your chest, hands under your knees. Inhale and flex your toes. As you exhale, draw the biggest circles that you can with your big toes. Repeat 5 times in each direction. This exercise can also be done seated or standing.

KNEE HUGS
From a standing position, pull up and hug each knee alternately, pulling it toward your chest. Repeat 5 times for each leg.

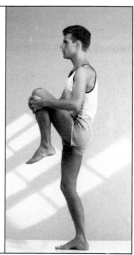

CHOOSING A PROGRAM

To find out your current fitness level, assess yourself by completing the tests on pages 12–15, then use the guidelines on this and the following pages to help you set up and maintain your own exercise program. It is important to choose an activity that you enjoy.

Aerobic exercise is one of the keys to improving and maintaining fitness and well-being. There are several means of aerobic conditioning: the "big three" are running, swimming, and bicycle riding. Walking is a good starter for runners, and if your current fitness level is low, you would not be able to start on the running program without completing a walking program first. Other aerobic programs you can try in this section, and use as alternatives on selected days if you wish, include stair climbing, aerobic dancing, skipping rope, and using a rowing machine.

About the programs
The programs for running, swimming, and bicycle riding, outlined on the following pages, give distances and times for beginners, intermediate, and advanced performers, and for men and women. The walking program, opposite, takes you from beginner stage to a level that is equivalent to about week four of the running schedules.

The swimming program is structured differently, since not everyone has the same natural ability at swimming. The beginners' program is for those who are not good swimmers. If you are beginning a training program but have been a moderately good swimmer in the past, try starting on the intermediate program.

The bicycling and running programs are designed to be interchangeable. You can also alternate them with aerobic dancing, skipping rope, and using a rowing machine. If you wish to interchange any program with swimming, however, it is wise, because of the different skills involved, to advance in both programs at the same pace concurrently.

Using the programs
Before you start any program, have the necessary medical checks (see pages 100–101), take note of your resting pulse rate (see pages 12–13), and warm up (see pages 106–107). If you are not used to exercise, be sure to start with the appropriate beginners' program.

The times in each program are to be used as guides; check yourself once or twice a week. The important element in these schedules is a steady increase in distance covered and, therefore, of energy expended. Time is, of course, a guide to energy expenditure in programs such as rowing. In these programs it is speed that is the optional extra.

If you are a beginner, do not start off too fast. You cannot get fit in a week, but you can get a long way toward it in a month. Work at your own pace. If you feel stiff the day after exercise, change activities or simply do some warm-up exercises instead to give your body a chance to recover; resume your program the next day.

Exercise at a time of the day that is most convenient, but preferably not until two or three hours after a meal. Never exercise if you feel ill or have a cold or fever. Do not start training again until you are free of symptoms, and keep your distance down to half your normal level for a week. For every day's exercise you miss, backtrack at least two days in the program. If you wish to exercise more than five times a week, be sure to make your extra sessions slow. Although you should feel physically stretched by the programs, you should not exercise to the point of pain or exhaustion. Keep a check on your pulse and do not exceed the safe maximum. **If you feel dizzy, or in pain, stop at once.**

Anyone below 35 should be able to work through the programs without trouble. If you are over 50, progress at about half the recommended rate, spending two weeks at each stage instead of one. If you are aged 35 to 50, attempt the first half of the beginners' program on a weekly basis, then cut back to a twice-weekly progression.

Once you have completed the beginners' running and bicycling schedules, 20 to 30 minutes at the level of the last week three times a week is enough to maintain fitness. For swimming, aim to complete a 1,000-yard swim three times a week. For walking, allow 60 to 75 minutes a session.

Natural ability does impose some restrictions on achievement beyond the beginner stage. When you feel you have reached your own limit, stay with that stage and measure your improving fitness by the decrease in your resting pulse rate, an increase in the time in which you reach your safe maximum pulse, and improved recovery times after exercise (see pages 12–13).

The 16-week walking program is well within the capabilities of anyone who can walk one mile. Start off walking at your own pace. For the first eight weeks, targets are offered in terms of either time or distance, but you will find that your pace increases naturally as you progress. If by week five or six you cannot walk two miles in 30 minutes, stay at the two-mile level and increase your pace before continuing to the next level.

To maintain an adequate level of fitness after completing this program, you will need to walk a minimum of five miles three times a week. If you are confined to your house or to an office, you can use stair climbing as an alternative.

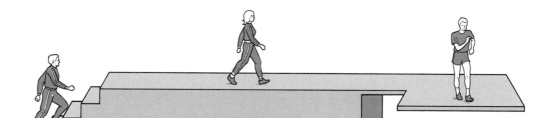

Stair climbing
The program below is a brisk one but is within most people's capabilities. If you are not fit, start more slowly, then increase your time and/or rate each week. The set rate of climbing includes the time for descents. So if you have 15 steps in your flight of stairs, you need to go up and down four times a minute to achieve the rate of 60 steps a minute.

Steps per minute	Time spent climbing/ mins
40	2
40	4
50	4
50	5
60	6
60	7
60	8
60	9
60	10
70	10
70	11
70	12

WALKING PROGRAM

Week	Distance/ miles	Time/ mins		Repeats/ week
1	1	or	15	5
2	1¼	or	20	5
3	1½	or	23	5
4	1¾	or	26	5
5	2	or	30	5
6	2	or	30	3
	2½	in any time		2
7	2½	or	30	3
	3	in any time		2
8	2	or	30	4
	any distance	in	60	1
9	2	in	28	4
	any distance	in	60	1
10	2	in	27½	4
	any distance	in	60	1
11	2½	in	35	4
	any distance	in	60	1
12	2½	in	34	4
	4	in	58	1
13	3	in	42	4
	4	in	58	1
14	2	in	27	3
	4	in	56	2
15	2	in	26½	3
	5	in	75	2
16	2	in	26	3
	5	in	70	2

Racewalking
This is a form of high-speed walking that is becoming increasingly popular as a means of achieving aerobic fitness. The speed of this type of walking is such that many people would find it more comfortable to run, but it imposes a discipline on body performance that you might find stimulating. The amount of energy used in racewalking is similar to that consumed in running, and more groups of muscles are exercised, so that mile for mile (at the speeds given below) it has a better training effect.
As a guide, use the walking program but aim to walk each mile in 9 to 10 minutes.

Hiking
Any long walk for pleasure or exercise can be a hike but, like walking, if it is to be part of your aerobic fitness program, it must be done briskly for at least 20 minutes. Take your terrain into consideration when you plan your hike, remembering that steep grades increase the intensity of your workout. Use the walking program chart as a rough guide on how to increase your workout.

BICYCLING

To undertake the bicycling programs on these pages, it is not necessary to possess a flashy, 10-speed bicycle. Bicycling is an efficient form of transportation. It demands less energy to move a moderate weight over a given distance than any other method. With a good bicycle, almost all your effort is used against air resistance or drag, not in forward propulsion.

This drag increases in proportion to the relative wind speed, so that an increase in wind or bicycle speed will create extra resistance; to reduce this effect, racing cyclists adopt a crouching position. The gradient also affects the level of effort that is required; even the mildest of gradients can double the amount of work.

Since the terrain and the relative wind speed make such a difference to bicycling energy levels, the times and distances in this program are a less accurate guide than they are in the running or swimming programs. The basic rule for beginners is to go by time rather than distance and to keep up a reasonable level of effort. You should be working hard enough to sweat a little, but easily enough to continue a conversation. Keep a check on your pulse and do not exceed the safe maximum.

Most modern bicycles have gears, and beginners are inclined to start in too high a gear. Try to increase your pedaling speed as much as possible in the early stages. As you progress, vary the terrain to include some work on hills.

With the intermediate program, add a one-minute interval (a short burst of high-level exertion) half way through and at the end of each 20 to 30 minutes' training. During each interval, bicycle as fast as you can (within the bounds of safety). Warm up before an interval and recover slowly after it. In the advanced program, gradually increase the time and frequency of the intervals; aim for four intervals of two minutes each at the beginning of the advanced program and build up to five intervals of two and a half minutes each.

THE EFFECT OF THE WIND

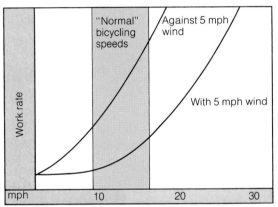

Each small increase in wind resistance imposes a huge strain on the cyclist. The graph shows the levels of energy needed to cycle when facing a 5 mph wind. The cyclist must work nine times as hard bicycling into—that is, against—this light wind as when bicycling with a wind of the same speed.

EXERCISE BICYCLES
Use an exercise bicycle in your health club or at home to gain and maintain a high level of aerobic fitness. These bikes range from basic versions, which depend on your manual manipulation of tension and speed, to the new high-tech models, which are computerized.

For your at-home choice, look for comfort and durability. Choose a bike that has a chain drive and flywheel. It must be stable, with a reasonable range of saddle and handlebar adjustments. To avoid the need for stopping in order to increase the level of work, make sure that you can adjust the tension mechanism while in motion. This mechanism varies the stiffness of the pedals and indicates your progress on a graduated scale.

Health clubs can afford to keep up with the latest technology in the fitness industry. Sophisticated models are computerized so that you can enter your vital statistics or choose a program that will allow the mechanism to vary your workout. It can give you information on your fitness level and even the number of calories you are burning.

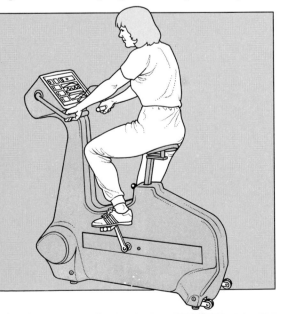

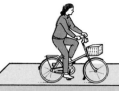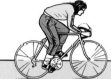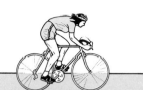

BICYCLING PROGRAM

Beginners				Intermediate				Advanced			
Week	Distance/ miles	Time/ mins	Repeats/ week	Week	Distance/ miles	Time/ mins	Repeats/ week	Week	Distance/ miles	Time/ mins	Repeats/ week
1	any distance	10	5	1	5 10	20 55	3 2	1	6 12	21 50	3 2
2	2 any distance	12 15	3 2	2	4 8	16 40	3 2	2	7 12	25 —	3 2
3	2 3	11 18	3 2	3	5 10	20 50	3 2	3	8 20	30 —	3 2
4	3 any distance	17 25	3 2	4	6 12	24 —	3 2	4	5 10	17 40	2 3
5	2 5	10 30	3 2	5	4 10	15 48	3 2	5	4 15 30	13 58 —	2 2 1
6	3 any distance	16 35	3 2	6	7 12	28 58	3 2	6	6 15	19 —	3 2
7	3 6	15 38	3 2	7	5 10	18 45	3 2	7	7 15 30	22 54 115	2 2 1
8	3 any distance	14 40	3 2	8	7 15	26 —	4 1	8	8 15	26 —	4 1
9	3 7	13 42	3 2	9	4 12	14 53	3 2	9	4 15 30	25 52 —	2 2 1
10	4 any distance	18 45	3 2	10	6 20	22 —	4 1	10	10 20 30	32 70 110	2 2 1
11	4 8	17 45	3 2	11	5 10	17 42	3 2	11	8 20	24 67	2 1
12	5 10	22 60	4 1	12	3 5 30	10 17 —	2 2 1	12	10 20 30	30 65 105	2 2 1

People have always run, but in recent years jogging and running have become almost a national pastime. There are many reasons for this new popularity: running—and its slower form, jogging—is convenient, affordable, flexible maintainable, satisfying, and produces numerous psychological as well as physiological benefits.

Anyone who is reasonably fit can enjoy jogging or running, and most people are probably attracted to it initially because of its convenience. It doesn't require advance booking or a special location, so you can always fit it in with your schedule, anytime, anywhere, even when you travel; many hotels throughout the world are tuned in to the needs of their running guests and may have prepared maps of the locale to help you plan your route. Once you've made your initial investment in high-quality running shoes (see pages 182–183), this sport need not burden your budget. Remember that good shoes and a careful warm up are needed to prevent injury to the hamstring (see pages 136–137). Health permitting, there is no reason why you cannot continue the sport for your entire life.

Running and jogging increase strength in the legs and lead to improved functioning of the cardiovascular and respiratory systems. They also are excellent calorie-burning activities. The number of calories that you burn per minute is dependent on your weight and the speed at which you move. However, the sport will raise your basal metabolic rate (see pages 70–71) not only while you are doing it, but also for up to eight hours afterward, which is good news for dieters.

You will also derive other pleasures from running, not the least of which is the satisfaction that you have taken time to do something positive for yourself. Long-distance runners even experience what is commonly known as "runner's high," a euphoria that might be caused by the stimulation of endorphins, a chemical, similar to morphine, that is found in the body (see pages 158–159). Even if you don't run long enough to get "high," you will still find that jogging and running consistently will help you to cope better with the stresses and frustrations of everyday life. If you eat, drink, or smoke too much, it is worth trying running as a substitute.

How to begin

Before beginning this or any other aerobic activity, you must first be sure to check with your doctor. If you decide to add this sport to your life, discipline is essential if you are to be successful at it. Let your program become a habit like brushing your teeth: in other words, don't think about it, just do it. Your ultimate goal is to exercise at least three times a week, for at least 20 minutes each time within your target heart range (see pages 12–13).

Evaluate where you are on the fitness scale so that you can establish realistic and attainable goals. If you are at a minimal fitness level and come to this activity from a sedentary lifestyle, it is best to begin your routine by walking. When you can walk three miles in less than 45 minutes, you are ready to begin to jog and, later, to run, although some people choose never to increase their pace.

The three variables to consider when planning

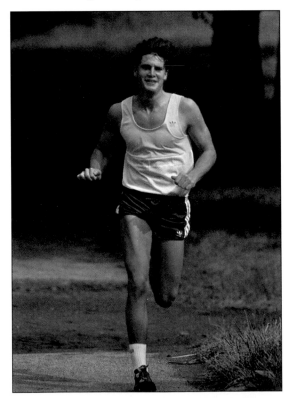

Jogging is one of the most popular types of aerobic exercise today. Many people jog in pairs, but it also often suits people who prefer to exercise alone or can exercise only at times that are not convenient for other people.

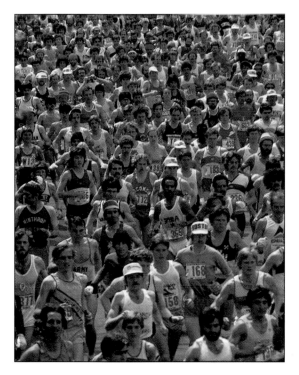

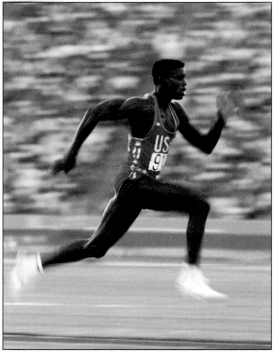

There's lots of company when you are running in a marathon. Among these everyday athletes are men and women from a wide variety of backgrounds and range of abilities. The message is that you can achieve a great deal in terms of aerobic fitness if that is your ambition.

Sprinters such as Olympic gold-medalist Carl Lewis are the ultimate anaerobic, explosive athletes. Overall body shape and the physiology of the muscles are important considerations in selecting world-class athletes for training but do not matter for individuals seeking an effective fitness strategy.

a program are frequency, duration, and intensity. By manipulating these factors you will build endurance, and progress to higher levels of fitness. If you have engaged in physical activities but are new to jogging, you might want to begin with a 20-minute session, interspersing jogging and walking until you feel comfortable about dropping the walking and only jogging for that length of time.

Where to run

Look for stable and smooth surfaces to run on when you plan your route. Avoid slanting places because their unevenness will put you off balance and cause stress on one side of the body, which can lead to injury. If you do run on a graded surface, go back the way you came to ensure you balance the body's stress. Try to choose low-traffic areas, and if you must run with cars and trucks, make sure that you face oncoming vehicles for safety. If you run at night, outfit yourself with brightly colored clothing or reflective running gear and try to find a course that is well lit. Avoid slippery wet or icy surfaces.

Before and after

Always make the warm up and cool down part of your program (see pages 106–107), and practice the stretching and strengthening exercises (see pages 126–135, 142–147) suited to jogging and running. To check how you are landing against your running surface, examine how your shoes are wearing. If one side is considerably more worn, you might need inserts to correct this problem. When you first begin, or when you intensify your program, you might experience soreness or discomfort. This is your body adjusting to a new level of activity. The soreness will abate if you work out on alternate days and treat yourself to warm, soothing baths afterward.

The running program below should produce an acceptable level of fitness by the beginning of the intermediate stage, and a run of three miles three times a week will maintain fitness. The men's advanced program should eventually enable you to run a full marathon in about four hours. The women's leads to a marathon time of about four and a half to five hours.

When you begin running, you should quickly fall into a style that suits you. A good running posture will make your workout easier and safer. Run smoothly in an upright position without leaning too far forward, and keep your ribcage lifted out of the waist. Relax the upper body by keeping your head high and dropping your shoulders. Your arms should be relaxed, with

MEN'S RUNNING PROGRAM

Beginners				Intermediate				Advanced			
Week	Distance/miles	Repeats/week	Time/mins	Week	Distance/miles	Repeats/week	Time/mins	Week	Distance/miles	Repeats/week	Time/mins
1	1	5	—	1	2	3	17	1	3	2	24½
					3	2	—		8	3	70
2	1	5	12	2	2½	4	22	2	4	2	33
					any distance	1	45		8	3	—
3	1	3	11	3	2	4	—	3	4	3	32
	1½	2	20		4	1	35		8	2	68
4	1	3	10½	4	3	4	26	4	7	4	58
	1½	2	18		any distance	1	55		10	1	—
5	1	3	10	5	2½	4	—	5	4	2	31
	1½	2	16		5	1	44		7	3	—
6	1	3	9½	6	3	4	25½	6	4	1	30
	2	2	22½		any distance	1	65		6	4	49
									10	1	—
7	1½	3	15	7	2½	4	21½	7	3	1	23
	2	2	22		7	1	63		7	4	58
8	1½	3	14	8	4	4	34½	8	5	3	—
	2	2	20		any distance	1	75		8	2	66
									10	1	—
9	1½	3	14	9	2½	4	21	9	3	1	22
	2½	2	26		5	1	44		8	4	64
10	1½	3	13	10	4	3	34	10	6	2	47
	2½	2	24		any distance	2	60		8	3	—
									10	1	80
11	1½	3	12½	11	3	3	25	11	3	1	21½
	3	2	30		5	2	—		7	3	55
									12	1	—
12	2	3	17½	12	4	3	34	12	4	3	29
	3	2	27		8	2	—		8	3	62
									15	1	—

elbows slightly bent, wrists lower than elbows, and fingers slightly curled. Carry your arms slightly away from your body and let them swing easily. Run with a heel-first action, making a clawing action as the rest of your foot hits the ground and pushing off from the ball of your foot at each stride. Start with small strides and alter them until you find your natural, most comfortable stride length. Breathe regularly, emphasizing the exhalation.

Test whether you are running within your capabilities by keeping a check on your pulse (see pages 12–13) and by always breathing easily. You should be able to talk as you run.

Wear proper shoes for running, and absorbent clothes (never rubber) suited to the weather.

WOMEN'S RUNNING PROGRAM

Beginners				Intermediate				Advanced			
Week	Distance/ miles	Repeats/ week	Time/ mins	Week	Distance/ miles	Repeats/ week	Time/ mins	Week	Distance/ miles	Repeats/ week	Time/ mins
1	1	3	—	1	2	3	17½	1	3	3	27
	1½ (Walk/jog)	2	—		3	2	—		4	2	—
2	1	3	13	2	2	4	17½	2	4	5	36
	2 (Walk/jog)	2	—		4	1	—				
3	1	5	12½	3	2½	4	23	3	3	3	26
					4	1	—		6	2	54
4	1	5	12	4	2½	4	34	4	4	4	35
					any distance	1	40		8	1	—
5	1	3	11½	5	2	3	17	5	3	4	25
	1½	2	—		4	2	—		5	2	45
6	1	3	11	6	2½	4	22	6	4	4	35
	1½	2	18		any distance	1	50		10	1	—
7	1	2	10½	7	2	3	—	7	4	4	34
	1½	3	17½		5	2	45		8	1	—
8	1½	5	16½	8	2½	4	21½	8	5	3	45
					any distance	1	60		8	2	—
9	1½	3	16	9	2	3	17	9	3	3	24
	2	2	22		4	2	36		8	2	72
10	1½	3	14	10	2½	4	21	10	3	1	23
	2	2	21		any distance	1	65		5	4	44
									12	1	—
11	1½	2	13½	11	3	3	28	11	3	4	22½
	2	3	20		5	2	44		6	1	—
									12	1	108
12	2	3	18	12	3	4	27	12	3	3	22
	2½	2	24		7	1	63		8	2	70
									15	1	—

SWIMMING

Swimming is an excellent way of getting plenty of aerobic exercise in a short space of time. And being able to swim well has the added advantage that it might help to save your own or someone else's life. Because the work you are performing when you swim is against water resistance rather than against gravity, the risk of injury to body muscles and joints is low.

If you look at a group of people in a pool, you will notice how markedly they differ in their swimming capability. The programs on these pages are designed to take account of this enormous variation in natural swimming ability.

Use the programs according to the general guidelines given on page 108, and remember to wait at least one hour after eating before you enter the water.

If you are already a competent swimmer, and especially if you can swim the front crawl continuously for 100 yards or more, start with the intermediate program. The same applies if you are adept at back crawl, which is almost as fast as front crawl when swum well and has a breathing technique that is much easier to master. Its chief disadvantage is the degree to which it reduces your ability to see other swimmers.

MEN'S SWIMMING PROGRAM

	Beginners				Intermediate				Advanced		
Week	Distance/ yards	Repeats/ week	Time/ mins	Week	Distance/ yards	Repeats/ week	Time/ mins	Week	Distance/ yards mixed strokes	Repeats/ week	Time/ mins
1	50	3	—	1	200	5	5	1	500	2	13
									500	3	11
2	50	2	—	2	200	3	5	2	500	2	12
	100	2	—		300	2	8		500	3	10
3	100	2	—	3	300	5	$7\frac{1}{2}$	3	500	2	12
	150	3	—						800	3	17
4	150	2	—	4	300	3	7	4	800	2	20
	200	3	—		500	2	13		800	3	$16\frac{1}{2}$
5	250	3	—	5	400	5	10	5	800	2	20
	300	2	13						800	2	16
									1,100	1	—
6	300	5	12	6	500	5	12	6	800	2	19
									1,000	2	21
									1,100	1	—
7	300	3	11	7	500	3	10	7	1,000	2	24
	400	2	—		700	2	16		1,100	2	25
									1,400	1	—
8	400	5	15	8	600	5	12	8	1,000	2	24
									1,400	3	31
9	400	3	14	9	600	3	$11\frac{1}{2}$	9	1,000	2	23
	500	2	—		800	2	17		1,400	3	30
10	500	5	19	10	700	5	14	10	1,000	2	23
									1,450	3	32
11	500	3	16	11	800	5	$16\frac{1}{2}$	11	1,000	2	22
	600	2	—						1,600	3	36
12	600	5	22	12	800	3	16	12	1,000	2	21
					1,000	2	22		1,800	3	40

As you progress through the program, you should aim to include more and more lengths of front or back crawl. You will probably need to do this to achieve the times set in the schedules, but the programs do not specify mixed strokes until you arrive at the advanced section. In this section you should spend an equal amount of time on each of your chosen strokes—ideally front crawl, back crawl, breaststroke, and butterfly if you can manage it. Whatever stage you are at, keep a check on your pulse rate, twice during each session and at the end (see pages 12–13), and do not exceed the safe maximum.

The programs are given in terms of yards. Ask the pool attendant the length of the pool (if it is not already marked) or pace it out at approximately one large stride per yard. Count the lengths as you swim, and do not cheat.

To avoid the crowds at public pools, try swimming early in the morning or late in the evening. You could also consider joining a club, which would offer coaching as well as reserved pool times. Protect your eyes from chlorinated or salt water with goggles, and wear a swimsuit that will not cut into you or slip off when you are swimming or diving.

WOMEN'S SWIMMING PROGRAM

Beginners			Intermediate				Advanced			
Week	Distance/ yards	Repeats/ week	Time/ mins	Week	Distance/ yards	Repeats/ week	Time/ mins	Week	Distance/ yards mixed strokes	Repeats/ week	Time/ mins
1	50	3	—	1	200	5	5	1	500	2	14
									500	3	11
2	50	2	—	2	200	3	5	2	500	2	13
	100	2	—		300	2	8		500	3	10
3	100	2	—	3	300	5	$7\frac{1}{2}$	3	500	2	13
	150	3	—						800	3	18
4	150	2	—	4	300	3	7	4	800	2	21
	200	3	—		500	2	13		800	3	17
5	250	3	—	5	400	5	10	5	800	2	21
	300	2	14						800	2	16
									1,100	1	—
6	300	5	13	6	500	12	20	6	800	2	20
									1,000	2	21
									1,100	1	—
7	300	3	12	7	500	3	11	7	1,000	2	26
	400	2	—		700	2	16		1,100	2	25
									1,400	1	—
8	400	5	16	8	600	5	$13\frac{1}{2}$	8	1,000	2	26
									1,400	3	32
9	400	3	15	9	600	3	13	9	1,000	2	25
	500	2	—		800	2	19		1,400	3	30
10	500	5	20	10	700	5	15	10	1,000	2	25
									1,450	3	32
11	500	3	18	11	800	5	$17\frac{1}{2}$	11	1,000	2	24
	600	2	—						1,600	3	36
12	600	5	24	12	800	3	17	12	1,000	2	23
					1,000	2	24		1,800	3	40

EXERCISES IN WATER

Water exercises have become increasingly popular in recent years as people have come to realize the enormous benefits that can be attained while they stay cool and relaxed in the pool. A structured workout in the water will not only improve your cardiovascular health, and tone and strengthen your muscles, but will do it with little risk of injury. The buoyancy of the water eliminates stress on the vulnerable joints so you can work your body through its full range of motion. The water bears your weight, cushions impact, and protects your spine.

Physical therapists and other rehabilitation specialists have always used water exercise therapeutically. The disabled, for example, can perform movements in the water that they cannot execute on land. The obese find that the support of the water allows them to exercise safely and for longer periods. Doing stretching and strengthening exercises in the water is safe even for those recovering from injuries and is often a good way to stay in shape during recovery. Use water exercise as a companion activity to any sport. Even if you don't know how to swim, you can reap benefits from, and have fun with, water workouts.

Getting ready

Choose a swimsuit that fits well, is not binding, and moves easily as you move. In an outdoor pool, you are being exposed to the sun's rays, so protect yourself by wearing a water-resistant sunscreen and goggles in the water, and a sunhat and sunglasses when you are by the poolside.

Check the temperature of the pool water. Water that feels too cold after you have been in it for a while will cause your muscles to tense and tighten; water that is too warm will make you drowsy. And be sure to wait at least one hour after eating before you enter the water.

Swimming programs

By following the charts on pages 116–117 you can create a swimming program that will gradually build your endurance. Remember to vary intensity, duration, and frequency in your workout. Combine sprint swimming (swimming your fastest for short periods of time) and aerobic swimming (building your time up to at least 20 minutes without concern for the number of laps) to derive maximum benefits for the respiratory and cardiovascular systems.

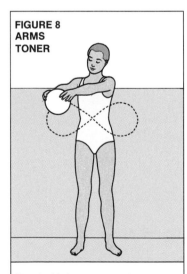

FIGURE 8 ARMS TONER

Stand with feet apart, arms extended straight in front of you holding a ball. Breathing rhythmically, draw large underwater figure 8's. Repeat 10 times.

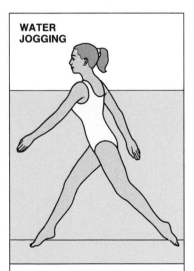

WATER JOGGING

Make continuous strides, extending arms and legs as far as you can and breathing rhythmically.

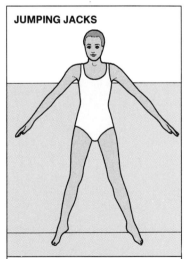

JUMPING JACKS

As on land, jump and inhale while you extend arms overhead and spread legs wide apart. Exhaling, jump and bring arms to your sides, feet together. Repeat 15 times.

Nonswimmers

If you are a nonswimmer or insecure about being in the water, begin by wearing a comfortable life jacket, and keep your feet on the pool floor and your head well above water. Use the pool ladder, the edge of the pool, or a cooperative friend for support. Familiarize yourself with the water by bobbing up and down at the shallow end of the pool. Take a deep breath, then bend your knees and submerge your face. Start to exhale as soon as your face touches the water; straighten your knees and come to the surface. Repeat the movement, gradually going lower, until you feel more confident.

Jogging and fast walking in the water are aerobic activities that you can perform and still keep your feet on the ground. Stay at the shallow end and take long strides across the width, using your arms to propel you through the water.

Stretching and strengthening

Stretching in the pool for the first time can make you believe in magic. You seem to be able to go farther with ease into each position than you could on land.

Try the stretching exercises on pages 126–131 in water. Almost all movements can be adapted to the pool. For instance, you can perform lunging stretches with your feet on the pool floor or against the wall. Use the pool ladder creatively to increase your repertoire of stretches. Try circling the shoulders, wrists, ankles, and hips in the water to feel the relaxing stretch.

Use the water's resistance to increase your muscle strength and tone. Remember to keep your fingers pressed tightly together and your hands cupped while they go through the water. Any movement of your arms through the water will build strength. Keep them fully submerged and extend them in each direction, taking the longest route between two points and drawing underwater circles as large as you can. Abdominal and leg muscles benefit from the same broad movements through the water.

Use props such as kickboards, balls, and water weights to vary your workout and increase intensity. The basic flutter kick done with ankle weights while holding on to a kickboard or the side of the pool is one of the best exercises for toning and firming buttocks and slimming thighs.

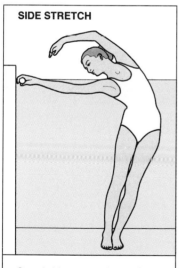

SIDE STRETCH

Stand sideways to the pool wall holding onto the edge with arm fully extended, and feet flat on the pool floor. Inhale as you extend the outside arm overhead. Exhale as you lean hips away from poolside. Do 10 times each side.

WAIST TONER
With your back against the poolside, arms along the edge, bring your knees to your chest. Extend your legs straight ahead. Inhaling, move legs to one side. Exhaling, move legs to front and withdraw to chest. Repeat 10 times, alternating sides.

TOTAL BODY STRETCH
Hold on to the pool edge with your hands. Bend your knees and press your feet against the poolside as you inhale. Exhaling, move hips back. Repeat 10 times.

Plenty of opportunities exist for indoor aerobic training.

Although a rowing machine cannot duplicate the sensation of actual rowing, it provides an acceptable substitute and puts the same range of muscles through their paces. The rowing program aims to build up your work level gently.

Skipping rope was first popularized by boxers and has now been recognized by other sports people as a most convenient form of aerobic training. It needs no equipment beyond an ordinary jump rope and can be done almost anywhere. Start off with a basic rocking skip with the same foot leading, then with alternate feet leading,

before progressing to double jumps, one-foot hops, and other variations.

Aerobic dance, a highly effective and for many the most enjoyable form of exercise, has the added advantage of improving strength and flexibility. Having learned the basics at formal classes, you can use the schedules to build up your fitness level in your own home.

As with all aerobic exercise programs, follow the general guidelines on page 108. Keep a check on your pulse and do not exceed the safe maximum (see pages 12–13). These programs can be interchanged with the beginners' and intermediate running and bicycling programs.

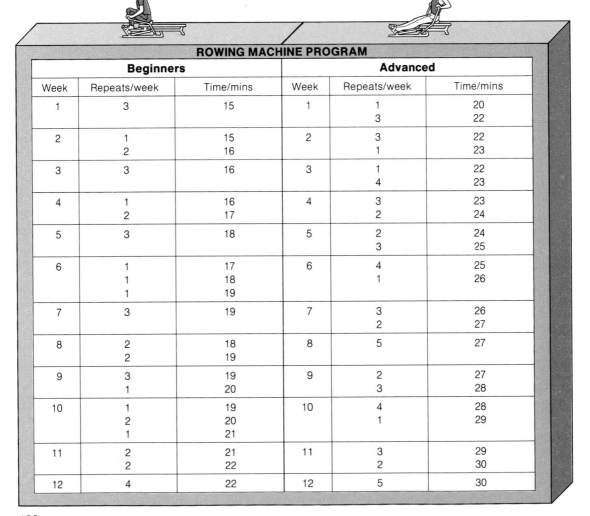

ROWING MACHINE PROGRAM					
Beginners			**Advanced**		
Week	Repeats/week	Time/mins	Week	Repeats/week	Time/mins
1	3	15	1	1 3	20 22
2	1 2	15 16	2	3 1	22 23
3	3	16	3	1 4	22 23
4	1 2	16 17	4	3 2	23 24
5	3	18	5	2 3	24 25
6	1 1 1	17 18 19	6	4 1	25 26
7	3	19	7	3 2	26 27
8	2 2	18 19	8	5	27
9	3 1	19 20	9	2 3	27 28
10	1 2 1	19 20 21	10	4 1	28 29
11	2 2	21 22	11	3 2	29 30
12	4	22	12	5	30

SKIPPING ROPE PROGRAM

Beginners			Advanced		
Week	Repeats/week	Time/mins	Week	Repeats/week	Time/mins
1	3	5	1	5	10
2	3	$5\frac{1}{2}$	2	5	$11\frac{1}{2}$
3	4	$5\frac{1}{2}$	3	5	12
4	4	6	4	5	13
5	4	$6\frac{1}{2}$	5	5	14
6	4	7	6	5	15
7	3	7	7	6	15
	1	6			
8	4	8	8	6	16
9	4	9	9	6	17
10	4	10	10	6	18
11	5	11	11	6	19
12	5	12	12	6	20

AEROBIC DANCE PROGRAM

Beginners			Advanced		
Week	Repeats/week	Time/mins	Week	Repeats/week	Time/mins
1	3	3	1	4	15
2	3	4	2	2	15
				2	18
3	3	5	3	4	18
4	3	6	4	4	19
5	4	6	5	4	20
6	4	7	6	4	20
7	4	8	7	2	20
				2	22
8	4	9	8	4	22
9	4	10	9	3	22
				2	25
10	4	12	10	5	26
11	4	14	11	5	28
12	4	15	12	5	30

Fitness has become big business. Scores of different devices can be found in health clubs and gyms, and are sold with the promise that used in your own home they will act as mainstays in your quest for fitness. The destiny of most such equipment is to gather dust in a garage or attic. The best of home equipment, including exercise bicycles (see pages 110–111), can be used for strength training and incorporated into an aerobic fitness schedule. A beginners' and an advanced rowing machine program is provided on page 120, and an assessment of the usefulness of other popular equipment is given on these pages.

Rowing machines

The rowing machine provides a wider range of exercise than many other activities. It works the major groups of muscles in the back, arms, shoulders, abdomen, and legs. Because it is a non-weight-bearing activity, it is a safe and efficient means to achieve aerobic fitness.

Mini trampolines

These trampolines are designed to make it easier and more fun to jog indoors, on the spot. They do produce a sensation reasonably akin to real running, but unless you are housebound or live in an area where the weather is not conducive to outdoor exercise, they are probably not worthwhile. However, they can do no harm and are a less expensive alternative to a treadmill.

Treadmills

The treadmill—a moving belt on which the participant walks or jogs—is an essential part of the sports physiologist's equipment and has been successfully adapted for club and home use. Treadmills are obtainable powered and unpowered, and, obviously, unpowered ones are much less expensive. Many models incorporate equipment for measuring the way in which your pulse rate changes as you exercise.

Sit-up benches

These devices are particularly useful for strengthening abdominals. There are two types shown here, but both use the same principle: you lie on your back on a raised, sloping board. Your feet are tucked under a strap or behind a bar. This gives you some leverage and helps you to pull yourself up into a sitting position.

Leg and arm stretcher

This piece of equipment can be screwed into a wall or a door jamb, and is used to strengthen and stretch your arms and legs. You stand next to the device and fasten your leg or arm to a flex attached to a movable weight. By extending your limb sideways, you pull against the weight.

Chinning bars

These are bars that you fix between the posts of a door and use for strength training. Useful and inexpensive, they allow you to exercise the muscles in the arms and chest. They rely on the principle of using your own body weight for strength training and are safe as long as you can find a secure position in which to fix them.

Chest expanders/grip developers

Spring chest expanders are an inexpensive, effective, and safe way of building up the arm muscles in an isokinetic way (see page 98). However, push-ups and chin-ups using your own body weight are better and more effective.

Grip developers are sprung isometric devices held in the hand. However, isometric exercise is less beneficial to the heart than aerobic exercise and can raise the blood pressure.

Weights

Until the late 1970's any sort of strength training involving the use of more than your own body weight meant the lifting of free weights. Today, however, weight-lifting devices have been incorporated into many sorts of gym equipment, such as the leg and arm press machines. Free weights remain a favorite among body builders and competitive weight-lifters, but they can easily cause injuries. For this reason, it is not safe to use them unless you are under expert supervision. There are also weights that you can attach to your hands and ankles to intensify exercise routines.

Home multi-purpose gyms

These pieces of equipment, incorporating devices such as the weight bench, leg raise/dip bar, lat bar, weight pulley, leg pulley, and neck developer, aim to provide isokinetic strength training to all the muscle groups in the body. Because the equipment is subject to a great deal of strain, it must be manufactured to high standards and will therefore, be expensive.

Rowing machine
A rowing machine is an excellent way to strengthen and tone the upper body. On most machines you can measure your progress and increase the resistance as you get stronger.

Treadmill
This offers you a means of running indoors or in your garden. It is particularly useful for exercising in spells of bad weather.

Sit-up bench 1
The simplest sit-up bench is equipped with a strap beneath which the feet are restrained. The angle of the bench can be altered to increase the degree of difficulty of the exercise. As with other such equipment, it is wise to consult your doctor before you begin an exercise schedule. Stop if you are in any pain.

Mini trampoline
This can be used for jogging by both children and adults.

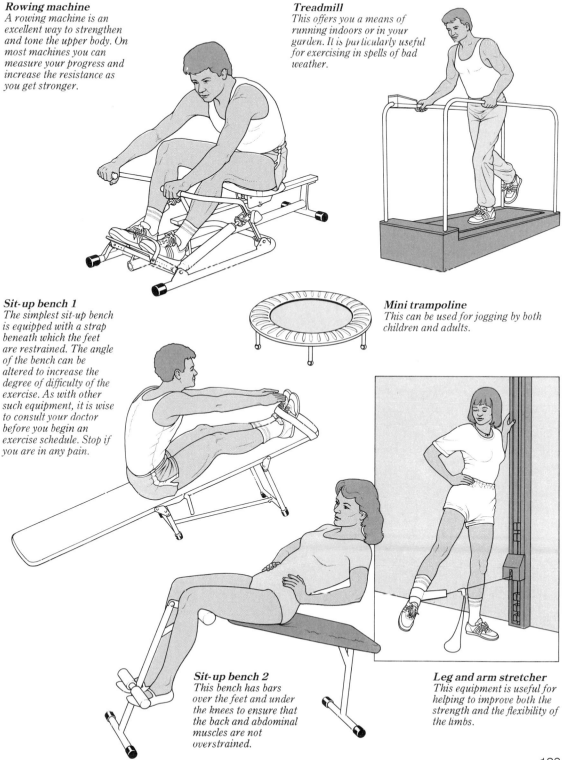

Sit-up bench 2
This bench has bars over the feet and under the knees to ensure that the back and abdominal muscles are not overstrained.

Leg and arm stretcher
This equipment is useful for helping to improve both the strength and the flexibility of the limbs.

HOME GYM

It is easy to find reasons not to exercise: it's too expensive, too far away, too time consuming. But all you have to do is look around your own home with a creative eye and a home gym will reveal itself to you in a very short time. Working out regularly at home does away with all the excuses that can stand in the way of a successful fitness program. People often convince themselves that just by virtue of spending a good deal of money on special exercise equipment they will become fit. Exercise equipment is excellent for those who can afford it, but only if they use it. Before you invest money in machines for home use, why not try to use ordinary household objects, at least for a test. It will be convenient, inexpensive, and can be fun for your family and friends. Along with the fitness benefits, think how impressed everyone will be by your ingenuity.

As with all exercise, consider safety first. Be sure all objects and furniture that you use are sturdy and in good repair and that the weights you choose are manageable. Beware the rug that slips, the towel that rips, and the five-pound bag of sugar that splits! If possible, designate an area in your home that can be used specifically for exercise. Otherwise, choose a spot that is free of obstruction, properly ventilated, and private. Set aside a time of day when you can exercise without interruptions, and turn on your phone answering machine if you have one. Plan your program realistically, with short- and long-term goals in mind. Keep track of your progress so that you will know when it is time to move on to more sophisticated gear or heavier weights. Use a full-length mirror as a friend and guide to help you decide which parts of your body need attention. Refer to pages 126–135 for specialized tips on stretching and strengthening.

Remember that each time you travel, you can look at your temporary environment as a challenge. See what ordinary objects you can find to continue your fitness program away from home.

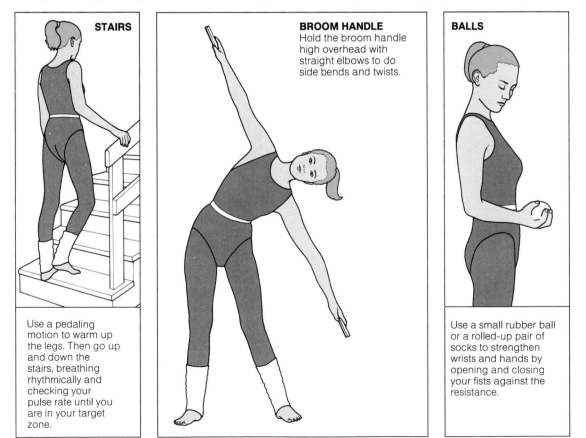

STAIRS

Use a pedaling motion to warm up the legs. Then go up and down the stairs, breathing rhythmically and checking your pulse rate until you are in your target zone.

BROOM HANDLE
Hold the broom handle high overhead with straight elbows to do side bends and twists.

BALLS

Use a small rubber ball or a rolled-up pair of socks to strengthen wrists and hands by opening and closing your fists against the resistance.

CANS

Use 1-lb cans of vegetables as hand weights. Hold a can in each hand and do arm exercises.
1. Bend arms, holding cans at shoulder level. Straighten and bend arms alternately.
2. Start with arms down at your sides. Keeping arms straight, raise them out to the sides and above your head. **3.** Start with your arms parallel in front of your body. Raise alternate arms to head height.

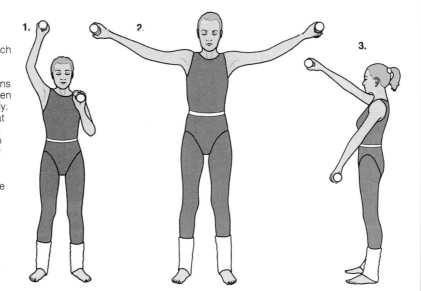

TOWELS

1. Hold a bath towel firmly at both ends and use the resistance of the material to increase your stretch as you lift the towel overhead. **2.** Sit on the floor with a partner, legs wide apart, feet touching. Each grasp one towel end and rock forward and back in unison.

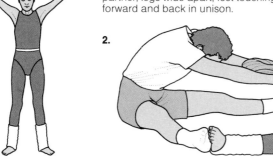

SOFA OR DRESSER

Use a sofa or dresser to help with sit-ups (see page 132). Hook your toes under the furniture and bend your knees as you roll up to a sitting position.

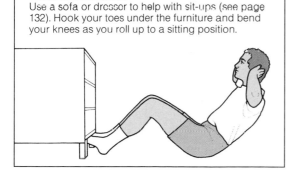

BAG OF SUGAR

Place a 5-lb bag of sugar in a bag with a handle and hook it around your ankle. Inhale. As you exhale, slowly extend the leg straight in front of you. Lower your leg slowly as you inhale.

STRETCHING

A regular program of stretching exercises will help you to attain and maintain the flexibility that you need for everyday activities and make you more graceful and "at home" in your body. From adolescence onward, the body's joints have a natural tendency to lose mobility. By putting the main joints of your body through their full range of motion daily, you can help keep them in good working order and possibly delay or diminish the pain of arthritis later.

A stretching routine lengthens and loosens your muscles, helping them to relax. Because blood is sent to the working muscles, when you are preparing for activity it makes sense to limber in particular the muscle groups that you will be using. Stretching can be targeted for the specific sports that you play (see pages 128–131).

Do all stretching slowly and evenly, using the weight of your body and your breath to relax (not pull) into your stretch. Ballistic stretching, or bouncing, is not recommended. Instead, go into position, hold it for approximately 10–20 seconds, and breathe regularly and fully. This will produce the same effect as bouncing, but without the risk of injury.

You can do the exercises shown here any time you choose. Be aware that you will stretch farther in the afternoon or evening, after your body has been moving for a while, than first thing in the morning. Plan to do stretching before and after any activity. Take the temperature of your environment into consideration. Warmth increases the benefits of flexibility exercises, so avoid extremes in temperature and wear layered clothing if you are exercising in chilly weather.

Stretching is a noncompetitive activity. Don't compare your stretch to others around you. Work at your own pace to get the most benefit from the routine you have chosen.

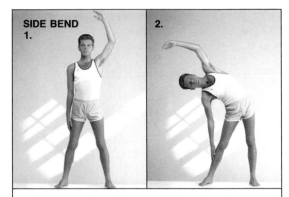

SIDE BEND
1.
2.

1. Stand with feet wide apart, right hand resting on your right leg, left arm raised overhead. Inhale. **2.** As you exhale, bend toward the right, letting your right hand slide down your leg and your left arm hang over your left ear. Hold, breathing fully for a count of 5. Contract abdominal muscles as you come up. Repeat on the other side. Do 3 times each side.

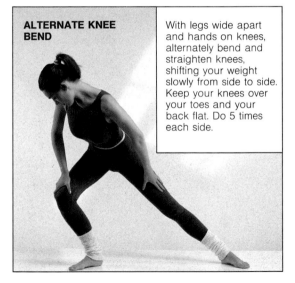

ALTERNATE KNEE BEND

With legs wide apart and hands on knees, alternately bend and straighten knees, shifting your weight slowly from side to side. Keep your knees over your toes and your back flat. Do 5 times each side.

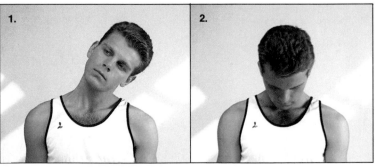

HEAD ROLL
1. Bend your left ear toward your shoulder. Keep both shoulders relaxed. **2.** Slowly drop your head forward into your chest. Roll right ear toward right shoulder and continue around. Repeat 3 times in each direction. Don't roll your head all the way back; you risk injury.

1.
2.

CAT STRETCH

1. Sit on your heels, head and shoulders dropped forward. **2.** Raise hips high in line with knees as you slide your chest and arms forward. Keep hips still and press chest down gently. Breathe fully and hold for a count of 10. Sit back on heels. Repeat 3 times.

1.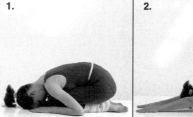

2.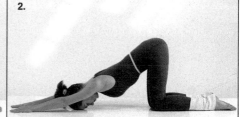

LEG STRETCH

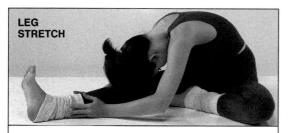

Sit forward on the floor with one leg extended. Inhale and raise both arms. As you exhale, stretch over your extended leg as far as is comfortable. Breathe deeply for 10–20 seconds, allowing your head to hang forward. Repeat, changing legs.

DOUBLE KNEE ROLL

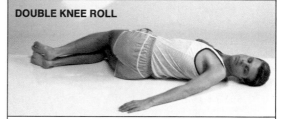

Lie on your back with knees bent into your chest, arms relaxed out to the sides. Bring your knees to the floor on one side, turn your head the opposite way. Hold for a slow count of 5, allowing your arm and shoulder to hang back. Repeat 3 times each side.

LUNGE STRETCH

Stand with one foot against a wall, palms at shoulder height pressing in. Stretch the other heel back and lean hips in toward the wall as you breathe for a count of 10. Feel the stretch in the calf and Achilles tendon. Repeat on the other side.

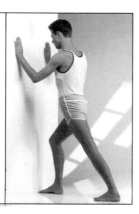

INNER THIGH STRETCH

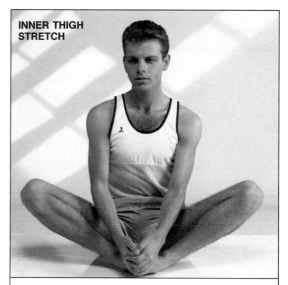

Sit forward on both buttocks, soles of your feet together, hands clasping your toes. Take a full breath. As you exhale, contract your abdominal muscles and press your knees toward the floor. Hold for a count of 5, then release. Repeat 3 times.

QUAD STRETCH

Steady yourself against a wall or chair with one hand. Bend the opposite leg back and grasp your ankle with your free hand. Try to align your knees and don't arch your back. Hold and feel the upper thigh stretch as you breathe for a count of 10. Repeat on the other side.

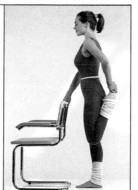

Specific sports and activities put stress on particular parts of the body. Therefore, in addition to a general flexibility program, use stretching exercises designed for those potentially vulnerable areas. Starting your sport slowly will help to warm up the muscles. See pages 106–107 for general warm-up exercises.

Use the exercises on these and the following pages to plan a program for your individual needs. Each exercise is coded for the sport for which it is relevant. Remember always to breathe fully and to use your body weight to relax into each position. Trying to stretch too far will tense and shorten your muscles instead of relaxing and lengthening them.

KEY

B = biking	K = skiing
G = golf	R = rowing
J = jogging/	T = tennis
running	W = swimming

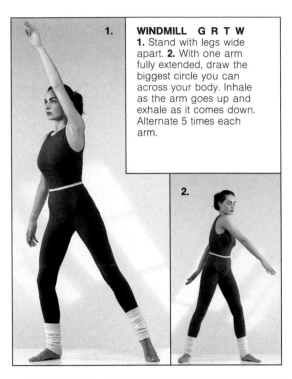

1. **WINDMILL G R T W**
1. Stand with legs wide apart. **2.** With one arm fully extended, draw the biggest circle you can across your body. Inhale as the arm goes up and exhale as it comes down. Alternate 5 times each arm.

2.

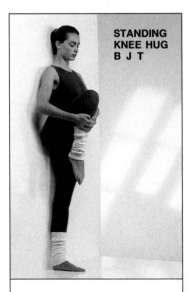

**STANDING KNEE HUG
B J T**

Stand with buttocks against the wall and slowly hug one knee as close to your chest as possible. Hold for 10 seconds while you breathe. Repeat 3 times on each side.

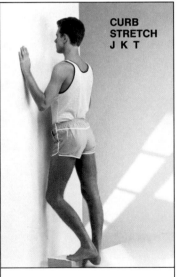

**CURB STRETCH
J K T**

Place your toes on the edge of the curb (or a phone book if indoors) and let your heels drop slowly. Steady your upper body with your hand while you breathe. Bend one knee and then the other in a slow pedaling motion for 30 seconds.

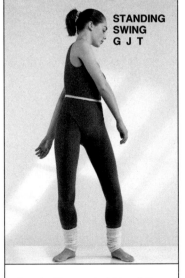

**STANDING SWING
G J T**

Stand with your feet hip width apart, knees slightly bent. Swing your arms freely from side to side and watch where you're going. This is good for getting out the morning "kinks."

LEG UP STRETCH B J

1. Stand with one leg supported at a lower-than-waist height, foot flexed. Reach up and over the extended leg to the farthest comfortable point. **2.** Grasping the leg firmly, slowly bend and straighten the knee. Feel the stretch in your hamstring muscle. Change legs and repeat. Do 3 times on each side.

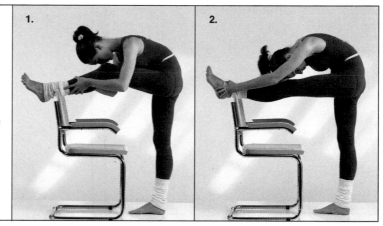

DEEP LUNGE B J K T

Crouch down with your feet behind your hands; bend the left knee forward keeping the heel down and stretch the right leg straight back. Slowly shift your weight forward and back, and feel the stretch in your hip and calf. Repeat on the other side.

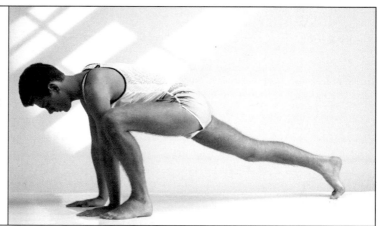

UPPER BODY STRETCH G K T W

1. Stand with feet hip width apart and bend left knee. Lift and bend left elbow back. **2.** Grasp the left elbow with right hand and slowly circle the upper body in each direction 3 times. Repeat on the other side.

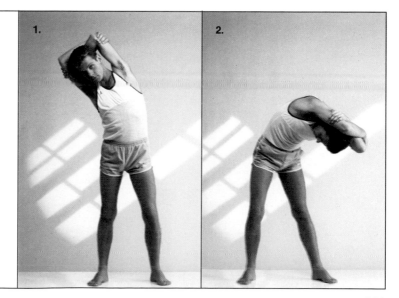

When going through your stretching routine, it is important to remember that the adage "no pain, no gain" is a myth. It is neither necessary nor beneficial to experience pain while doing these exercises. Pain means that your body is telling you that you are either doing something that is incorrect or inappropriate.

On different days and in different seasons you might need to do different stretches or do them in different ways. You might experience some mild discomfort while you stretch, especially if you haven't used a muscle or muscle group for a while. This is your body complaining, but the discomfort will ease with regular stretching. Start slowly and increase the stretches gradually as you find your flexibility improving.

KEY

B = **biking**	**K** = **skiing**
G = **golf**	**R** = **rowing**
J = **jogging/**	**T** = **tennis**
running	**W** = **swimming**

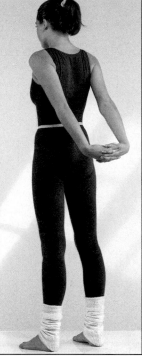

SHOULDER STRETCH
G J R T W
Stand with feet hip width apart and clasp hands behind buttocks. Roll your shoulders back and lift hands away from buttocks as high as you can, keeping your elbows straight. Slowly twist from side to side, breathing regularly and relaxing the neck.

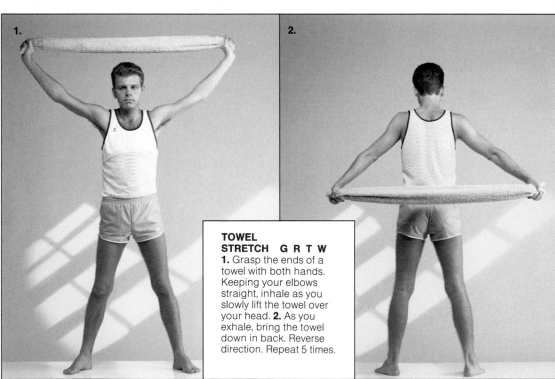

1.

2.

TOWEL STRETCH G R T W
1. Grasp the ends of a towel with both hands. Keeping your elbows straight, inhale as you slowly lift the towel over your head. **2.** As you exhale, bring the towel down in back. Reverse direction. Repeat 5 times.

HIP CIRCLES G J K T

Stand with your legs wide apart, toes turned out, hands on hips. Keep your knees slightly bent and move your hips as if you were scraping the inside of a bowl. Repeat 5 times in each direction.

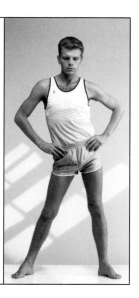

SKIER'S SQUAT B J K T

Stand with your feet wide apart, toes turned out, heels down, buttocks against the wall. Keeping your hands on your knees, slowly slide down toward the floor. Stop when your heels start to lift off the floor. Hold and sway your hips gently from side to side as you breathe. Slide up to release. Repeat 3 times.

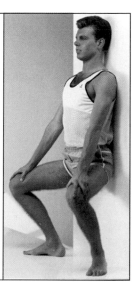

CHAIR BACK STRETCH B G J K R T

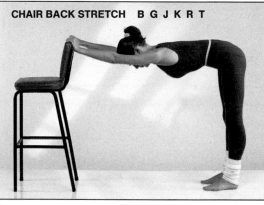

Lean forward and support your hands on a higher-than-waist-height chair back, table or ledge. Keeping your knees straight and heels down, exhale and press your chest toward the floor and flatten your back like a table. Inhaling, shift your weight slightly forward to release. Repeat 5 times.

ROCK AND ROLL J K T W

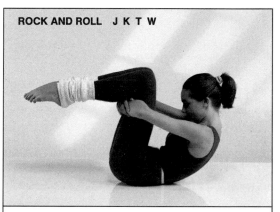

Lie on your back and hug your knees into your chest. Lift your head and shoulders and tuck in your chin as you roll forward and back. Roll back only as far as your shoulders. It is best to do this exercise on a padded surface.

LEG ROCK B G J K

1. Sitting forward on the buttocks, cradle your right leg with knee bent in both arms until you feel a stretch in your hip joint. **2.** Gently rock the leg from side to side for 10 seconds. Repeat the exercise on the other side.

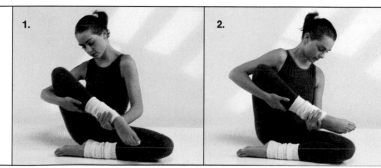

Strength training is not essential to fitness, but being strong will undoubtedly help you to build up your endurance and aid your aerobic training. There are also a number of good reasons why you might want to build up your muscle strength as well as improving your aerobic endurance. What is important is to go about strength training in the correct way. Otherwise, you may harm yourself.

Muscle strength can have a striking effect on your appearance. Your posture is better if you are strong. This not only looks more attractive than a weak, slumped posture, but does much to protect your back from common ailments. Since, volume for volume, muscle is heavier than fat, you might gain some weight but actually be slimmer as your proportion of body muscle increases.

In many sports, both aerobic and anaerobic, strength is a positive advantage to performance. In rowing, windsurfing, and swimming, strength of the upper body muscles is essential to success. In football and ice hockey, leg strength is critical. Upper and lower body strength is helpful to racket games and to martial arts such as judo.

Another bonus of strength training is that if you are strong for your size, you will be more likely to stay active longer. This will, in turn, keep you aerobically fit for longer and help to prolong your life. If you simply wish to improve your strength for its own sake, remember that strength training will not in itself make you fit.

How to train for strength
The simplest and probably the safest way to train for increased strength is to use your own body weight. Push-ups and chin-ups are good for improving the strength of both your arms and your shoulders. Runners and people who play sports such as soccer, which concentrates on lower body activity, might find such exercise particularly worthwhile, since running is good for strengthening the legs and back but does little for the upper part of the body. Before you begin, do some warm-up exercises (see pages 106–107).

Even if they have done no strength training, most men are able to do a few push-ups. If this is so, then training is simply a matter of building up the number. Lie face-down on the floor, with your legs together and your hands flat on the floor beneath your shoulders. Straighten your arms, pushing your body off the floor and keeping it straight. Then lower your body back into the starting position. When you can repeat this 20 or more times with ease, raise your feet on a box or low stool. This increases the work that your arms have to do.

Beginners usually find push-ups difficult. If this is so, keep your knees on the ground and simply use the upper part of your body for the push-up.

Chin-ups are the reverse of push-ups. In these you use your arms to pull yourself up high enough to reach your chin over a bar. (This usually needs to be done in a gym, but you can buy bars for use at home—see pages 122–123.) If you cannot manage more than two or three repeats, modify the exercise by lying under a lower bar, placed at the level of your chest. Keeping your heels on the floor and your body straight, grasp the bar and pull yourself up.

To strengthen the abdominal muscles, the easiest exercises to do are sit-ups. Lie on your back with your legs bent and feet held by a partner or under a firm support. With hands behind your head, raise your trunk toward your knees; then return to your starting position. Repeat 10 times. Other exercises for the abdominals are on pages 142–143.

To derive the benefits from strengthening, as from other exercises, and avoid stressing the body, you must breathe regularly and correctly. Many people who are beginning to exercise for the first time have a tendency to hold their breath while exerting themselves. Concentrate on exhaling audibly on each effort and inhale as you return to the starting position.

PUSH-UPS 1.

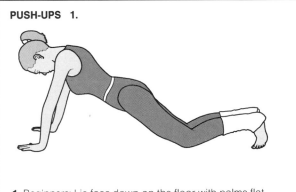

1. Beginners: Lie face down on the floor with palms flat. Inhale. As you exhale straighten your arms and push your body up, keeping your knees on the floor.

CHIN-UPS

1. Use two identical sturdy chairs, firmly anchored, to support a strong broom handle or chinning bar. Lie under the bar and grasp it with an underhand grip. Point your toes, support with your heels, tighten your abdominals, and as you exhale pull yourself up, aiming your chin for the bar. Inhale on the way down. **2.** Place a chinning bar at chest level in a doorway. Tighten your abdominals, exhale, and keep your body straight as you pull up your chin toward the bar.

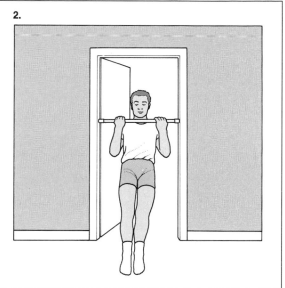

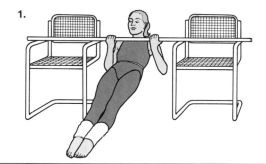

DIPS

Use two chairs that are stable and won't move for dips to strengthen your triceps. **1.** Suspend yourself between the chairs, elbows straight, heels on the floor.
2. Inhale as you lower yourself almost to the floor. Exhale as you press up and straighten the elbows.

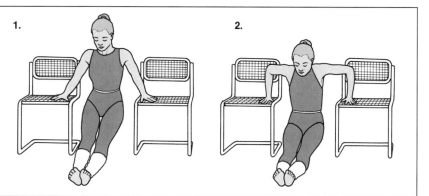

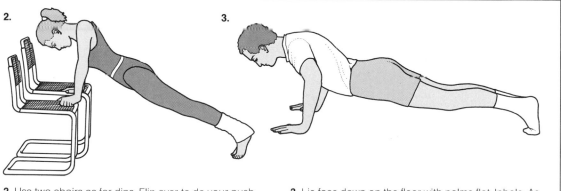

2. Use two chairs as for dips. Flip over to do your push-ups, making sure to keep your body in a straight line and not allowing your back to sway.

3. Lie face down on the floor with palms flat. Inhale. As you exhale straighten your arms, pushing your body up. Inhale as you return to starting position.

The best and safest sort of strength-training equipment is that in which the weights are fixed, rather than free, and are moved by pulleys of various kinds. The introduction and development of such equipment in recent years has done much to reduce the many injuries that people used to suffer when using free weights for strength training.

The most sophisticated equipment available puts each muscle group in the body through its complete range of movement with little risk of injury. If you use free weights or even a fixed pulley to put muscles through their entire movement range, the muscles are subjected to considerable strain at the extremes of their range—for example, when holding free weights straight overhead. This is because they are working at a mechanical disadvantage. Variable resistance equipment, however, such as that made by Nautilus and Universal, automatically alters the load on the muscles as the operator carries out a range of movements. This means that the load is least when the muscles are at the greatest mechanical disadvantage.

Variable resistance equipment, which many gyms and health clubs now provide, has the added advantage that the exercising muscle can be put under adequate, but not excessive, tension during its relaxation phase. This prevents muscle-shortening and the consequent diminishing of flexibility that accompanies it. As with other types of exercise, it is essential to warm up before beginning work on variable resistance equipment.

If you are considering using a gym for strength training, make sure that you choose one that not only has a full range of variable resistance equipment, but also provides close supervision, particularly for beginners. Look, too, for other facilities, such as equipment that is specially designed to measure your aerobic fitness (see pages 100–101, 104–105).

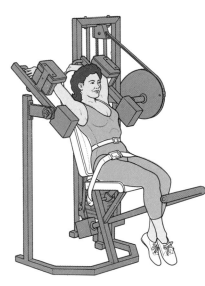

Note: Always adjust the weight and tension of these machines to fit your body size and strength.

Abdominal machine
The abdominal machine strengthens the rectus and other abdominal muscles. Inhale and as you exhale, pull body weight forward into a "crunch" position. Inhaling slowly, return to starting position just before the weights touch.

Pullover
This machine strengthens the upper back, chest, and shoulders. Keep lower back pressed into the cushion to avoid arching your back. Inhale. As you exhale, pull elbows down. Inhaling, slowly resist weights as you return to "elbows up" position.

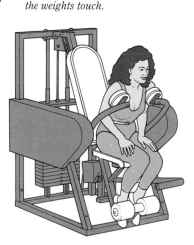

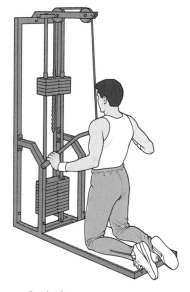

Latissimus
This station strengthens the upper and middle back muscles. As you exhale, press down on the bar handles. Inhale as you resist the rising weight.

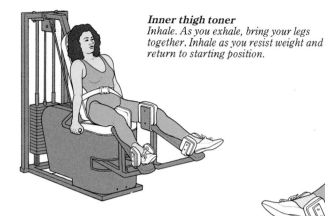

Inner thigh toner
Inhale. As you exhale, bring your legs together. Inhale as you resist weight and return to starting position.

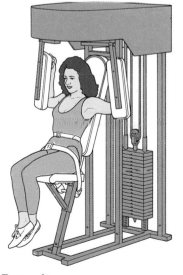

Thigh and knee
This machine strengthens the quadriceps muscles on the front of the thigh. Keep your chin close to your chest to avoid straining your neck. As you exhale, raise feet to a fully extended position. Inhale. Resisting the weight, lower your feet as you exhale.

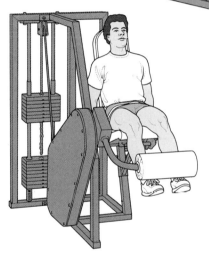

Outer thigh toner
In a stable and comfortable position, inhale. As you exhale, slowly and smoothly open your legs as wide as you can. Return to starting position, focusing on the slow, smooth reverse movement, tightening muscles.

Bench press
This machine strengthens arm and shoulder muscles. Keep the back of your neck pressed onto the bench. Inhale. As you exhale, tighten your abdominals and press up. Inhale as you resist the weight slowly lowering.

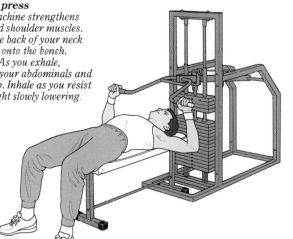

Pectorals
This machine strengthens the pectoral muscles on the chest. Inhale. As you exhale, bring your elbows together. Inhaling, resist the pressure as your arms open.

PREVENTING INJURIES

As you begin to exert your body in new ways, the risk of injury increases. Although there is no guaranteed method to keep you injury-free, there are precautions that you can take to minimize your risks. Anyone, even the most highly trained athlete, can sustain an injury on any given day, seemingly without explanation. However, if you take the time to learn about your body and train it well, you are much less likely to be thwarted by aches, pains, strains, and sprains. Choosing a sport or activity that suits your body type and build helps to prevent injury.

Men and women are equally vulnerable to sports injuries. These injuries usually, but not always, reflect the natural tendency of men to be stronger, especially in the upper body, and for women to have greater flexibility. This is not to say, of course, that men cannot be flexible and graceful, or that women cannot develop great strength. However, it is by understanding these characteristics and by evaluating your own strengths and weaknesses that you can guard against problems.

The factors that you should consider to prevent injury are: stretching and strengthening, training and coaching, and equipment and facilities.

Stretching and strengthening

To perform your sport at maximum efficiency, you need to prepare by lengthening and toning your muscles and building strength. Each time you use a muscle, it becomes slightly "injured" and shortens in the "healing" process. Stretching counteracts this natural shortening. Regardless of your level of strength, stretching will help your muscles to resist stress. Stretch and warm-up exercises also increase the temperature of your muscles and gradually prepare them for harder work (see pages 106–107 and 126–131).

Strength training improves your muscles, ligaments, tendons, and even your bones. The key to becoming strong is to work your body to its safe capacity. You can train for a specific sport by using weights or the objects that you use when you play—such as a tennis racket or golf club. Focus on building strong muscles around the joints that receive the most strain in your sport.

Training and coaching

Knowing the correct way to perform an activity is an excellent defense against injury. A good instructor has the experience and knowledge to observe your movements with a perspective you can never have. Video equipment can also be helpful for giving you feedback.

Many people learn about sports and other physical activities from books, magazine articles, and training manuals. If this is your only option, try to associate with other devotees who can give you tips based on their experience or education, and ask them to observe your movements to gain a different viewpoint.

Equipment and facilities

Poor equipment and inadequate facilities can sabotage your safety. There is a wide selection of equipment from which to choose. Magazines devoted to individual sports abound, as do feature articles and advertisements that will tell you what is being manufactured. Buy the best equipment you can afford and make sure that you are paying for quality of materials and workmanship, not just fashion and frills.

Where you perform is as important as how. You should consider the following variables.

● **Surface:** A good, resilient surface can help cushion the shock that travels through the joints and spine each time your feet make contact with the ground. Indoors, look for a sprung wood floor in aerobics areas and tracks. Outdoors, choose grass, composition, clay, or manmade tracks for your workouts. The urban athlete can compensate for concrete surfaces to a certain extent by choosing shoes with extra cushioning.

● **Temperature and air quality:** Take the temperature into consideration when you plan your workouts. Muscles that are cold pull more easily. In winter, wear layered clothing and take a longer time to warm up and stretch. Try to avoid extremes in temperature, making seasonal adjustments when necessary. Exertion during the heat of a summer day can lead to heat stroke or dehydration. Drink plenty of water, wear "breathable" clothing, and cover your head. Especially in urban areas, check the weather reports on air quality and pollution level.

● **Lighting and space:** Good lighting is essential. If you can't see something adequately, you might trip over it or run into it. Space is equally important. Investigate the activity area itself and note factors such as pool depth and length, and fences around playing fields.

Treatments

Consult a doctor immediately if you sustain a serious injury. Milder injuries might heal by themselves, but see a doctor if the pain persists after a few days. Immediate treatment for injuries should follow the acronym RICE.

The most common injuries sustained by both men and women during exercise and sports activities are indicated in this illustration.

Rest the injured area.
Ice the injured area with ice in a towel to prevent swelling.
Compress the injured area if possible with a towel or bandage to prevent swelling.
Elevate the injured area above the level of the heart to help drain fluid that might collect.

When the pain subsides, try working gradually and gently back into activity.

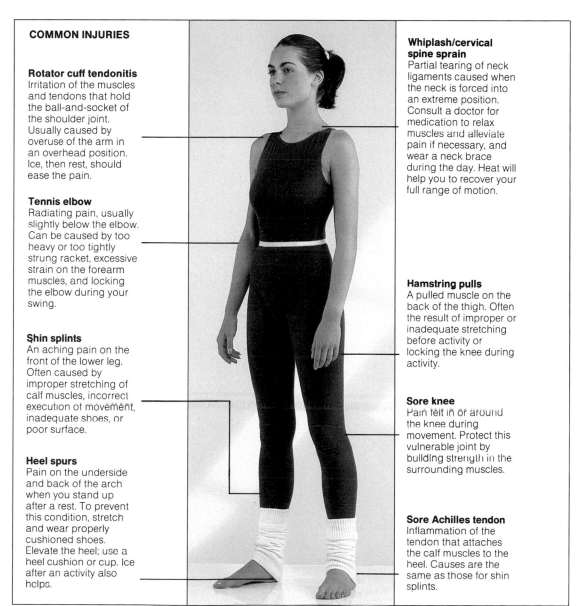

COMMON INJURIES

Rotator cuff tendonitis
Irritation of the muscles and tendons that hold the ball-and-socket of the shoulder joint. Usually caused by overuse of the arm in an overhead position. Ice, then rest, should ease the pain.

Tennis elbow
Radiating pain, usually slightly below the elbow. Can be caused by too heavy or too tightly strung racket, excessive strain on the forearm muscles, and locking the elbow during your swing.

Shin splints
An aching pain on the front of the lower leg. Often caused by improper stretching of calf muscles, incorrect execution of movement, inadequate shoes, or poor surface.

Heel spurs
Pain on the underside and back of the arch when you stand up after a rest. To prevent this condition, stretch and wear properly cushioned shoes. Elevate the heel; use a heel cushion or cup. Ice after an activity also helps.

Whiplash/cervical spine sprain
Partial tearing of neck ligaments caused when the neck is forced into an extreme position. Consult a doctor for medication to relax muscles and alleviate pain if necessary, and wear a neck brace during the day. Heat will help you to recover your full range of motion.

Hamstring pulls
A pulled muscle on the back of the thigh. Often the result of improper or inadequate stretching before activity or locking the knee during activity.

Sore knee
Pain felt in or around the knee during movement. Protect this vulnerable joint by building strength in the surrounding muscles.

Sore Achilles tendon
Inflammation of the tendon that attaches the calf muscles to the heel. Causes are the same as those for shin splints.

THE BACK

The back is the focus of almost all physical movement, a marvel of engineering that can bend, twist, and bear weight. Although the back is a powerful structure of muscle, bone, and elastic disks, its very flexibility makes it vulnerable to injury, a situation aggravated by today's increasingly sedentary lifestyle. Millions of working days are lost every year because of back pain; except for colds and flu, it is the most common cause of absenteeism in the workplace. To remain strong, the back needs exercise.

The anatomy of the spine

The spinal column provides strength, stability, and flexibility to the whole body. It consists of 33 small interlocking bones, the vertebrae, stacked one on top of the other. One end of the spinal column supports the head; the other end is anchored to the pelvis, a solid ring of bone that links the top and bottom halves of the body.

Twelve pairs of ribs are attached to the spinal column and curve around to the breastbone, forming a protective cage for the lungs and heart. Four groups of muscles, those of the back itself and of the abdomen, the pelvis, and the neck, support the spine and prevent the body from falling forward. When any of these muscles, particularly the abdominal muscles, is weak, the spine becomes unstable and back pain follows.

Running through the spinal column like a thread through a string of beads is the spinal cord, a dense network of nerves that transmits signals from the brain to the rest of the body.

The flat, bony vertebrae are separated by disks. Each disk consists of a semi-rigid ring of cartilage enclosing a jellylike center. Spinal disks absorb

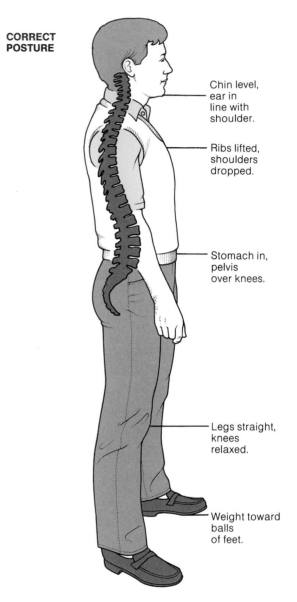

CORRECT POSTURE

Chin level, ear in line with shoulder.

Ribs lifted, shoulders dropped.

Stomach in, pelvis over knees.

Legs straight, knees relaxed.

Weight toward balls of feet.

Stand sideways in front of a full-length mirror and follow these five steps for correct posture.
1 Place your weight forward toward the balls of your feet.
2 Keep your legs straight; but don't lock your knees.
3 Pull your stomach in and line up your pelvis over your knees.
4 Lift your ribs and drop your shoulders. If your shoulders are rounded, the pectoral muscles on your chest need stretching.
5 Hold your chin level and line up your ear with your shoulder. The trapezius is the most important muscle in the neck region, forming the back of the neck and upper shoulders. It needs to be stretched and strong to prevent your neck from curving forward.

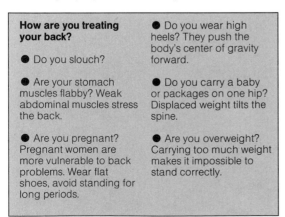

How are you treating your back?

● Do you slouch?

● Are your stomach muscles flabby? Weak abdominal muscles stress the back.

● Are you pregnant? Pregnant women are more vulnerable to back problems. Wear flat shoes, avoid standing for long periods.

● Do you wear high heels? They push the body's center of gravity forward.

● Do you carry a baby or packages on one hip? Displaced weight tilts the spine.

● Are you overweight? Carrying too much weight makes it impossible to stand correctly.

What to do about back pain

● Never exercise when your back hurts.

● Try not to slouch or overarch your back; both can result in back pain. Consider Rolfing or the Alexander Technique (see pages 314–316).

● Sitting exerts more pressure on your spine than standing or lying down. If you sit for long periods, relieve the pressure by occasionally walking around or lying down.

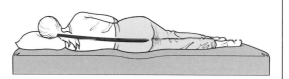

It is best to sleep on your side or on your back. On your side, bend your knees as much as is comfortable. If you suffer from backaches, place a pillow between your knees to alleviate pressure on your back and keep your body from twisting as you sleep.

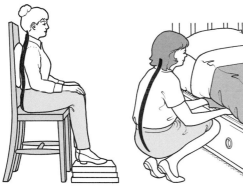

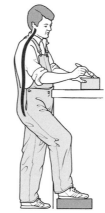

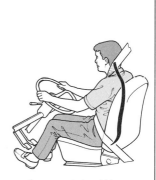

Sit well back in a chair, with a small pillow behind your shoulder blades. Place your feet on a 6-inch-high pile of books to bend your knees to a 90° angle.

When bending down or lifting anything, always bend your knees, separate your feet about shoulder width apart, and keep your back straight.

If you must stand for long periods of time, place one foot on a stool or box to prevent stressing the pelvis. The work surface should be at elbow height.

A car seat should be tilted back slightly so that your knees are higher than your hips. The seat should be close enough to the wheel to let your arms bend.

shock and distribute mechanical stress to the body. Tough ligaments hold the column of vertebrae and disks in alignment. As long as the spinal column is kept in balance, the disks remain flat; but if the spine gets out of alignment, the disks become wedge-shaped and vulnerable to injury. Subjected to a heavy load, a weakened disk can slip out of place or extrude its soft center. Anyone at any age can have back trouble, but severe degenerative back problems can often be avoided with proper care and exercise.

Furniture for a healthy back

Since you spend approximately one-third of your life in bed, your mattress should be comfortable—firm enough to support your body but yielding enough not to distort the body's natural curves. Replace your mattress every 10 years, or when it starts to sag or get lumpy. Before buying a new mattress, test it in the store. Kick off your shoes and lie on it in different positions. If you and your spouse have different requirements, buy individual mattresses. An orthopedic mattress or even a board placed between the mattress and the box spring can help a painful back. Many people find platform-style beds to be helpful.

There is no such thing as a perfect chair, but low, soft seating is the bane of back sufferers. When buying a chair, test it for firmness and for support of your lower back. The ideal chair back is angled backward about 5 to 10 degrees.

When working at a table, try to have the surface at elbow height to allow your back to remain straight and unhunched. A typewriter table is the exception to the rule; it should be somewhat lower.

BACK EXERCISES

More than 90 percent of back pain is caused by muscle weakness in the back or the abdomen, or both. You can cure back pain and prevent it from recurring by doing the exercises on these pages.

You can start on a gentle daily stretching and strengthening program if you have no serious spinal problems. If you have suffered problems, use these exercises only after consultation with your doctor. Give any back pain immediate attention.

It is vital that you distinguish between the feeling of exertion and pain when you exercise. Pain is a signal from your nerves that what you are doing is wrong for you. When you get such a signal, do only mild exercises that feel comfortable. Try the side slide, knee hug, and pelvic tilt.

When you no longer have any pain, you can continue to exercise to strengthen your back muscles. To make exercises and sports productive and safe you must have a constant awareness of your body alignment. When your body is aligned, its parts centered over one another like building blocks, you feel fit and look good. It is easy to keep the blocks aligned when your muscles are strong and stretched. You need to build correct alignment and good posture into the unconscious patterns that move you through the day and to reinforce it by strengthening the muscle groups that sustain it. Use the exercise called curling against a wall to practice standing in perfect alignment.

Your abdominal muscles are the core of your fitness. The rectus is an oblong muscle running vertically from the pubic bone to the breast bone that helps to support your trunk and keep your tummy from sagging. The oblique muscles form diagonal bands that crisscross at the navel. The transverse muscle is a horizontal band across the waist. Feel these muscles tighten when you do the curl back and diagonal crunch exercises.

Exercises for stamina are also valuable. Start these more rigorous activities slowly and always warm up before the activity and cool down afterward (see pages 106–107). Use the fundamental hamstring stretch shown here, and see pages 126–131 for more stretches.

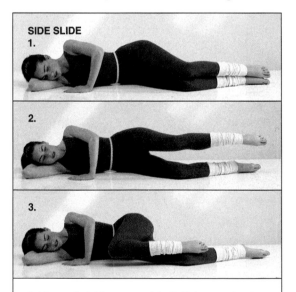

SIDE SLIDE

1. Lie comfortably on one side. **2.** Raise your top leg to the level of your hip. **3.** Gently bend your knee toward your chest, slide your leg back to starting position; hold still and feel the weight of your leg, then let it drop. Wobble to loosen your body. Repeat 3 times each side.

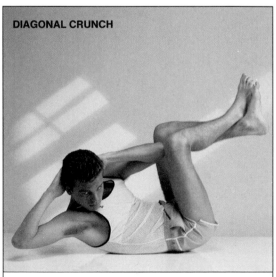

DIAGONAL CRUNCH

Lie on your back, hands behind your head. Bring your knees to your chest, turn them out to the sides and cross your feet at the ankles. Inhale. Exhale slowly as you raise your trunk and move the left elbow as far as you can to the right knee; then repeat with the right elbow and the left knee. Keep the abdominals pulled in tight and the knees at right angles to the waist at all times. Do a total of 10 times.

HAMSTRING STRETCH
1. **2.**

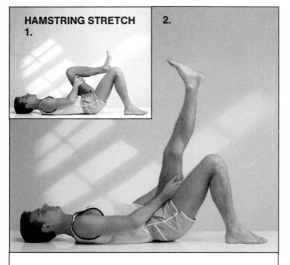

1. Lie on the floor, knees bent. Hug one knee to your chest. **2.** Stretch your leg up toward the ceiling. Using both hands, gently press your leg toward your face. Do not bounce. Flex your foot. Bend your knee, drop your foot to the floor, slide your leg down, and wobble it to loosen. Alternate legs 5 times each.

CURLING AGAINST A WALL
1. **2.**

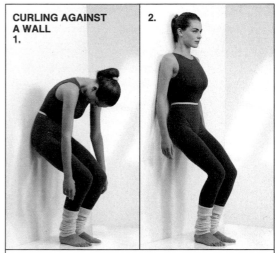

1. Stand with your knees bent, buttocks against wall, feet 6 inches from wall. Drop your head and shoulders. **2.** Pull your stomach in as you slowly roll up by pressing one vertebra at a time against the wall.

CURL BACK
Sit with knees bent, feet flat on the floor hip width apart. Exhale as you role back slowly; stop before your waist touches the floor. Set your stomach muscles to hold position for a slow count of 5, then inhale as you pull forward to the starting position. Press in lower abdomen to release lower back and sway gently before repetition. Repeat 5 times.

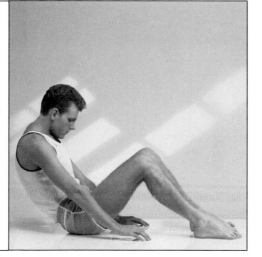

KNEE HUG

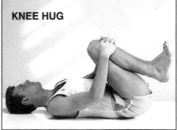

Lie on your back, knees bent and together, hands hugging knees gently. Press your knees toward your chest and sway gently. Do this when you feel stiff in your lower back and need to stretch and relax your muscles.

PELVIC TILT
Lie on your back, knees bent. Pull all your stomach muscles in toward your navel; feel your concave stomach with your hand. Squeeze your buttocks together to "set" this position. Do not lift, although your buttocks will automatically lift slightly and you will feel a tilting up of the pelvis. Hold for a slow count of 5, but do not hold your breath. Release, pause, and repeat 5 times.

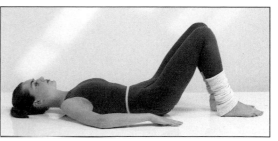

EXERCISES FOR THE ABDOMINALS

Everybody has certain areas that need special attention. On these and the following pages are exercises for three areas to help you to achieve a body of which you can be proud. You will find a firm, padded floor is the most comfortable surface for doing these exercises.

Abdominals

A common desire among people of all ages is for a flatter stomach. A protruding midriff results from flabby, soft abdominal muscles that are not exercised. This is a perfect example of "If you don't use it, you lose it."

When you resolve to "flatten your stomach," you will pay attention to three distinct sets of muscles that crisscross at your navel. They are the upper abdominals, lower abdominals, and the oblique (diagonal) muscles. In order to achieve the look you want, you must isolate each muscle group and do specific exercises that strengthen and tone it. Along with the satisfaction of a firm abdomen, you will have the added benefit of

ALTERNATE LEG STRETCH
(all abdominals)
Lie on your back. Bend your right knee to your chest. Lift your head and shoulders off the floor. Grasp your ankle and knee as you stretch the left leg 2 inches off the floor. Alternate bent and straight legs. Watch that your abdomen stays flat and breathe regularly. Repeat 10 times.

CURL-UP (upper abdominals)
Lie on your back with your knees bent, one hand on each knee. Inhale. As you exhale, slowly curl your head, shoulders, and upper back off the floor as you reach toward your knees. Your goal is to clear your shoulder blades off the floor. Inhale as you roll back. Repeat 10 times.

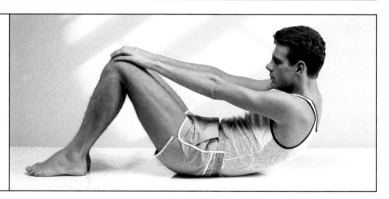

ROLL BACKS AGAINST THE WALL
(upper abdominals)
1. Sit on the floor near the wall with your feet against the wall, your knees bent, and your calves parallel to the floor. Cross your arms at chest level. Inhale. **2.** As you exhale, slowly roll back, tucking in your chin. Stop just before your waist touches the floor, pulling your stomach in tight. Inhale as you curl up to the starting position. Work up to 10 repeats; if you are a beginner, do not overstrain yourself.

1.   2.

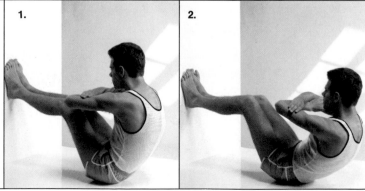

helping to maintain a healthy back. When the abdominals are toned and tight, the back muscles can lengthen and relax.

For the best results, follow these guidelines while exercising.

● Breathing is very important. Always inhale to relax and prepare the body for movement, and exhale on the effort, pulling in the abdominals.

● Check that you are performing correctly by looking down at your belly and seeing that it becomes flatter rather than rounder. Abdominals strengthen by pulling in, not pushing out.

● Alignment (proper placement) of your body during exercise will allow you to get the most from your efforts without injury. Pay close attention to the instructions for checking your placement.

● To make sure you are focusing on the correct muscle, you must mentally command the abdominals to contract, and consciously relax other "helpful" muscles, such as those of the legs, back, neck and upper arms.

ALTERNATING CRUNCH (obliques)

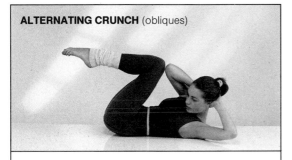

Lie on your back, knees into your chest. Clasp your hands behind your head, elbows forward. Inhale to prepare. As you exhale, lift the upper body and touch opposite elbow to knee. Breathe regularly, alternating sides. Do 10 times on each side.

SIDE LEG LIFTS (lower abdominals)

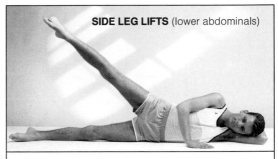

Lie on your side, drawing your stomach in firmly. Inhale to prepare. As you exhale, slowly move your leg up and down, imagining a heavy weight on your ankle. This is known as resistance; raising and lowering the heavy leg will make the abdominals work hard and get strong. Do 10 times each side.

REACH-UP (all abdominals)
1. Lie on your back, with legs raised and hands on bent knees. Inhale.
2. As you exhale, lift your head and shoulders off the floor and reach your arms and legs toward the ceiling. Inhale as you roll back to the starting position. Work up to 10 repeats.

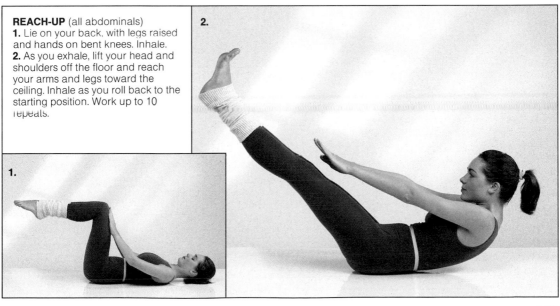

EXERCISES FOR HIPS AND THIGHS

Some qualities are genetically determined, but even those people who have inherited a predisposition to heavy hips and thighs can reduce inches as they firm these areas. The following exercises concentrate on rounding and lifting the buttocks, reducing the "saddlebags" on the outer thigh, toning and firming the inner thigh, and strengthening the quadriceps muscles on the front of the thigh. Extra dividends for working these muscles are easier bicycling, running, and stair climbing, and added strength for other sports.

Proper placement is particularly important for these exercises because they are difficult to do and your body will tend to take the line of least resistance. Always keep the abdominals pulled in while you do them to prevent rolling and swaying in your pelvis. If possible, get a friend to check your alignment. If you can't do all the recommended repetitions at first, it is better to do fewer correctly and increase as you get stronger.

OUTER THIGH LEG LIFT

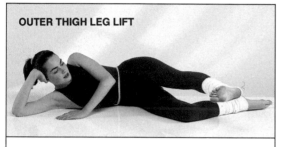

Lie on your side with your head on your hand. Bend both knees to a right angle to your body, checking the alignment of your hips. Stretch the top leg straight, foot flexed with the toes in line with your waist. Inhale. As you exhale, lift the top leg as high as you can without rolling back. Inhaling, slowly lower the leg almost to the floor and repeat 15 times. Change sides and repeat.

BUTTOCKS TIGHTENER

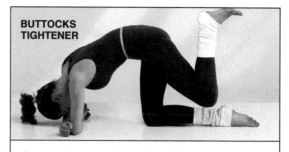

On your elbows and knees, head down, keep your back rounded as you stretch a leg straight back. Keep your stomach in and your buttocks tucked under as you bend your knee, foot flexed. Inhale to prepare. As you exhale, press your heel toward the ceiling. Breathe regularly as you continue pressing 25 times. Feel the tightening in your buttock. Repeat on the other side.

QUAD LIFT

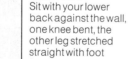

Sit with your lower back against the wall, one knee bent, the other leg stretched straight with foot flexed. Hold the bent knee. Inhale. As you exhale, tighten the upper thigh muscle and lift the straight leg as high as you can. Inhale, lowering the leg almost to the floor, and repeat 10 times. Change legs and repeat.

BUTTOCKS LIFTER

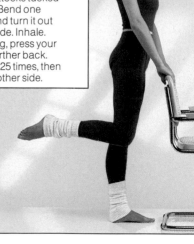

Stand straight with your hands resting on a chair. Keep your hips parallel to the chair, stomach in, and buttocks tucked under. Bend one knee and turn it out to the side. Inhale. Exhaling, press your knee farther back. Repeat 25 times, then on the other side.

FACE-DOWN LEG LIFTS

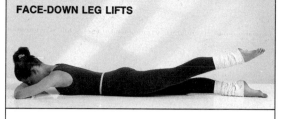

If you are weak or have back pain, start with this buttock-tightening exercise.

Lie face down with your forehead resting on your hands. Keep your stomach pulled in, hips pressing downward. Inhale. As you exhale, lift one straight leg up only as high as comfortable. Do 10 gentle lifts. Repeat on the other side.

INNER THIGH LEG LIFT

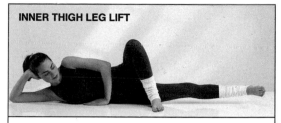

Lie on your side with your head on your hand. Cross the top leg over, keeping the knee up and foot flat. Do not roll forward or back. Keep the bottom leg straight with foot flexed. Inhale. Exhaling, lift the bottom leg up by squeezing the inner thigh muscle tightly. Keeping the leg off the floor, continue breathing regularly and raise and lower it 25 times. Repeat on the other side.

FOUR-PART OPEN AND CLOSE

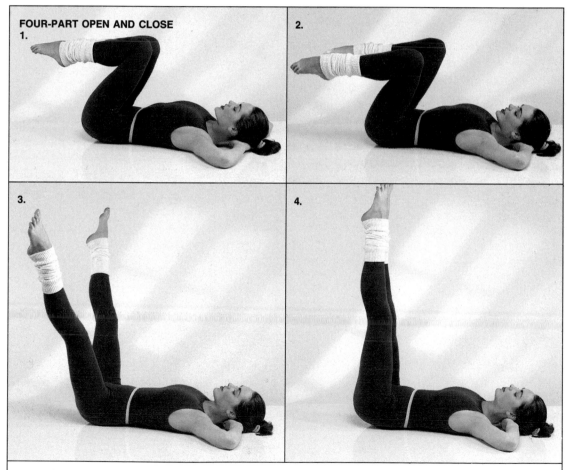

1. Lie on your back with hands clasped behind your head. Bring your knees into your chest above your waist. **2.** Inhale as you open the knees. **3.** Exhale as you extend legs wide apart. **4.** Inhale to bring the legs together straight and exhale to bend the knees. Feel the resistance to make hip and thigh muscles tighten and work hard. Repeat 10 times.

EXERCISES FOR THE UPPER BODY

By being aware of your posture and regularly practicing the exercises below, you can not only combat conditions of aging, such as a hunched back, flabby upper arms, and sagging shoulders, but you can feel more energetic. Improving your upper body strength and posture will make you look better and lighter, and help you to perform everyday activities with ease. If you play tennis or other racket sports, you should see an improvement in your game as well.

Upper body exercises can be done effectively both on strength-training equipment (see pages 134–135) and by using the weight of the body itself to strengthen weakened muscles. Remember the resistance principle—imagine you are pushing against or holding a heavy weight—and you will get results.

Always be aware of the total body when you perform these or any other exercises. Don't make the common mistake of arching backward when what you really want to do is to lift your ribcage out of your waist. Be aware, too, of how you use your body throughout the day. The workplace, for example, is often the scene of much stress and body strain. Do you ever feel the tension in your neck and shoulders after a long phone conversation? Chances are that you have been hunching the receiver between your ear and shoulder. Try the shoulder circle exercise shown here to release upper body tension.

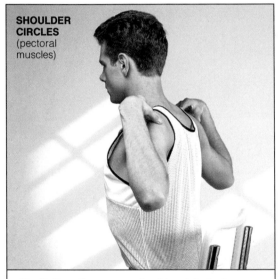

SHOULDER CIRCLES (pectoral muscles)

Sit with fingertips on your shoulders. Inhale. As you exhale, lift the shoulders and circle them as far back as you can, until you feel the shoulder blades squeeze together. Press down to complete one circle. Pause and repeat 10 times.

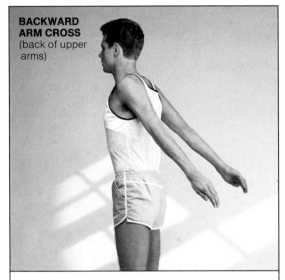

BACKWARD ARM CROSS (back of upper arms)

Standing straight with shoulders rolled back and down, chin dropped, and stomach tucked in, stretch arms straight back as high as you can. Inhale. As you exhale, think of crossing your arms at the elbows. Repeat 25 times, breathing regularly.

NECK ROTATION (upper back and neck)
Lie on your back with knees bent, feet flat on the floor. Inhale. As you exhale, stretch the back of your neck, bring your forehead forward, and lift your head 1 inch off the floor. Turn your head over the left shoulder until the ear touches the floor. Return to center and put your head down, letting it roll a few times side to side. Repeat 3 times on both sides.

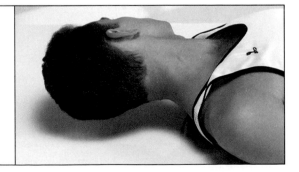

ARM FLEX (back of upper arms)
1.

2.

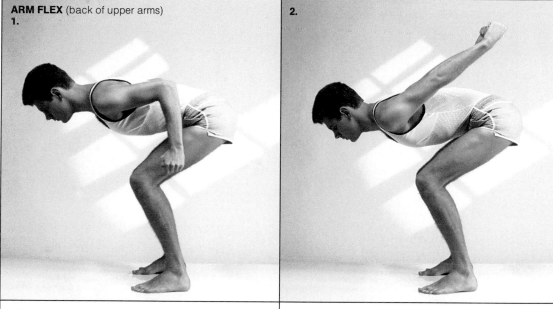

1. Bend your knees and bring your chest and head down. Bring your bent elbows in tight to your body and inhale. **2.** As you exhale, straighten and lift your straight arms to the ceiling. Inhale as you bend. Keep the upper back flat and support it with the abdominal muscles. Repeat 25 times.

OVERHEAD ARM PRESS
(upper back and arms)

1. Standing straight or sitting on the edge of a firm chair, bend your arms at right angles. Inhale. **2.** As you exhale, imagine pushing up a heavy weight and straighten your arms. Inhale as you bend your arms. Repeat 10 times.

1.

2.

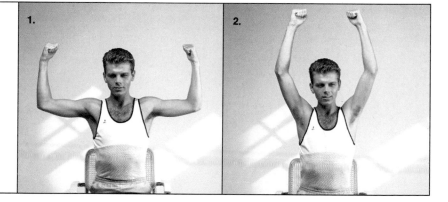

CHEST LIFT
(upper back, neck, and pectoral muscles)

Lie face down with hands behind your head. Inhale. As you exhale, lift the head, chest, and shoulders. Keep elbows open, stomach in, and feet down. Hold for a count of 5, and repeat 3 times.

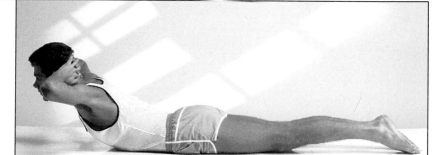

147

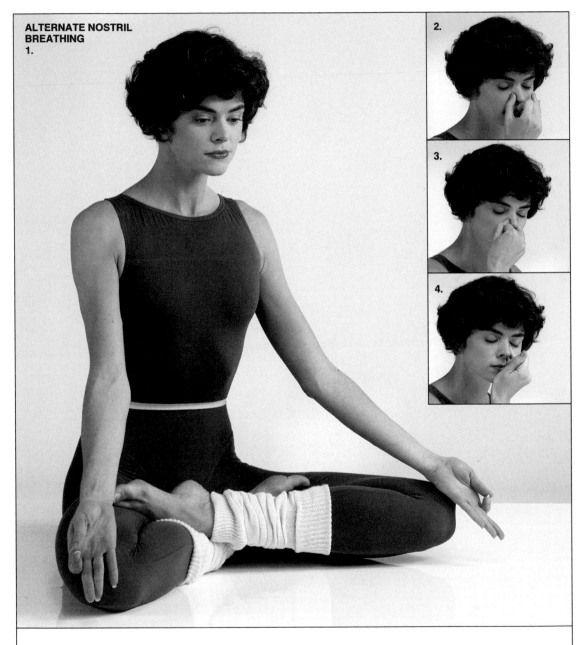

ALTERNATE NOSTRIL BREATHING

1.

2.

3.

4.

Alternate nostril breathing has an immediate tranquilizing effect on the mind. **1.** Sit in the lotus position or simply with your back straight, and eyes and mouth closed. **2.** Shut the right nostril by pressing the side with the right thumb. Keep the next two fingers bent and the last two fingers together and straight. Breathe in through the left nostril until the lungs are comfortably filled. **3.** Close the nose for a few seconds, using the last two fingers to press in the left nostril. **4.** Release the right nostril and exhale slowly, then breathe in on the right to fill the lungs.

Again close the nose, this time reapplying the thumb. Hold for a few seconds. Release the left nostril, breathe out slowly and immediately breathe in again.

Repeat the entire sequence 5 times, finishing with the final out-breath on the left side.

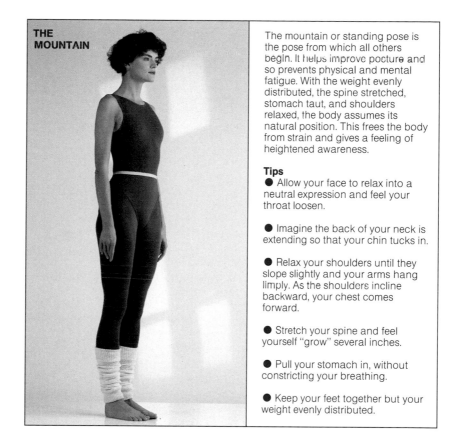

THE MOUNTAIN

The mountain or standing pose is the pose from which all others begin. It helps improve posture and so prevents physical and mental fatigue. With the weight evenly distributed, the spine stretched, stomach taut, and shoulders relaxed, the body assumes its natural position. This frees the body from strain and gives a feeling of heightened awareness.

Tips
● Allow your face to relax into a neutral expression and feel your throat loosen.

● Imagine the back of your neck is extending so that your chin tucks in.

● Relax your shoulders until they slope slightly and your arms hang limply. As the shoulders incline backward, your chest comes forward.

● Stretch your spine and feel yourself "grow" several inches.

● Pull your stomach in, without constricting your breathing.

● Keep your feet together but your weight evenly distributed.

Yoga (from the Sanskrit word for union) has been practiced for thousands of years in the East and embodies many different systems. The one that is best known in the West is *hatha* (*ha* = sun, *tha* = moon) yoga, which focuses on the mastery of the body and the breath. The yoga postures and breathing exercises are designed to help people to achieve harmony through balance, as well as improved flexibility, release from stress, and a new body awareness. Yoga is an excellent adjunct to any physical activity, for it teaches the integration of body, mind, and spirit.

It is best to learn from a qualified teacher. However, if you have no access to a class, you can still derive many benefits from the exercises shown here and also in the many books on yoga that are now available.

Breathing
By practicing the breathing exercises, you can retrain your respiratory system to function more efficiently. Learning to breathe correctly feels odd at first, but will come easily after a few weeks of practice and will allow you to gain more benefits from the yoga postures.

First become conscious of the lower, middle, and upper lobes of your lungs. Feel the breath draw deep down into your chest, slowly filling up, without strain, to just under the shoulder blades. Then breathe out fully from the bottoms of your lungs up. The out-breath is as important as the in-breath and clears the lungs of accumulated toxins. While walking, breathe out for double the count that you breathe in.

The corpse pose
The so-called corpse pose can be the kiss of life if you are short of sleep or feeling tense, and is a good resting pose between more strenuous postures. Lie on your back, with your feet in a V-shape, arms by your sides. With eyes closed, breathe in for a count of 6, hold for 3, breathe out for 6, and hold for 3. Repeat the cycle for about 10 minutes, stretch, and get up.

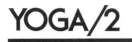

Some people have not tried yoga because they have seen photographs of practitioners in advanced poses that seem impossible to achieve. However, most of the beginning postures are simple and attainable by anyone of any age. If you have a physical condition that you feel might prevent you from performing a certain pose, check with your doctor; show him the instructions and follow his advice.

Attitude

The key to the benefits of yoga practice is attitude. Approach your practice with an open mind, understanding that you will progress at your own pace. Yoga is not a competitive activity. It helps you to "tune in" to yourself and in that sense is a physical meditation. Concentrate on executing the movements, emphasizing proper placement and breathing. Never force an exercise or try to pull or push yourself into position. Instead, use your breath and the weight of your body to ease into position.

If you become distracted, don't try to fight off your thoughts. Instead, gently bring your focus back to your breathing pattern and how your body feels as it relaxes into position.

Conditions and equipment

Practice the postures shown here in a well-ventilated room, preferably where you will be free of noise and distractions. Always use a mat, or a towel on a carpet, to cushion your body. Sections of rug with rubber backing are ideal for yoga; rugs without backing will slip and slide dangerously on polished floors. Wear loose-fitting clothing, preferably in a natural fiber, such as cotton, that moves with your body. Avoid binding waists or any garment that interferes with your breathing. Bare feet are best for yoga; they help with traction and encourage you to use your feet and toes in making contact with the floor as you attain your balance. If you have a full-length mirror, use it to gain perspective. Check your alignment from the front and sides.

Practice

Combine the limbering exercises on pages 106–107 and 126–131 with your yoga program. Head

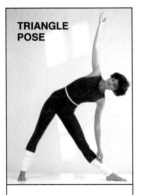

TRIANGLE POSE

Place feet more than hip width apart with the left foot at right angles to the right. Put the left hand on the left leg and stretch the right hand up as you inhale. As you exhale, let the left hand slide down the leg until it stops. Look up to the right hand as you breathe in this position. Hold for 1 minute. Repeat on the other side.

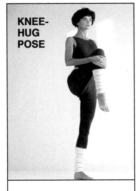

KNEE-HUG POSE

Standing erect, focus your eyes on a stationary object in front of you. Lift the right knee into your chest and grasp the knee with both hands. Keep the ribs lifted out of the waist. Hold for 1 minute. Repeat on the other side. (Beginners: Do this near a wall for security.)

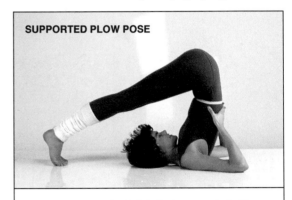

SUPPORTED PLOW POSE

Lying flat on your back, inhale. As you exhale, lift your head off the floor to help lift straight legs up and over your head. Support your back with your hands and **keep the weight across your shoulders, not on your neck**. You should be able to breathe easily in this position for 15–30 seconds initially. Don't try to force toes to the floor.

Place your palms flat on the floor and slowly roll down your back, letting the legs hang over your head until your lower back touches the floor. Lift your chin into your chest to help lower the legs straight to the floor. If you have any pain in your back, bend your knees.

rolls, arm swings, and foot pedaling are all good preparatory movements for yoga. You will soon come to know how much limbering you need.

Because the main goal is balance and harmony, each posture in your program should be followed by a posture that reverses it. Thus, any position that you assume bending forward should be followed by arching backward; any left-sided stretch should be followed by the same stretch on the right.

Be realistic when you plan your program. Regular practice will be beneficial.

FULL BODY STRETCH

Lie face down, arms stretched above your head. As you inhale, stretch your right arm and leg as far as possible away from each other, tucking the pelvis forward into the floor. Exhale as you release. Repeat 3 times on each side.

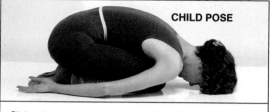

CHILD POSE

Sit back on your heels, forehead resting on the floor in front of you, hands near your ankles. Allow elbows and shoulders to drop heavily as you breathe fully for 1 minute.

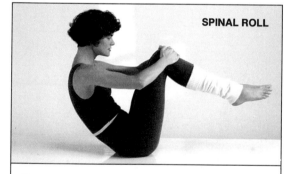

SPINAL ROLL

Bring your knees tight into your chest, tuck your chin in tight, and clasp your hands around your knees. As you breathe, gently roll forward and back on the spine. **Do this only on a mat, or cushioned floor.**

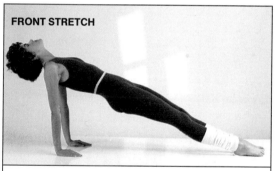

FRONT STRETCH

Sit straight, hands behind your hips, fingers pointed in. Inhaling, lift the pelvis toward the ceiling, pointing your toes and stretching your chin up. Hold for 15–30 seconds, breathing deeply and fully.

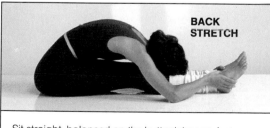

BACK STRETCH

Sit straight, balanced on the buttock bones, feet flexed. Inhale as you reach up. Exhaling, stretch forward, keeping knees straight. Grasp the legs or toes, dropping head forward. Breathe deeply and hold for 1 minute.

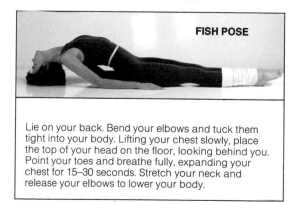

FISH POSE

Lie on your back. Bend your elbows and tuck them tight into your body. Lifting your chest slowly, place the top of your head on the floor, looking behind you. Point your toes and breathe fully, expanding your chest for 15–30 seconds. Stretch your neck and release your elbows to lower your body.

The Sun Salutation is a posture series that combines a number of traditional yoga positions. Whereas most yoga postures are meant to be held for a period of time, in this program you are meant to hold each position for only a moment before moving smoothly onto the next. This series is designed to be performed at sunrise, when the day is new and the air is fresh and energizing. However, no matter what your schedule, the Sun exercises will help restore your vitality, increase and maintain your flexibility, and tone your muscles. Use them either at the beginning of a longer program or as a complete activity.

Even beginning students can perform the movements that constitute the Sun Salutation, although at first progressing from one posture to the next might feel awkward. As you acquaint yourself with the positions, take the time to adjust your hands and feet to conform to the directions here. Initially, if your muscles are tight and the moves are unfamiliar, you might have to stop to reposition your limbs. If a position causes pain, ease up and try to adjust yourself to a point of comfort. Remember the difference between pain and stretch, and be sensitive to the messages that your body is giving you.

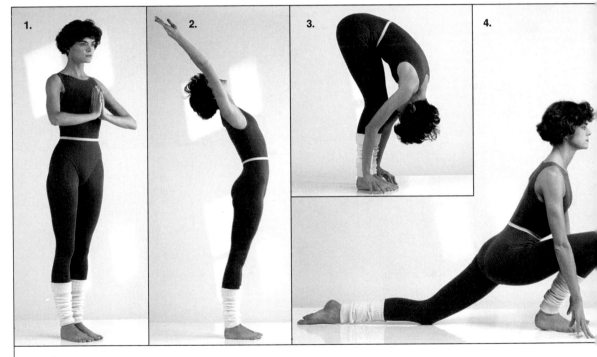

THE SUN SALUTATION

1. Stand erect, balanced on the soles of your feet, palms together. Feel the top of your head connected to the ceiling.

2. Inhale, stretching your arms high, and bend back. Keep your arms close to your ears, and don't let your head hang back. Focus on stretching through the front of your body; if you feel a pinch in your lower back you are bending too far.

3. As you exhale, bend forward, knees softly bent. Place fingertips beside toes.

4. Inhale, extend the left leg back, left knee on the floor, chest and head lifted.

5. Hold your breath as you extend the left leg back into a "push up" position, and support yourself with your abdominal muscles.

6. Exhale and bend your knees to the floor, chest down between your hands, chin on the floor.

7. Inhale as you slide your chest forward into the Cobra position, lifting your head and chest up, eyes straight ahead. If you have any pain in your back, bend your elbows more

and make sure your shoulders are pressed down, away from your ears.

8. Curl your toes under and as you exhale, push back on your heels, buttocks in the air, head down.

9. Inhale and slide your left foot forward between your hands, right knee on the floor, head and chest lifted.

10. Exhale and slide the left foot forward, feet together.

Inhale and slowly roll up, stretch up, and bend back as in the second position. Exhale back to the first position.

The program is designed to be done fairly rapidly, but at first take all the time you need to stretch as far as possible into each position. Focus your attention on the smoothest way to move from one position to the next, remembering that the object of this and all yoga exercises is to use your breath and body weight rather than strength and tension to achieve your goal. Be aware of the transitions and changes in level and you will soon become comfortable with the series. With practice, you will find yourself going farther with greater ease and you will naturally move more quickly through this compact program.

When you begin to practice the Sun Salutation, two full repetitions will be adequate. As you get more comfortable and familiar with the series, add two more cycles, gradually adding two until you can do 12 easily. Alternate your series, beginning first with the right foot, then with the left. Find your own rhythm and stick to it, increasing the rate of performance only when you feel ready. Properly done, this series will increase your heart rate and you will perspire. Concentrate on the breathing pattern indicated in the captions, and be careful that you do not hold your breath unnecessarily.

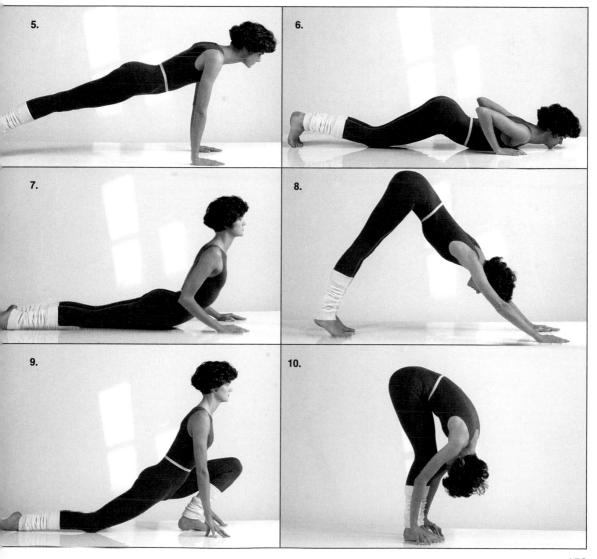

5.

6.

7.

8.

9.

10.

FAMILY FITNESS

Fitness and good health habits that are ingrained in family life will probably stay active for as long as you live. The support of those around you is an important ingredient both in beginning and maintaining a healthy lifestyle, so it makes good sense to think creatively about how you can involve all the members of your family in a fitness routine.

Consider the times that your family spends together as opportunities to do something active. Participating together in a sport or game is a chance for you to learn from and teach one another in a positive atmosphere of support and camaraderie. Fitness activities done together have a double benefit. You each get to improve personally while having fun with those you love.

Both adults and children learn best by example. If you are involved in an activity that you enjoy, the best way to get your family members to join you is to show them by your enthusiasm how you feel. Don't make the mistake of trying to force your partner or your children to participate, but let them know that you are ready, willing, and able to teach them and help them when they ask. Share with your family the reasons why you began and continue your fitness program, how it makes you feel, and the benefits you receive from your regular workouts. Provide them with the information that helped you to make your decision and be available to answer questions and give assistance.

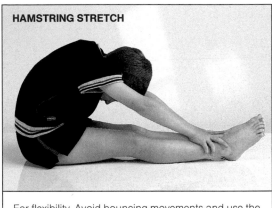

HAMSTRING STRETCH

For flexibility. Avoid bouncing movements and use the weight of the body and deep breaths to relax into the position. The child should grasp his legs as close to the ankles as possible, drop his head, and breathe deeply to a count of 10. Leg strength will naturally improve with sports activities.

Getting children fit

Don't count on your children's school to bear the total responsibility for their fitness. No matter how good or bad the physical education system is, you will still want to take an active part in ensuring that your children are getting a well-rounded program that will provide a good basis for their adulthood.

Competitive sports are often stressed in school,

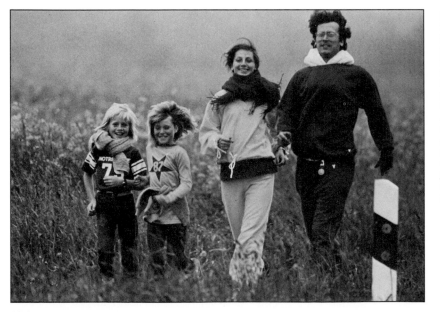

Children adopt the habits of their parents, whether these are good or bad. This makes it important to introduce children to the value of physical fitness and regular aerobic exercise at an early age. Children should be encouraged to try a wide selection of sports and activities rather than concentrating on just one or two. This will promote the development of strength, flexibility, and eye-hand and eye-foot coordination as well as muscular endurance.

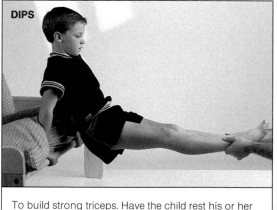

DIPS

To build strong triceps. Have the child rest his or her hands on a ledge or park bench. You hold the ankles firmly. The child should inhale as he lowers his buttocks below the level of the bench, and exhale as he pushes up to a straight arm position. Dips can also be done with heels resting on the ground.

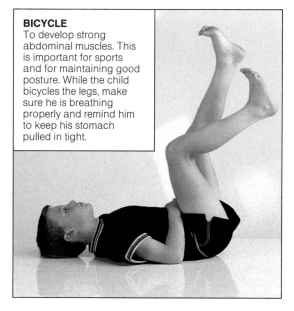

BICYCLE
To develop strong abdominal muscles. This is important for sports and for maintaining good posture. While the child bicycles the legs, make sure he is breathing properly and remind him to keep his stomach pulled in tight.

leaving out those children who either cannot or choose not to participate. You can be important in providing alternative activities that will help to build self-confidence and self-esteem in your children. Look to local YMCA's or community centers for classes or teams that might appeal to your children. If you belong to a club or team, other members might have children who would be interested in joining a junior league under adult supervision. One way of enabling the whole family to get fit is to take out family membership in a sports center or health club with a variety of facilities. Such clubs usually offer coaching facilities for adults and children. Think of planning a family vacation around some mutually enjoyed sport, such as tennis, canoeing, sailing, or skiing, for example. Activities such as swimming, bicycling, and walking, or using a hiking trail are easy to organize on a family basis. Children from the age of 10 can start on the beginners' parts of the programs on pages 108–111 and 116–117.

Your children's fitness level will steadily improve with practice, conditioning, and good coaching. Expose your children to as many sports and activities as possible to provide a broad spectrum from which to choose. Start to help children develop skills of eye-hand coordination by playing simple ball games with them at an early age. All sports are easier to learn when you are young, so the more skills you can introduce,

the better. At different stages of development, children will gravitate to different activities. Try your best not to judge which sports your children should or should not attempt. Boys and girls should be given equal opportunities to explore and develop to their fullest potential.

Children naturally try the sports and activities that they see their parents doing, and so today more kids are running, weight training, and bicycling seriously than ever before. Teenagers in particular enjoy seeing the improved muscular definition and strength gained from these sports. In addition, it helps them to improve in other activities, such as tennis, basketball, and gymnastics.

The same rules of safety apply to children and adults but, as the parent, you should keep a watchful eye on your children's programs to make certain that goals are realistic and progress is well monitored. Research on children's participation in various sports is constantly being undertaken. To keep up to date on what is safe, ask your local librarian to recommend journals that report on the research on risks, cardiovascular efficiency, skeletal changes, growth patterns, hormonal changes, and other physiological and emotional effects of rigorous, sustained activity. Consult your children's doctor and discuss any questions about how your children should proceed with their fitness training.

KEEPING IT GOING

Tips for keeping it going

● Plan a regular program and follow it.

● Keep track of your progress.

● Measure your improvement.

● Evaluate and redefine your goals as you progress.

● Add music to your workout.

● Look in the mirror and note changes.

● Enter and train for a "fun run" or a race such as a half (or even a full) marathon.

● Train with a friend.

● Add plenty of variety to your training routine.

● Train with someone more experienced than yourself to provide extra stimulus.

● Try some interval training in each session.

● Join a club or group.

When you have started and maintained a fitness program for any length of time, you should be aware of the many physiological and psychological benefits that come with regular exercise. Keeping the program going, particularly in times of pressure or stress, is a challenge. When times are rough, people tend to return to their old ways of coping. This is the point when many grow lax or even abandon their fitness routine. In fact, this is when you should devote more, not less, energy to yourself.

When you start a fitness program, you will probably be spurred on by enthusiasm. There may well come a moment, however, when that first enthusiasm begins to wane. Ask yourself whether the activity that you chose originally was convenient, affordable, and enjoyable? If not, what can you choose to replace it that will more closely meet your needs? Sometimes what you need is companionship to renew your interest. Investigate clubs or leagues where you will meet others with similar interests.

The benefits in health and the improvements in how you look and feel have been hard won. If you abandon your program, the amount of progress that you made over two weeks can be lost in the same amount of time. If you cannot participate in your regular sport because of injury, season, or finances, find a viable alternative.

There are many ways in which you can add stimulus to your training. Use some of the tips suggested here or seek out a fitness trail like the one shown opposite. If one does not exist where you live or work, perhaps you can suggest it to your company or town council, or you and your family can create one in your own backyard.

Interval training

Interval training can make an exercise program more fun and can help to build up your speed.

The basic type of interval training is to exercise at maximum capacity for short bursts interspersed with periods of rest or low-level activity. To produce the maximum effect on your "sprint," or fast-twitch, muscle fibers, these bursts of speed need last for only 40 seconds. As you progress, you can build them up to 2 to 5 minutes, while keeping going slowly between each. This will build up speed in the context of endurance.

As you get fitter, you can cut down the time spent on rest or low-level activity between bursts.

Runners might find it helpful to mix their interval training with stretching exercises (see pages 126–131).

*A **good way** to keep track of your progress, re-establish long- and short-term goals, and notice trends is to keep a daily chart of your workouts. This sample will give you an idea of how to arrange one. Decide which factors you want to monitor, then make the chart and leave it in a convenient place. Average your progress regularly. You might want to make a graph of the averages for easy reading.*

FITNESS RECORD

DAY		JAN	FEB	MAR	APR	MAY	JUN	JUL	AUG	SEPT	OCT	NOV	DEC
1	TIME												
	DIS												
2	TIME												
	DIS												
3	TIME												
	DIS												
4	TIME												

FITNESS COURSE

Many parks and open spaces now have fitness courses, or *parcours*, built into them. These courses provide not only some extra interest and incentive to keep you going, but also a valuable additional range of exercises.

The idea of the fitness course is that you start off on a marked run with exercise stations placed about every 100 yards. The exercises are designed to help build up strength and improve flexibility and balance, as well as to improve your level of aerobic fitness.

A well-planned course, such as the one below, will usually begin with simple warm-up exercises, progress to a range of strenuous activities, then end with groups of exercises that help you to cool down (see pages 106–107). The instructions at each station should suggest the number of repeats to be done by participants at different levels of fitness. **Stop at once if you are in pain or feel ill**.

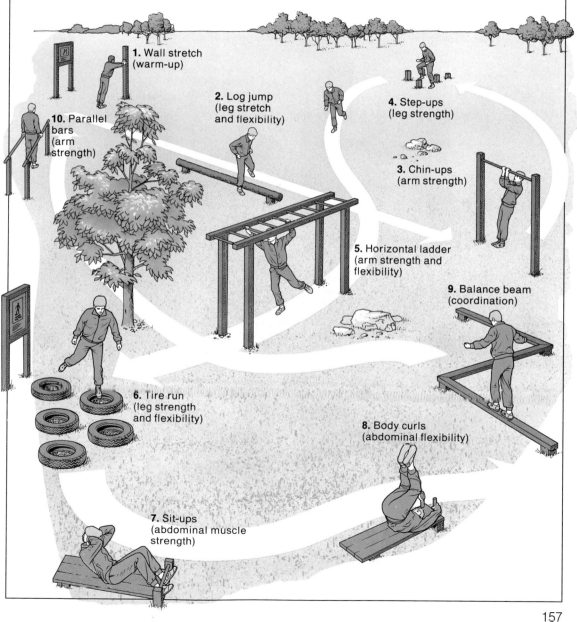

1. Wall stretch (warm-up)

2. Log jump (leg stretch and flexibility)

3. Chin-ups (arm strength)

4. Step-ups (leg strength)

5. Horizontal ladder (arm strength and flexibility)

6. Tire run (leg strength and flexibility)

7. Sit-ups (abdominal muscle strength)

8. Body curls (abdominal flexibility)

9. Balance beam (coordination)

10. Parallel bars (arm strength)

COMPETITION

Aerobic exercise is undoubtedly the way to improve your physical fitness. It can, however, become addictive. This addiction is useful in the sense that it keeps people exercising and thus maintains fitness. But it can also make people obsessive about their sport, to the detriment of other areas of their lives.

In one Canadian survey it was shown that runners have a higher divorce rate than nonrunners. And, in an article published in the *New England Journal of Medicine* in 1983, three doctors from the University of Arizona put forward a well-argued case that obsessive running in men in their thirties and forties is the male counterpart to anorexia nervosa in women.

In physical terms, obsessive participation can endanger your health (and possibly your life) if it means that you run in extreme weather conditions or when you are ill.

The reason why exercise has such powerful psychological effects seems to lie in a group of chemicals produced by the body called endorphins. These chemicals, which bear a close similarity to the powerful and potentially addictive painkiller morphine, were discovered in medical research into the cause of narcotic addiction. They are found in the highest concentrations within the brain and nervous system, where there are special receptors that ensure that the endorphins react on certain nerve cells.

Exercise, according to one theory, acts to increase the levels of endorphins in the brain. This could explain why hard endurance training, which might appear both painful and exhausting, is in fact enjoyable. The phenomenon of "runner's high," in which athletes feel euphoric and capable of effortless exertion, almost certainly depends upon endorphin release. Another theory is that their release is linked to the production of the hormone epinephrine (adrenalin), which is involved in the fight or flight reaction (see pages 268–269).

Endorphins have physiological as well as psychological effects. They interact closely with the pituitary gland, for example, and can interfere with its function of controlling hormonal output.

Competition

At all levels of sport, and at all ages, competition is an important element. This is because it provides goals for people to aim at and gives training a tangible purpose. At the same time, people may use their will to win as a way of preserving their personal identity.

At its best, competition creates a positive drive that makes people perform at their best and achieve new goals. At worst, the need to win overtakes them, depriving them of the perspective that allows them also to enjoy "playing the game." Be sensitive to yourself in relation to your sport. Always keep in mind the reasons why you began, and be wary when the need to win overshadows your desire to benefit from the activity.

One of the great advantages of the running boom has been that it is now possible to train for, and participate in, events in which there is no need to beat the person next to you. In such events, it is more likely that you will team up with someone in a joint attempt to complete the course in a reasonable time so that, in fact, you are competing against no one but yourself. In events such as the New York and Boston marathons, the proportion of entrants with serious thoughts of winning is probably less than one percent of the total field. Remember that the desire to win at all costs can do more than make you disappointed. It can reduce rather than increase your sense of well-being and mean that you do not get the maximum benefit from exercise.

In hot weather, dehydration and heat exhaustion are the major risks to exercisers. Remember that high humidity, because it prevents evaporation of sweat from the skin and thus lowers the effectiveness of the body's cooling mechanism, is as dangerous as a high air temperature.

If you wish to exercise in hot conditions, choose the coolest part of the day, such as the early morning or late evening. If you are running or bicycling, search out as much shade as you can. Remember that it takes time for the body to acclimate to hot conditions. Keep a steady, slow pace and take plenty of breaks for rest and drinks. Wear light, reflective clothing, avoid the use of rubber "exercise suits," and wear a hat. After you have finished exercising, drink plenty of water to replace the lost fluids.

In cold weather, remember that the wind can provide an additional, unwelcome chill factor, as can being wet through to the skin. As a general guide, it is safe to exercise in temperatures down to −25°F, as long as you are properly protected.

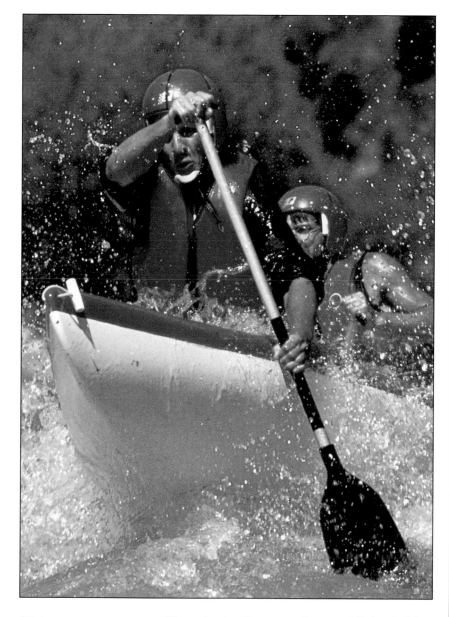

Mishaps are an occupational hazard in many kinds of competitive sports, but are unlikely to deter the keen participant. What is important is to keep the prospect of severe injury or illness in perspective. Obsession can place your health and happiness at risk.

Wear plenty of separate layers of light clothing, and keep your head covered (20 percent of body heat is lost from the head). Protect any exposed areas of the skin with petroleum jelly. If it is raining, sleeting, or snowing, make sure that your outermost layer of clothing is waterproof but allows for the escape of water vapor. Warm up indoors before you begin. When you have completed your period of exercise, change out of any wet clothes immediately.

Even if it is a race, STOP exercising if you:

● Feel pains in the chest, or any severe discomfort

● Feel sick.

● Feel extremely hot.

● Experience difficulty in breathing.

● Have an intense headache.

● Feel dizzy or disoriented.

● Cannot think clearly.

● Cannot move in a straight line.

● Feel nauseated.

● Lose sensation in any part of the body.

Reduce your level of activity if:

● It is very hot or cold.

● You are short of time.

● You are under considerable pressure at home or at work.

● You begin to feel uncomfortably tired while exercising.

Do not:

● Suddenly do much more exercise than you are used to.

● Enter a competition without adequate training.

● Enter a competition if you are unwell, even if you have trained for many months beforehand.

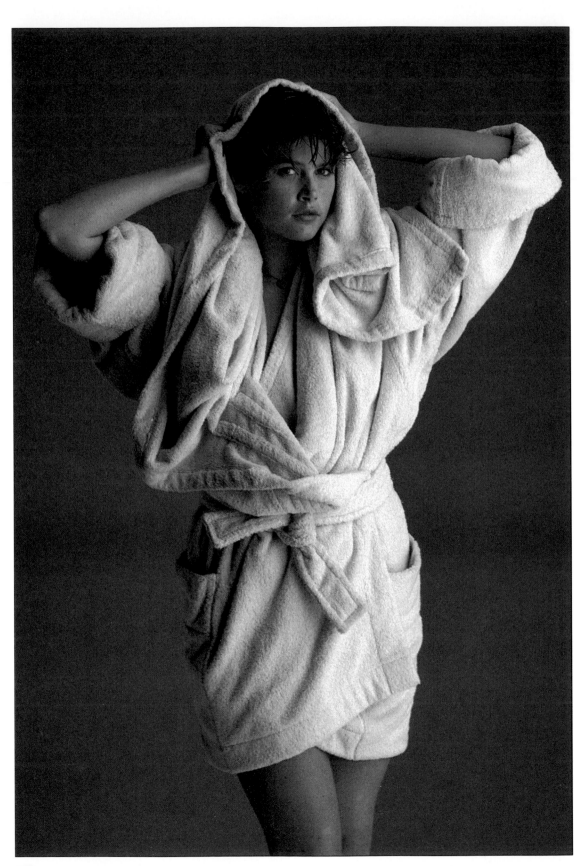

HEAD TO TOE

A finely tuned body in good working order from top to toe promotes and reflects a sense of well-being. If you treat your body with respect, you actively encourage a feeling of vibrant health, energy, and confidence.

You may not always be completely happy with the way your body looks. With self-control most people can regulate some aspects of their physical appearance, such as excess weight. You must, however, learn to live with those elements that you cannot change, such as height, skin color, and hair texture—and even turn them to your advantage—instead of wasting time and energy worrying about them. The secret is to capitalize on good points and make whatever improvements are possible.

Understanding how your body works, and knowing how to take care of it on a day-to-day basis, are two of the keys to fitness and well-being. Such body care includes looking after your skin, whatever its type, and protecting it from the extremes of heat and cold; caring for your hair, again according to type; keeping hands and nails well-groomed; and looking after teeth and gums. Advice is included here, also, on keeping eyes and ears healthy. These delicate organs need regular care and attention if they are to serve you well for life.

This chapter focuses, therefore, on the most important areas of self-care. To help you keep fit and healthy from head to toe it also indicates when professional help might be beneficial or necessary.

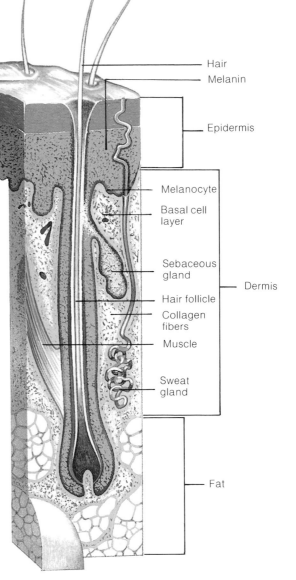

SKIN LAYERS

All skin has the same basic structure. Your exact skin type is governed by your sex, your age, your genetic make-up, and your environment.

Hair
Melanin
Epidermis
Melanocyte
Basal cell layer
Sebaceous gland
Dermis
Hair follicle
Collagen fibers
Muscle
Sweat gland
Fat

The skin is the largest of all the body organs, and the one of which you are most aware. Waterproof and self-repairing, this impervious body-covering is a reflector of health and well-being. It controls body temperature and eliminates some wastes through the sweat glands. The nerves in the skin endow the body with its senses of touch, pressure, and pain. In sunlight the skin makes vitamin D, essential for healthy bones. In addition, the skin reflects your emotions: fear makes it pale, cold, and clammy, while the blush is an unmistakable sign of embarrassment.

The way the skin works

The skin is structured in layers, and grows from the inside out. At the bottom is a layer of fat of varying thickness. Above it are the dermis and the epidermis or outermost layer. At the junction of the dermis and the epidermis is a basal layer of cells that divide, grow, mature, and gradually die, moving all the time through the epidermis to the surface. At the surface, all that remains of these cells is a layer of tough material called keratin, which is thickest in the body areas subject to the most wear and tear, such as the palms of the hands and soles of the feet. Keratin prevents water loss and is impervious to many harmful chemicals and to bacteria.

Melanin, the pigment that gives skin its color and acts as a natural sunscreen, is produced by melanocytes within the basal cell layer. Everyone has the same number of melanocytes. What varies is their melanin-producing ability—the more melanin, the darker the skin.

Hair is made in the dermis, and hairs, which are made of keratin, grow outward in follicles through the epidermis. Hairs are lubricated by oily, water-repellant sebum made in the sebaceous glands. These glands are particularly active and prone to infections such as acne in adolescence, but they become less productive in middle age. Sweat is made in sweat glands in the dermis and also exudes onto the skin surface.

Elastic tissues in the skin, the collagen fibers, give the skin its resilience. These tissues lose their elasticity with age, which causes the skin to wrinkle. Beneath the dermis, the fatty layer acts as insulator and cushion. In areas such as the face, muscles under the fat enable the skin to move.

Caring for the skin

Body skin takes good care of itself. Surprisingly, superficial dirt does not interfere with the skin's

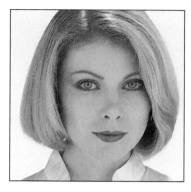

Dry skin
Fair skin is sometimes dry in childhood, but dryness is more often a problem in mature skin.

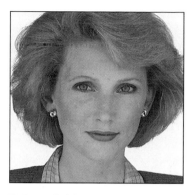

Balanced skin
Balanced skin, with a peachbloom glow, is rare. More common is a combination skin, a mixture of dry and oily.

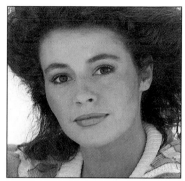

Oily skin
Most teenagers have an oily skin due to overproduction of sebum. Darker skins are often more oily than fair ones.

Do you have dry skin?
- Does your skin feel tight?
- Is it fine textured?
- Does it flake, chap, and peel easily?

Do you have balanced skin?
- Is your skin even in texture?
- Are the pores visible but not obvious?
- Is your skin soft, not flaky to the touch?

Do you have oily skin?
- Are the pores clearly visible?
- Do you often get pimples?
- Does your skin shine?

---

proper functioning—it does not, for instance, prevent sweat being released, nor does it block the hair follicles. And any proteins, vitamins, or other nutrients applied directly to the skin are not absorbed by it beyond the outermost layer.

Bathing, showering, and washing with soap to get rid of dirt, grease, and body odor undoubtedly make the skin look and feel good. Soap can, however, lead to allergic reactions, causing itching, soreness, and possibly a rash. Stop using any product that causes such a problem and choose a hypoallergenic product instead.

Soap dries out the skin, stripping it of its protective sebum and making it taut. After washing, therefore, you will feel more comfortable if you apply a moisturizer to relubricate the skin. Men often have oilier skin than women, and can use a lighter moisturizer. Frequently these are sold as after-shave products, but men with dry skin should use an all-over moisturizer after showering or bathing. Elderly people find that their whole skin has become drier and more delicate. In addition to using a moisturizer, it is often a good idea to bathe or shower only three or four times a week instead of every day.

Facial skin is the most vulnerable and fragile of all body skin. Treat it carefully and with the products suited to its degree of dryness or oiliness. This aspect of your skin can change as you age, so from time to time reassess it and the products you use. The area around the eyes is especially sensitive and can be damaged by aggressive application and removal of make-up.

Whether or not they use shaving cream, men should wet their faces with hot water before shaving because it softens the beard and makes shaving less irritating to the skin.

Make-up

Today there is such a vast and bewildering array of cosmetics that it can be difficult to choose which to use. Have fun experimenting with color and texture, but do not pay a lot for packaging unless you will use the product over and over.

Always apply make-up to a clean skin, and use a moisturizer if your skin is not oily. If you have a sensitive skin or allergies, it is best to use hypoallergenic cosmetics.

Removing make-up at night is essential. Treat your face gently, and use cleansing lotions and creams, which are more efficient than soap for removing make-up. Astringents and toning lotions remove traces of cleansing lotions and excess oil.

The problem of acne

Acne is a skin disorder most often associated with adolescence, but it can also be a problem in your twenties and thirties. It occurs when the sebum from an overproductive sebaceous gland thickens and combines with dirt and dead cells to block pores or hair follicles. It is important to keep the skin's oiliness to a minimum by washing several times a day with a soap specifically formulated for acne or oily skin, such as a transparent glycerine soap. Baby soaps, perfumed, and richly lathering soaps are not good for acne sufferers.

Exfoliation—removing the top dead layer of cells—with a mechanical sponge, face mask, or washing grains and granules can be helpful because it loosens the blockages and removes deep seated dirt and bacteria. It also prevents the accumulation of fatty deposits on the skin. Be sure that any acne treatment you buy is suited to your skin type or you could make the condition worse instead of better. If you have severe acne, consult your doctor or a dermatologist, who might prescribe antibiotics.

When a person no longer suffers from acne, superficial acne scars and wrinkles can be successfully treated by dermabrasion, which sands off the outer layer of the skin. Chemical peeling removes the skin by chemical rather than mechanical action, and chemabrasion is a combination of the two. In all cases, treated individuals must stay out of the sun or use a complete sunscreen for six months to avoid changes in skin pigmentation.

Treating aging skin

Most people aspire to retard and counteract the basic signs of aging by various means. Aging skin frequently develops patches of peculiar pigmentation. Flat brown spots (lentigos) that look like large freckles are the result of skin maturation, exposure to the sun, and genetic factors. A dermatologist can remove them easily with a light application of liquid nitrogen, an electric current, or various chemical peeling agents. Sun-induced facial spider veins can also be treated with a fine electric needle.

As the collagen fibers lose elasticity with age, the skin becomes thinner and wrinkled. You can buy various collagen products to apply to the skin, but it has not been proved that collagen can penetrate the skin in sufficient amounts to restore

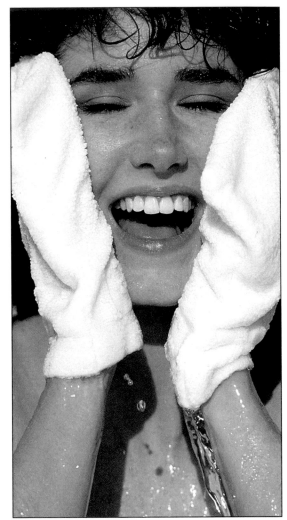

Washing mitts *are made of a synthetic material that gently exfoliates the skin.*

your own collagen tissue. Any topical preparation applied to the face may also lead to an adverse reaction. If you experience itching, redness, or blistering, stop using the product immediately. Consult a dermatologist if the symptoms persist for more than 24 hours.

Collagen fibers can be injected to fill out prominent and fine wrinkles, acne and other disfiguring scars, and contour defects. In the hands of a skilled dermatologist or plastic surgeon the procedure is simple, relatively painless, and produces immediate results. However, the

FACIAL EXERCISES

You can help to keep your facial muscles firm and help prevent drooping of your features by devoting just 6 minutes a day to these exercises. Do each action for 6 seconds and repeat it 10 times. It is important to keep the rest of the face relaxed while working on any specific area.

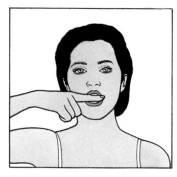

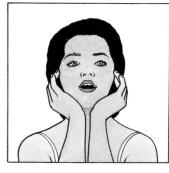

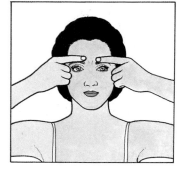

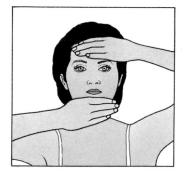

1. Horizontal forehead lines
Place the side of the forefingers gently but firmly against the forehead just above the eyebrows, allowing thumbs to rest lightly on cheeks. Raise the eyebrows against the resistance of the fingers.

2. Vertical forehead lines
Place the underside of the forefingers flat against the forehead just above the eyebrows. Pull gently toward the temples.

3. Mouth wrinkles
Place the hands flat on the cheeks with the fingertips touching the cheekbones and the wrists meeting. Gently pull toward the ears. Holding this position, say "you."

4. Droopy chin
Hold your head up straight, chin level, shoulders back and relaxed. Place your forefinger horizontally between your teeth. Push your tongue against the roof of your mouth while keeping your teeth touching your finger.

5. Neck 1
With your mouth half open, place your palms under your jaw and curve your fingers around to rest lightly on the side of your cheekbones. Try to open your mouth against the resistance of your hands.

6. Neck 2
Place one hand flat on your forehead and the other on your chin. Move your head forward against the resistance of your hands, keeping your shoulders straight and relaxed.

effects are not permanent, as the collagen will be absorbed by your body over a period of six to 18 months. You must also be tested for sensitivity before you can be treated.

Plastic surgery can remove loose or flabby skin on the neck and erase deep furrows on the forehead, but it cannot completely eradicate deep furrows between the nose and mouth. The effects of a facelift can be excellent, but they are not permanent; on the average they last for between five and seven years. Blepharoplasty, plastic surgery to remove folds of skin over and bags under the eyes, is also very successful and the effects are often permanent.

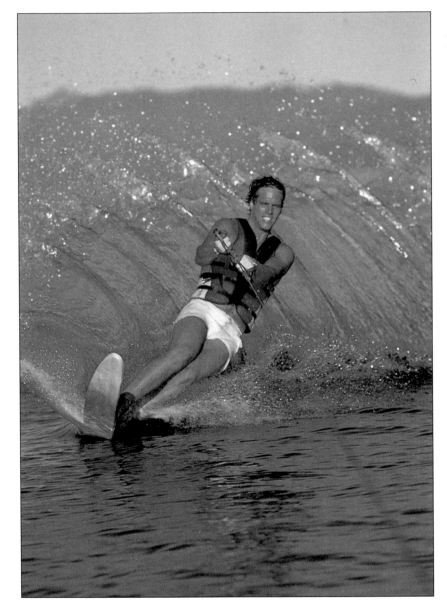

The skin needs to be protected by a sunscreen particularly when you are in or near water. You should continue to use a sunscreen even when you have developed a deep tan.

The skin is the body's automatic heat regulator. In response to an increase in temperature, whether it is generated internally through exercise or externally by the sun, the many thousands of sweat glands situated all over the body respond to messages from the "thermostat" in the hypothalamus deep in the brain. The sweat released onto the skin's surface cools the body as it evaporates. In cold conditions you have to protect the skin with clothing and barrier creams to prevent loss of body heat and minimize chapping—drying and cracking of the skin.

Stressful and emotional situations also trigger the sweat glands into action, particularly those glands that develop during adolescence in the groin and underarms. This sweat, however, contains pheromones, odors that are thought to be involved in sexual arousal. If you allow them to become stale, they are quickly broken down by bacteria and develop a pungent smell.

To prevent body odor developing, bathe or shower and change underwear and socks or pantyhose every day. Underarm deodorants help to kill the bacteria that collect there and antiperspirants contain certain metal salts that close up the sweat glands. Vaginal deodorants, however, are not advisable. Any offensive vaginal secretions demand medical attention and treatment.

Cotton is the best fabric for sports gear worn next to the skin, since it is absorbent and allows sweat to evaporate quickly. Choose non-constricting, stretchy clothes; avoid seams and fastenings that might rub, and wear layers that can be discarded as necessary.

Sun and the skin

Sunshine gives you a sense of well-being. You feel more relaxed and, with a glowing, golden tan, more beautiful. Overexposure to the sun, however, is dangerous. In the short run, excess water and salt loss can lead to overheating and dehydration. In the long run, it can cause skin damage and even cancer. Children are particularly susceptible to sunstroke, since, if unrestrained, they will spend considerable time running around in the sun, and particularly near water, which intensifies the effect of the sun's rays by reflection. Make sure that children are adequately protected, particularly their heads, by sunscreens and clothing, and monitor the time they spend in the sun.

Tanning is the skin's defense against the sun's harmful, ultraviolet rays. Melanin, the dark pigment made by the skin, acts as a screen to prevent burning. When the skin gets hot, it turns red and the blood vessels dilate. Increasing the blood supply to the surface of the skin helps to cool it down. If the skin becomes too hot, however, it will burn regardless of natural skin color or depth of tan. A clear fluid oozes into the skin and blisters bubble up. The outer layer of the skin stretches, hardens, and eventually peels, leaving a raw layer underneath.

Repeated overexposure to the sun and harsh weather conditions can age the skin prematurely, making it wrinkled and leathery. Because the hands, face, and neck are the areas of your body most often exposed to the elements, they are the first to show signs of aging. You can delay and minimize these effects by taking good care of your skin now.

A shining head of hair makes you look good and feel good, and it usually reflects a good state of health. The color and texture of hair are genetically determined but can change during life. Many blonde babies, for example, have darker hair as adults, while in later life, loss of pigment turns hair gray, and reduced oil production makes it drier and rougher.

Hair is composed of the dead material keratin. Deep within each hair follicle the root sprouts a strand of hair. The cells divide rapidly, so that head hair grows about half an inch a month, or even faster in warm weather. Each strand is composed of an inner shaft, containing the pigment that gives hair its color, and an outer cuticle. The cuticle is lubricated by sebum released by the skin's sebaceous glands (see page 162), and this gives it a sheen.

There are four different types of hair: scalp hair; underarm, pubic, chest, and facial hair; eyebrows and lashes; and the fine down of insulating body hair. The structure of the hair root, which is genetically determined, dictates whether a hair strand grows straight or curly.

A full head of hair consists of 100,000 to 120,000 hairs, but everyone loses between 50 and 100 hairs a day. A hair grows for between two and six years, and some people's hair can grow long enough to sit on. When the strand reaches full length, it rests for a few months before a new hair pushes it out. Fortunately, however, the growing and resting cycles are not synchronized in adjacent follicles. If a follicle dies, it cannot produce hair, and balding results.

Hair care

Like the skin, the hair can maintain itself in a healthy condition with little or no help. For comfort and cleanliness, however, you should brush and/or comb your hair daily, and shampoo and trim it regularly.

Although the hair is composed of dead material, you can still damage it by mistreatment (see panel, far right). It is also important to remember that the substances you put on your hair can be absorbed into the skin. Some people are allergic or very sensitive to the chemicals used in hair dyes. Always test a product on a small area before using it. Alternatively, use herbal and vegetable dyes, which are unlikely to irritate and can achieve many of the same effects as the harsher chemical hair dyes.

IS YOUR HAIR OILY OR DRY?			
Shampoo your hair as you would normally. After two days check on its condition.			
Appearance	**Type**	**Care guidelines**	**Special treatments**
Strands separate and stick to your head.	Oily	1. Shampoo as often as necessary, even if that means every day. 2. Use a mild shampoo. 3. Use very little shampoo. 4. Put a conditioner on the ends unless the hair is very oily. 5. Don't use too hot a hairdryer. 6. Don't brush or comb more than necessary.	To help reduce sebum production, use $2\frac{3}{4}$ pints of water with the strained juice of 1 lemon added for the final rinse after shampooing.
Tangles easily, brittle.	Dry	1. Shampoo your hair every 4–6 days. 2. Use a mild shampoo. 3. Use a cream conditioner after every shampoo, combing it thoroughly through the hair and leaving it on for a few minutes before rinsing. 4. Never brush your hair when wet, always comb gently. 5. Protect your hair from the sun, either with a hat or scarf.	Massage 2 tablespoons of warm olive or almond oil into your hair. Wrap your head in a warm damp towel or a plastic turban and keep it on for at least 30 minutes. Do this every 3–4 weeks.
Oily roots/dry ends (most common type).	Combination	Adapt the guidelines above for your own hair type.	

When caring for your hair

Do
● Choose brushes and combs with widely spaced and smooth-tipped bristles and teeth to avoid the risk of splitting hairs and scratching the scalp.

● Wash combs and brushes in shampoo or soap at least once a week.

● Always rinse your hair thoroughly.

● Use a conditioner to smooth the outer surface of the hair, which is roughened by washing.

● Apply extra conditioner when using a hairdryer, rollers, or tongs.

● Always try a temporary rinse first, before you risk using permanent color.

● Go to a professional colorist for permanent dyeing or bleaching.

● To disguise graying, try a semipermanent colorant, which lasts for six to eight shampoos.

WASHING, DRYING AND BRUSHING

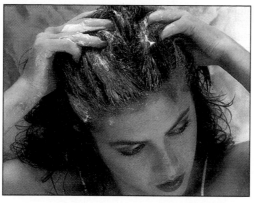

Massage shampoo into your scalp as you wash your hair, but rub gently if your hair is oily to prevent excess sebum production.

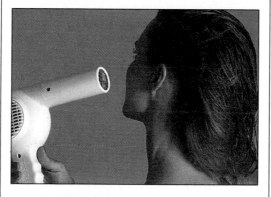

When blow-drying, take care not to burn your scalp or the skin of your neck. Remove metal necklaces, which conduct heat rapidly.

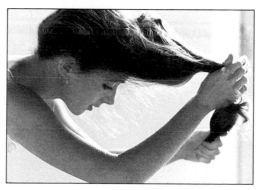

Brush your hair gently to avoid splitting the strands or pulling them out. Too much brushing and combing can exaggerate oiliness.

When caring for your hair

Don't
● Overbrush your hair; it may increase the greasiness of oily hair and break the ends of dry hair.

● Tangle the hair while washing it.

● Give dry hair two applications of shampoo.

● Rub too vigorously when drying; it may break and tangle the hair.

● Have a permanent bleach if all you really need are "highlights."

● Apply a permanent color until you have tested the solution on your skin for 36 hours to check for any adverse reactions.

Did you know?
● Brushing your hair 100 a times a day to make the hair shine does no good and may even damage the hair.

● Daily shampooing, although not strictly necessary, can do no harm as long as you use a mild shampoo.

● Static electricity is reduced by a conditioner.

● The hair is heavy when wet and up to 20 percent less elastic when dry.

● A permanent can give body to lank hair, but the chemicals can make it drier and more brittle.

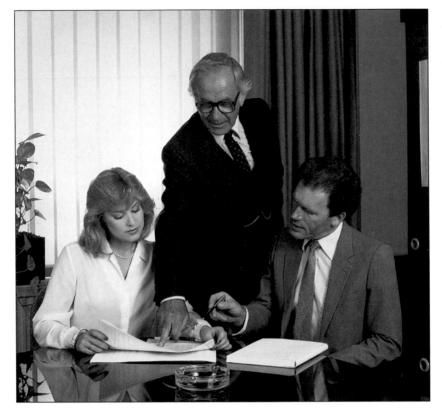

Baldness is accepted by most men as a natural part of the aging process. But if it is regarded as a threat to looks and esteem, it may well become a severe impairment to well-being.

Human hair helps to protect the head from the sun and prevents heat loss from the body, but otherwise it performs a largely cosmetic function. Most people take hair for granted, but a lack or excess of it can give rise to anxieties and, often, a considerable loss of self-confidence.

Hair problems

Pattern baldness, in which hair is lost successively from various parts of the scalp, is an hereditary male adjunct to aging that affects around 40 percent of all men. Women do not normally develop pattern baldness, but can experience generalized thinning of head hair from middle age onward.

All men lose some head hair after puberty, when the increased androgens (male hormones) cause the hairline to recede slightly over the forehead and temples. Those with an inherited predisposition to baldness also lose hair in the crown area. Men are 10 times more likely to be severely bald than women, but although some men do find going bald distressing, in general

women find the experience of losing their hair more traumatic.

Diffuse hair loss in women might occur after childbirth, if a contraceptive pill is being taken, or after acute physical or mental stress, such as fever or bereavement. This last reaction, which can also occur in men, is temporary, and hair should start to regrow within a few months. Excessive hair loss might be caused by a hormone imbalance or lack of iron, and can be medically treated.

Psychological stress can also trigger the occurrence of patches of baldness in children and young adults. Occasionally the patches coalesce into total loss of head or even body hair, but the hair that has been shed usually regrows within six to nine months.

Dandruff affects over 60 percent of the population. It is usually a mild form of eczema in which scales of dead skin flake from the scalp, but it is sometimes caused by psoriasis, a condition in which the skin cells multiply abnormally fast, forming larger, thicker, oilier flakes. The best treatment for dandruff is to wash hair regularly

Tips for men

Shaving
Change your shaving method if it gives you a skin rash. Consult your doctor if the rash persists.

● For a wet shave, use a really clean and sharp blade. Work with, not against, the grain of the hair, and shave the chin and upper lip first.

● Electric shaving works best when the hairs are stiff and dry.

Moustaches and beards
Allow up to six weeks for the hair to grow.

● Wash regularly with soap and water, and trim. Shape to suit your face. A drooping moustache disguises chubby cheeks or a square jaw. A beard may overemphasize a narrow forehead or hollow cheeks.

Thinning hair
There is no known prevention or natural cure for baldness. A drug, minoxidil, sometimes helps to halt its progress.

Wigs and toupees can improve appearance and therefore self-confidence.

Hair weaving connects new to natural hair and is an improvement on the toupee, but it also needs frequent adjustment.

Hair transplants are rarely satisfactory, since they depend on the continuing growth of transplanted hair follicles and might be of hair already destined to be permanently lost.

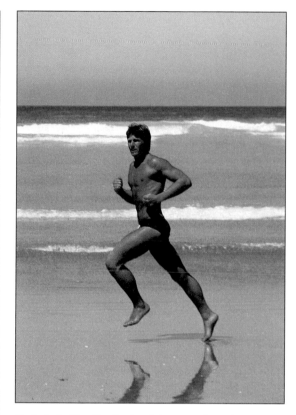

Body hair distribution in adult men varies widely. Some men have little or no hair on their chest or back while others are profusely endowed with hair. The difference is largely determined by heredity.

with a shampoo containing a selenium compound or coal tar extracts. If the problem is severe or persistent, you should consult your doctor.

Nits, lice eggs found on the shafts of the hair, do occur in clean hair. The minute lice that hatch cause intense itching. They can be killed with shampoos containing lindane.

Fragile, brittle hair is often the price paid for overexposure to the sun, frequent perming and bleaching, and using hairdryers and heated curlers. The best treatment is to give your hair a rest from such processes.

Unwanted hair
Excessive hair growth in women is caused by the overproduction of androgens or the skin's oversensitivity to natural levels of androgens. Most women control unwanted hair by one of the following: shaving, bleaching, electrolysis, waxing, abrasive pads, or the use of depilatory creams.

Tips for women

Shaving
Quick and easy. Shave legs, underarms, bikini line, but never hairs on breasts because it can damage the hair ducts and lead to infection. Shaving does not make the hairs grow back thicker or darker.

Depilatory creams
Chemicals dissolve hair, leaving a smoother, more lasting result. Test on a small area of the skin before first use of any product, in case you are allergic.

Waxing
Although painful, waxing lasts longer and leaves the skin soft and smooth. Best done by a professional, but home kits are effective.

Abrasive pads
Hairs do not regrow bristly. May destroy some hair follicles.

Plucking
Most effective on chin and eyebrows. Never pluck hairs from a mole; it can stimulate malignancy in certain types of mole.

Bleaching
Best for disguising facial hair. Always test on a patch of skin before use and rinse off thoroughly.

Permanent hair removal
Electrolysis causes a chemical reaction, and shortwave diathermy uses heat. Both *must* be performed by a trained operator; avoid home kits. Although skin is left temporarily red and sore, these are effective ways to remove facial hair.

THE EYE

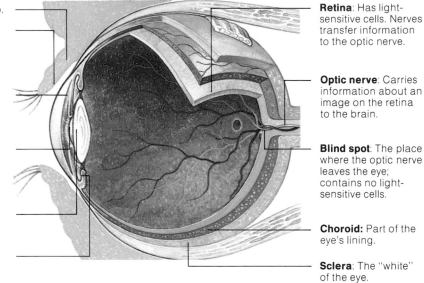

Eyelid: Protective flap.

Conjunctiva: The thin covering of the inner surfaces of the eyelids and exposed cornea.

Iris: The colored muscle that alters the amount of light entering the eye.

Pupil: A hole whose size changes with the action of the iris in response to the amount of light.

Lens: A flexible transparent structure used for focusing.

Ciliary muscle: Alters the shape of the lens for focusing.

Retina: Has light-sensitive cells. Nerves transfer information to the optic nerve.

Optic nerve: Carries information about an image on the retina to the brain.

Blind spot: The place where the optic nerve leaves the eye; contains no light-sensitive cells.

Choroid: Part of the eye's lining.

Sclera: The "white" of the eye.

Eyes are the most highly developed of the special sense organs. They feed in most of the information about your surroundings, reveal many of your inner feelings, communicate significant information to others, and reflect well-being. Your eyes need care, attention, and protection, particularly when the strength of the sun or the hazards of an occupation or sport demand it. Above all, they should be checked regularly for any problems with vision, especially in children.

The bones of the skull naturally protect the eyes, and the eyelids and lashes help to prevent grit from entering the eyes. The lacrimal gland lies above the inner corner of each upper eyelid and secretes tears, which are salty and antibacterial. When you blink, tears sweep across the eyes to keep them clean, lubricated, and free from infection. When you produce tears through crying, they drain into a channel that leads to the nose.

The eye is spherical, and is moved by three pairs of muscles working in unison. You see through the black opening in the front of the eye called the pupil. The muscles of the iris alter the size of the pupil to control the amount of light falling on the retina, which is at the back of the eye. Light-sensitive cells on the retina convey information to the optic nerve, which passes it to

The eye works like a pinhole camera. The object that is observed is focused on the light-sensitive retina, just as light-sensitive film is used in a camera.

the brain, where it is interpreted as vision. A transparent, elastic lens is attached to the ciliary body behind the iris and pupil. The muscles in the ciliary body enable the eye to focus on objects at various distances by causing the lens to become thicker or thinner.

Eye tests

Good eyesight can be maintained only by having regular eye check-ups. Most people go through life without any disease of the eye itself, but most need corrective lenses at some time. Early detection of any problem might make the difference between good eyesight and blindness.

In a typical examination the ophthalmologist determines how much a person can see without corrective lenses, and, if necessary, tries to improve the vision by selecting suitable ones. First he assesses how well the two eyes work together (binocular vision), then carefully examines the inside and outside of the eye. He will measure the pressure inside the eyes of all patients over the age of 40, and of younger people if they have a near relative with glaucoma, a condition in which there is a dangerous build-up of pressure in the eye. Next he will check the width, or field, of vision, and then color vision. One male in eight suffers from color blindness—difficulty in distinguishing between certain colors.

Normal sight is classified as 20/20, which means you can read letters of a fixed size on a chart at a distance of 20 feet. A measure of 20/32, for example, means that you can read only at 20 feet a line that someone with normal vision can read at 32 feet.

Eyestrain

Tired, sore eyes usually result from making the muscles around the eyes work too hard. Glare from the sun, snow, or a television set, for example, can make the eyes feel sore because of the strain of keeping the eyelids protectively screwed up. Poor lighting can also stress the eye muscles, so adequate light is important. No permanent damage can be done to the eye itself from prolonged study or close work, or from too much television viewing. If your eyes feel tired or sore, bathe them in warm water, with a little salt added, or, occasionally, use one of the commercially available eyewashes.

Eye problems

The following are common eye problems.

Nearsightedness (myopia): Distant objects appear blurred because the light entering the eye focuses in front of the retina, instead of precisely on it. This is corrected by concave lenses. Contact lenses (see page 174) might be preferable to eyeglasses since they give a wider field of vision.

Farsightedness (hypermetropia): Close-up vision is fuzzy, while distant objects are more clearly focused, because light rays focus behind the retina. This condition is corrected with convex lenses, which must be used for close work or, in some cases, constantly. Because focusing power diminishes with age, most people over 45 require glasses for reading.

Astigmatism (distorted vision): The result of an uneven cornea or lens. Slight abnormalities will go unnoticed, but more severe cases need to be corrected by lenses worn most of the time.

Lazy eye (amblyopia): Normal vision fails to develop in one eye, which is usually markedly long- or short-sighted. It is obvious as a "squint" and results from the brain habitually suppressing the image received by the defective eye; that eye then becomes "lazy." Treatment is most effective if carried out at an early age and involves patching the strong eye and, possibly, prescribing glasses. In severe cases an operation may be necessary.

Cataract: A condition in which the lens inside the eye becomes cloudy, so light reaching the retina is gradually reduced. More than 90 percent of people over the age of 65 have some sign of this disorder. An operation might be necessary to remove the diseased lens.

Other common eye problems include styes, which are caused by an infection of the eyelash follicles, and conjunctivitis (pink eye), an inflammation of the delicate lining of the eyelid, caused either by bacteria or viruses. These infections are highly contagious.

Even if your vision is not defective, regular eye tests are vital. Some serious eye disorders are symptomless in their early stages, but can be treated and cured if detected in good time. An eye test every two years is ideal, but you should report any sudden changes in your vision to your doctor or an eye specialist immediately.

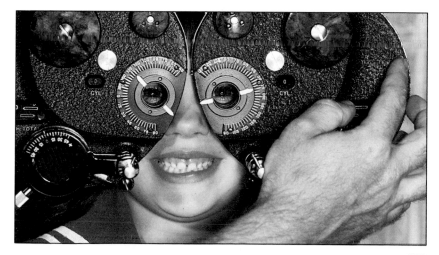

Eyeglasses

Use the following tips for choosing various types of glasses.

● Look for lightweight plastic frames that return to shape, even if you sit on them.

Sunglasses

● Polaroid lenses reduce glare but will make a car windshield appear blotchy.

● Photosensitive lenses adjust to the light intensity. However, they can be dangerous if you drive from bright sunlight, in which they will have darkened, into a dark tunnel, where your vision may be impaired until the lenses clear.

Mirrored lenses protect the eyes from reflected glare, and are particularly useful when skiing and sailing.

Sports glasses are specially designed and made with shatterproof lenses to protect the eyes during sports.

Protective goggles are essential in many industrial jobs, to guard against flying metal and reflected infrared and ultraviolet light.

Contact lenses have cosmetic appeal and provide better all-around vision than glasses. Although initial discomfort can occur, only a few people are unable to wear them. A specialist must be consulted for fitting. You should have a professional check-up once a year.

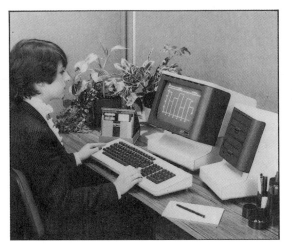

Working at a VDT or computer screen can make eyes feel tired. This is because muscles concerned with focusing are subjected to a heavy workload. Ideally, you should work at a screen for 20-minute stretches with a five-minute break between each, and do something completely different after two or three hours. Have your eyes tested if you have problems with tired, red, or itchy eyes, or with headaches. You may be suffering from a visual defect of which you are unaware.

CONTACT LENSES

Type	Description	Advantages	Drawbacks
Hard	Rigid plastic, fitting over part of cornea.	Good, clear vision. Last a long time. Can be repolished to remove scratches. Easy to handle and clean. Least expensive to buy and maintain.	Might be uncomfortable at first. Can distort the cornea if not perfect fit. Can be unsuitable for extremely sensitive eyes. Might have adverse long-term effects.
Soft	Look like drops of water. Made of a hydrophilic plastic polymer.	More comfortable initially than hard lenses and better for occasional use. Particularly good in dusty environments.	Can react adversely to high temperatures and pressures. High maintenance costs. Do not last as long as hard lenses.
Gas-permeable hard lenses	Rigid plastic that allows the passage of air.	Crisper vision than soft lenses. Allow more oxygen to reach the cornea than hard lenses do.	Often need soaking in special solution to remove accumulated proteins.
Extended-wear lenses	May be worn for 1 week to 3 months without being removed.	Useful for babies, small children, and the elderly.	Can be harmful to the eyes if not used with careful, regular professional supervision. Vision not as good as with hard or soft lenses.
Colored lens filters	May be worn if one or both eyes are damaged or to change eye color.	Useful for medical camouflage of eye damage. Do not affect vision.	

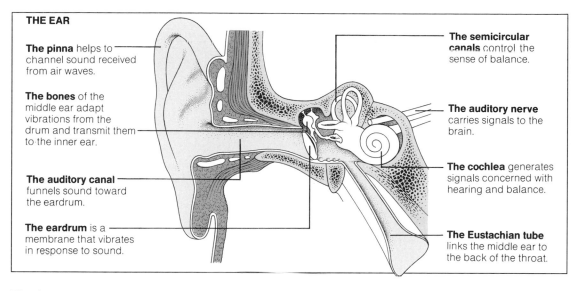

THE EAR

The pinna helps to channel sound received from air waves.

The bones of the middle ear adapt vibrations from the drum and transmit them to the inner ear.

The auditory canal funnels sound toward the eardrum.

The eardrum is a membrane that vibrates in response to sound.

The semicircular canals control the sense of balance.

The auditory nerve carries signals to the brain.

The cochlea generates signals concerned with hearing and balance.

The Eustachian tube links the middle ear to the back of the throat.

The human sense of hearing is developed long before birth. Recordings of sound within the uterus are known to be soothing to a newborn baby, who soon comes to recognize his own mother's voice. However, the brain's ability to translate nerve impulses into meaningful sounds, such as the rattling of a spoon against a cup or the complexities of a conversation, takes months and even years to develop fully. A child, therefore, needs to be brought up in a world of sounds, especially words, to develop his hearing and language facilities fully. Of course, that can be achieved only if the hearing is normal.

The ears are organs of balance as well as hearing. Impulses generated in the cochlea of the middle ear are sent to the brain and inform it of the body's orientation in space. This combination of functions explains why ear infections can be accompanied by dizziness. As with hearing, the sense of balance becomes less acute with age.

Care of the ears

The ears are normally efficient, self-cleaning organs that take care of themselves. The wax in the outer ear, which contains a bactericide, helps to trap dirt and potential irritants. Body warmth melts the wax, which travels outward with the help of movement of the hairs in the outer ear. Never poke the wax with any type of cotton swab, hairpin, fingernail, or other instrument; this can damage the eardrum and result in deafness. The most that you should do is wipe or wash only

The ear has three parts: the inner ear, which controls hearing and balance, deep within the skull; the middle ear, associated with hearing; and the outer ear, extending from the eardrum outward, which concentrates sound.

the outer ear with a washcloth.

If you suspect that a blockage of wax is affecting your hearing, arrange to see your doctor, who might syringe your ears with warm water. If you need to soften the wax for a few days before syringing, you can use warm olive oil or one of the products you can buy over the counter in the drugstore. Always protect your ears and those of your children from severe cold and sun.

Air travel

Give a little thought to your ears when you travel by air. The pressure in the middle ear is the same as atmospheric pressure because the Eustachian tube, an open, air-filled channel, links the middle ear with the back of the throat. The tube might narrow, however, with sudden changes in altitude, resulting in an alteration in pressure between the middle ear and the outside.

To keep the tube open during take-off and landing, try swallowing, sucking candy, or drinking. Alternatively, hold your nose and blow; you will feel a "pop" as the pressure equalizes. If possible, avoid flying when you have a cold or throat infection, since bacteria in the throat are more likely to enter the middle ear under these high-pressure conditions. A decongestant spray, used before a flight, should help to prevent pain.

The sense of hearing is essential to normal development. A deaf child cannot communicate his handicap to parents or teachers because he does not understand it. So any child with learning problems should have a hearing test immediately. If an infant does not startle at a loud noise, a mother might suspect impaired hearing or deafness, particularly if she contracted German measles (rubella) in the early months of her pregnancy (see pages 214–215).

The sense of hearing begins to deteriorate, although slowly, with advancing years. For this reason, it is sensible to have your hearing checked regularly (see pages 26–51). However, if you suspect at any time that your hearing is less than perfect, it is well worth having it tested by a specialist to see if it can be improved.

Hearing tests

Accurate hearing tests cannot be conducted until a child is two and a half to three years old. Rudimentary testing, however, can be done at any age. Between six and nine months, the normal baby begins to localize sounds and will turn his head to look for the source of a sound. From 18 months onward, the first formal hearing test can be given, since the child is old enough to respond in a meaningful way to various spoken words, commands, and test sounds.

The most common cause of deafness in young children is infection of the middle ear, which is caused by bacteria passing into the ear from the throat. The Eustachian tube becomes blocked, and, as a natural response to infection, fluid collects in the middle ear, thus impairing its efficiency. If the infection persists despite antibiotic treatment, a small hole can be made in the eardrum, the sticky fluid sucked out, and a tiny ventilation tube, or "grommet," inserted into the middle ear for a period of three to nine months. Children with grommets can go swimming if they wear walled earplugs and a cap that covers their ears completely, and do not dive or put their heads under the water.

Occasionally, a middle ear infection can cause the eardrum to burst and a sticky discharge to trickle from the ear. The severe pain of infection is relieved by the spontaneous perforation of the eardrum. Although the eardrum usually heals within a few weeks, the ear should be regularly looked at by a doctor for six to eight weeks and the

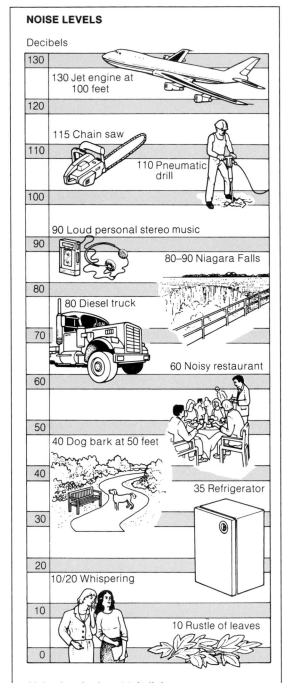

NOISE LEVELS

Decibels

- 130 Jet engine at 100 feet
- 115 Chain saw
- 110 Pneumatic drill
- 90 Loud personal stereo music
- 80–90 Niagara Falls
- 80 Diesel truck
- 60 Noisy restaurant
- 40 Dog bark at 50 feet
- 35 Refrigerator
- 10/20 Whispering
- 10 Rustle of leaves

Noise levels above 90 decibels can cause permanent damage to the ears and thus to the sense of hearing. The diagram shows the decibel rating of some common sources of noise whose potential danger to your hearing can be evaluated.

efficiency of hearing subsequently checked by a specialist.

The prospect for improving loss of hearing depends on its cause, and on the part of the ear that is affected. (The anatomy of the ear is illustrated on page 175.) If a wax or dirt blockage, poor vibration of the middle ear bones, or a permanently ruptured eardrum is causing poor sound conduction, the condition might be helped by medical treatment or a hearing aid. Hearing tends to deteriorate with age, but in recent years many younger people have suffered some hearing loss, partly due to the increased noise levels in the everyday environment.

Hearing and noise

Noise-induced hearing loss that has affected the cochlea is irreversible. The louder the noise, the shorter the exposure time needed to produce hearing loss. Noise arising from heavy machinery, pop concerts, and hi-fi and personal earphone stereo systems can all cause varying degrees of deafness.

Noise is measured in decibels. Sounds of about 10 decibels and above are audible to the human ear. Exposure to noise levels of more than 90 decibels can, however, result in permanent damage to the ears. Pop music in discotheques is usually played at sound levels well over 100 decibels. After 100 minutes of subjection to such extreme noise levels, hearing might not be restored to normal for 36 hours. If the exposure to this level of noise is repeated, hearing capacity will be diminished as a result of permanent damage to nerve cells.

A persistent ringing or buzzing in the ears usually indicates temporary damage. The most common result of damage is a reduced ability to follow discussions when several different conversations are going on at the same time. Firearms, fireworks, noise at work, particularly from heavy machinery, and noise at home, especially from electric tools, garden appliances, and motorbikes, can also adversely affect hearing. If you live or work in an environment that you think might be damaging your concentration or your hearing, do what you can to change it. If change is not possible, wear earplugs or protective earguards to prevent occupational deafness. In some cases compensation can be claimed for industrial injury to hearing.

TEETH AND GUMS

Teeth are an important aspect of your self-image, as well as playing a major role in speech, digestion, and your appreciation of food. Yet many people neglect to look after their teeth properly. Decay (caries) in the teeth, and receding, bleeding gums, with accompanying pain and bad breath can be prevented by understanding dental disease and by making an effort to clean the teeth and gums thoroughly after every meal, if possible or at least twice a day.

Diet and teeth

A healthy diet, with as little sugar as possible, is the basic rule for preventing dental problems. Eskimos rarely suffered from tooth decay until they adopted a high-sugar Western style diet. Likewise, during World War II, when sugar was scarce, there was much less tooth decay in Europe than there is today. Having a sweet tooth is a reversible habit but it is better to prevent children from developing one in the first instance. Remember that soft drinks contain a lot of sugar, so offer children water to quench their thirst and give them raw vegetables, bread, fruit, or nuts as snacks rather than candy or cookies.

The total amount of sugar consumed is, however, less important than the number of times that sugar enters the mouth. Sugar eaten at mealtimes is less damaging than, say, sweets sucked between meals. This is because, in the early stages of dental caries, it is possible for the saliva to repair the small amount of damage caused by the interaction of sugar and bacteria in the mouth. If the teeth are constantly bathed in a sugar solution, this repair process cannot occur.

The effects of fluoride

The mineral fluorine plays an important part in the prevention of dental decay, both during the development of teeth and after they have erupted. The most effective way of supplying people with fluorine salts—fluoride—is by adding fluoride to the public water supplies. Some cities and towns have fluoridated their water for more than 30 years, to good effect. And where fluoride exists naturally in the water supply, lifelong residents are found to be resistant to tooth decay in proportion to the fluoride level.

No harm has ever been demonstrated from drinking water fluoridated at the level of one part fluoride to every million parts of water (one part per million). Where fluoride levels reach three parts per million or more, white or brown marks might appear on the teeth (as can occur when children are given certain antibiotics). If the fluoride level is less than one part per million, your dentist might advise you to give your children up to 13 years of age fluoride tablets or drops. Fluoride toothpastes, mouthwashes, and paint applied by a dentist all help prevent decay.

Sticky dental plaque is the primary cause of both tooth decay and gum disease. Made up of millions of bacteria, plaque accumulates between the teeth and around the gum margins and feels rough to the tongue. When sugar is present, the bacteria produce acid, which dissolves a hole in the protective enamel surface; other bacteria then cause tooth decay.

A recently developed vaccine against these bacteria has been shown to reduce caries in animals by 75 percent. Clinical trials are now being conducted and may provide a breakthrough in preventing caries.

More teeth are lost through gum disorders than tooth decay. Again, plaque is the cause. It collects around the gum margin, inflames the gum, and eventually loosens the contact between gum and tooth. The gum shrinks away from the tooth, leaving a gap in which bacteria breed, and the tooth loosens. Regular and careful brushing, flossing, and massaging are the best forms of prevention, along with visits to the dentist and hygienist every six months.

Modern dentistry

Anesthetic injections, high-speed drills, and comfortable surroundings have made a visit to the dentist less daunting—an important factor, that may help to prevent unnecessary delays in getting cavities filled.

Today a natural-colored filling material is available for treating front teeth and fissure sealants, plastic coatings for crevices in the back teeth, are used to prevent dental decay in children. Badly damaged teeth can be capped or crowned, and a fixed bridge can also be made to hold new replacement teeth. Tooth-straightening (orthodontics) is best done between the ages of 12 and 16. It usually takes two years to complete, and invisible plastic braces help to make the treatment acceptable to young people who are at an acutely self-conscious age.

DENTAL CARE

To prevent gum disease and tooth decay from developing, make sure that you have the necessary equipment (right). Chew a disclosing tablet, available at most drugstores, and spread the liquid around the teeth with the tongue, then rinse. Use a dental mirror to see where the plaque is concentrated—indicated by an intense red or blue color. To remove plaque, floss regularly and clean the teeth at least twice daily with fluoride toothpaste, using both a standard and a single tuft, or interspace, brush.

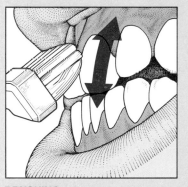

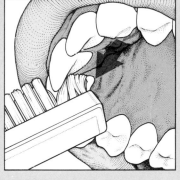

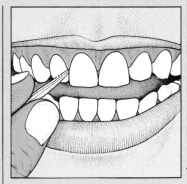

BRUSHING
Use a small soft or medium toothbrush and fluoride toothpaste. Keep the bristles at 45° to the teeth and brush up and down on all sides of each tooth.

Concentrate on a few teeth at a time and establish a routine to ensure you brush all around them. Begin with the inside surfaces, move to the chewing surfaces, then brush the outside of the teeth.

MASSAGING
Use wooden interspace sticks, an interspace brush, or rubber tip to massage the gums and remove plaque. Gently scrape between the teeth and at the gum margin, but never force an object between closely set teeth.

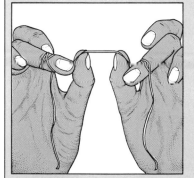

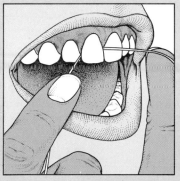

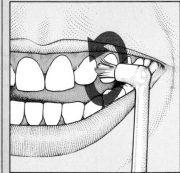

FLOSSING
Cut off a piece of dental floss or tape 18 inches long. Wind it around the middle fingers of both hands, leaving 4 inches between the two hands.

Gently push the floss between the teeth, rubbing it against the inner surfaces of each tooth, particularly at the back. Do not press too hard on the gums; if necessary ease the floss backward and forward.

Single-tuft brushes help to massage the gums and clean the more inaccessible gaps between teeth. Use a circular motion and pay particular attention to the molars.

HANDS AND NAILS

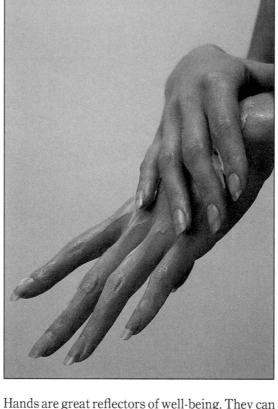

When washing your hands always rinse and dry them thoroughly. Wear gloves and barrier creams for dirty work. Rubber gloves can produce red, itchy, cracked skin, so plastic gloves are preferable. Your hands might sweat if you wear waterproof gloves for more than 15 minutes, so try to wear cotton gloves inside them. Gardening and other similar protective gloves are also advisable. Apply hand lotion often, especially over the knuckles and around the nails.

Hands are great reflectors of well-being. They can indicate the kind of work you do, your age, your degree of nervousness or self-esteem, and can show the first sign of certain illnesses and vitamin or mineral deficiencies. Yet the hands come in for a lot of rough treatment. They suffer the extremes of weather and temperature; they are immersed in water and garden soil, and subjected to irritants such as detergents.

Hands are great communicators. They emphasize your words and silently express your feelings through gesture and touch. The new world that is opened up through touching or being touched is an indefinable part of well-being. Everyone—but especially someone who lives alone—feels more relaxed with a pet to stroke.

Nail care

Each fingernail grows about half an inch every three months, and each toenail about a third of that rate. Growth varies with the individual, but it is a myth that the nail grows twice as fast if it is persistently bitten.

The nails

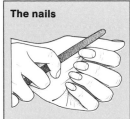

The nail is a plate of keratin. The cells grow from a root in the nail bed, where they divide rapidly. Blood vessels in the soft tissue beneath the nail nourish the nail bed, which is visible as a white crescent.

Nail care

● Keep nails short to stop them splitting and always use an emery board in preference to a metal nail file, which can cause splitting and flaking.

● File from the sides toward the center and avoid cutting or filing down the sides, which leads to ingrown nails. A painful infection can develop if the skin is pierced.

● Most nail problems are caused by abuse rather than dietary deficiencies. The best prevention and cure is to file them correctly, to avoid any obvious irritants or submersion in water, and to wear protective gloves and use hand lotions whenever necessary. Swollen fingers might be a symptom of heart disease, which needs medical attention. If you suffer from stiff fingers, exercise them as much as possible.

Although they are made up of the tough, dead material, keratin, fingernails enhance the sense of fine touch, adding dexterity to the fingers by enabling the hand to pick up tiny objects. Nail-biters are reminded every day of the clumsiness arising from the loss of this ability.

The condition of nails is a signal of general health, both psychological and physical. A severe or traumatic illness can cause nail growth to slow down temporarily, until a transverse furrow develops, which indicates the approximate date of the onset of the illness. Lack of iron can make the nails depressed and spoon-shaped. Contrary to popular belief, however, brittleness is not caused by vitamin or mineral deficiencies, and eating extra protein, gelatin, or cheese is of no use whatsoever in solving the problem.

The best cure is to keep the nails short and to apply hand lotion at night. Small white spots or flecks on the nails are probably caused by minor injuries to the nail bed rather than by any problems with calcium, and usually grow out with the nail.

All manual work damages the nails, which is another reason to keep them short and trim them regularly. Split edges of nails and brittleness are common among people who work with their hands in water and detergents or use harsh acetone nail polish removers. You should wear waterproof gloves if you are going to immerse your hands in water for more than a few seconds. Nail polish applied under the tip and on top of the nail provides an additional shield.

Discoloration of the nails has many possible causes, including smoking, ill-health, and some nail polishes. It cannot be removed, but will eventually disappear as the nails grow out.

Exercises for hands and wrists

To keep hands and wrists supple, exercise them regularly, for example, while watching television. Place the heel of each hand on your upper leg or the arm of a chair. Stretch your fingers and thumb out as far as they will go, then relax them. Repeat this 10 to 15 times.

To exercise the wrists, hold your arms out in front of you with your elbows straight. Point your fingers alternately toward the ceiling and the floor. Repeat this action 10 times. With your arms still outstretched, rotate your hands from the wrist, making five to 10 circles with each.

Cuticle care

Care of the cuticle at the base of the nail is important. Tiny painful tears in it can become infected. Push the cuticle back about once a month.

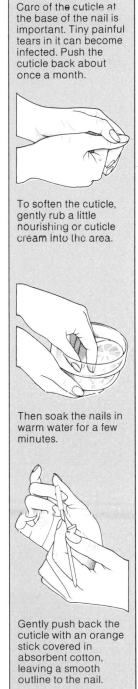

To soften the cuticle, gently rub a little nourishing or cuticle cream into the area.

Then soak the nails in warm water for a few minutes.

Gently push back the cuticle with an orange stick covered in absorbent cotton, leaving a smooth outline to the nail.

FEET

Most people are born with perfect feet, but four out of five develop some foot trouble later in life. Since, on the average, feet walk around 1,200 miles each year, often in ill-fitting shoes, socks, or pantyhose, few manage to escape discomfort.

When you are standing on both feet, each bears half your weight, but when you are walking or running, your whole weight is transferred alternately to one foot. The longitudinal arch, which transfers this weight from heel to toe, provides most of the upholding strength; while muscles, ligaments, and joints give the foot spring and elasticity. The big-toe joint is particularly vulnerable to stress, especially when the heel is raised by high-heeled shoes and when the sole of the shoe is made of a rigid material.

Shoes for children

Children's bones are soft, and if young feet are squeezed into badly fitting shoes, they can become misshapen for life. Wearing shoes before actually walking can weaken the muscles of the foot and reduce flexibility. When a baby first starts to walk, bare feet give the best grip on the floor. Do not put toddlers into shoes until they are walking well.

Socks or all-in-one stretch suits must accommodate the foot comfortably and should be checked regularly for size. If necessary, you can cut off the foot part of the suit and let the baby wear socks instead. Children should have the width and the length of their feet measured approximately every three months. Specialists in foot care recommend that shoes should be selected with a growing space of three-quarters of an inch.

Adult footwear

Shoes need to be flexible to promote a springing step; they must be supple, especially where the toe joints bend, but they should be firm in the arch. Shoes with laces or an adjustable strap are best because they hold the foot firmly to the back of the shoe, so preventing the foot from sliding forward and cramping the toes.

Shoes should be at least half an inch longer than the feet to allow the toes to move freely, and must be wide enough to allow toes to lie straight, without forcing them to the side. When buying shoes, always walk around in them in the store and try standing on tiptoe—if the heel slides off easily, the shoes are unsuitable. Shoes with low

heels impose less strain than those with high heels because they distribute the weight more evenly over the foot. Varying the height of heels from day to day helps prevent aching feet. Heels over two and a half inches high impose a great strain, so they should be worn for only a short time to avoid damaging the feet.

Always wear the correct shoes for sports. They must be roomy enough to allow the foot to expand when hot, and firm enough to prevent any injury through slipping.

Socks, pantyhose, and stockings of synthetic materials can be harmful because the fabric does not allow proper ventilation; feet can become hot and sweaty, thus creating a breeding ground for fungal infections.

RUNNING SHOES

A pair of running shoes should endure about 1,000 miles of running. Before you buy, test shoes with the socks you will wear. Choose shoes with tops made of natural materials such as leather or canvas, and layered cushioned soles, as shown below.
1. If you usually run on a road or sidewalk, a waffle-patterned tread helps to cushion the impact that travels up the legs to the spine.

2. A shallow zigzag is better for running on softer surfaces.
3. To ensure sufficient support, the sole must be flexible at the ball of the foot (pale pink), not at the arch (dark pink).
4. The heel back needs a firm collar to prevent sideways slip, while being flexible enough to avoid chafing. Shoes with rearfoot control and corrections for rolling in and rolling out over the arch are available.

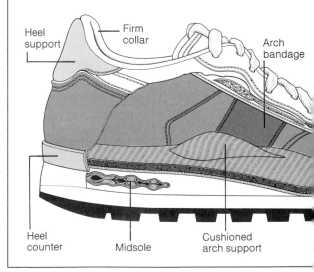

Heel support   Firm collar   Arch bandage

Heel counter   Midsole   Cushioned arch support

Podiatry, pedicure, and foot exercises

Podiatrists are trained to identify and treat common foot ailments, and provide a useful service, particularly for the elderly or infirm, who might be unable to look after their own feet.

A professional pedicure is a real treat and can prevent the build-up of hard skin on the heels and soles of the feet. Correct care of the toenails is equally important; always keep them short and cut straight across to prevent ingrown nails. Regular exercises are also beneficial; try spreading and curling the toes alternately, then flexing and pointing the whole foot. To improve the circulation and strengthen the small muscles of the feet, rotate the whole foot, then turn the soles inward and outward. Remember to walk barefoot as often as possible because it also helps strengthen the foot muscles.

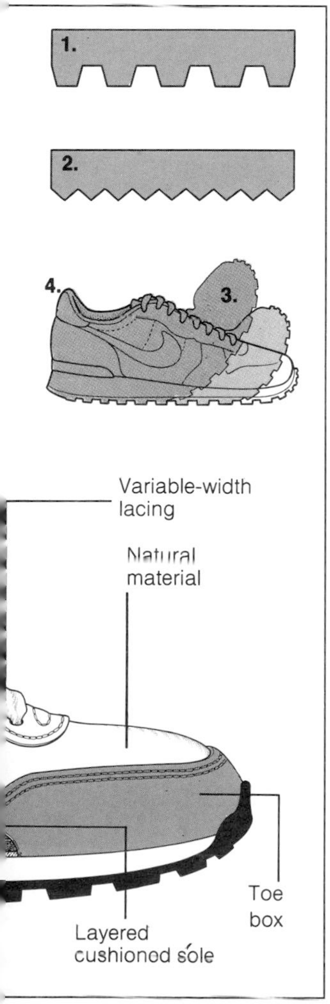

Variable-width lacing

Natural material

Toe box

Layered cushioned sole

COMMON FOOT PROBLEMS AND WHAT TO DO ABOUT THEM

The problem	The cause	What to do
Athlete's foot	A fungal infection between the toes, causing itching, soreness, and peeling. May also affect nails.	Wash the feet with soap and water once or twice a day. Dry carefully between the toes and use antifungal powder or cream. Change socks or pantyhose every day and wear cotton, not nylon, socks. Wear open sandals when possible.
Bunions	The fluid cushion around the big-toe joint becomes inflamed and thickened through wearing badly-fitting shoes. A tendency to bunions might run in families.	Wear shoes that do not crowd the toes. An operation will relieve the pressure.
Corns	Painful pads of thick, hard skin on the soles of the feet and tops of the toes, especially the little one. Caused by tight shoes.	Avoid tight shoes and change footwear often. In children corns are alarming signs of damage caused by shoes. Corn pads and adhesive bandages relieve pressure, but if it persists see a podiatrist.
Ingrown toenails	Pain, discomfort, and sometimes infection caused by a nail growing into the flesh at the sides of the toe.	Avoid tight shoes and socks. Never cut the nails away at the sides. Can be removed by a simple operation.
Verruca (wart)	An infectious wart on the foot. Common in children.	Try using special wart-removing preparations. If it persists, see your doctor or podiatrist.
Sweaty feet	Overproduction of sweat by sweat glands. A common problem.	Keep your feet clean and dry. Change socks or pantyhose daily. Avoid nylon socks and buy all-leather shoes. Choose sandals or open shoes if possible. Apply foot powder.

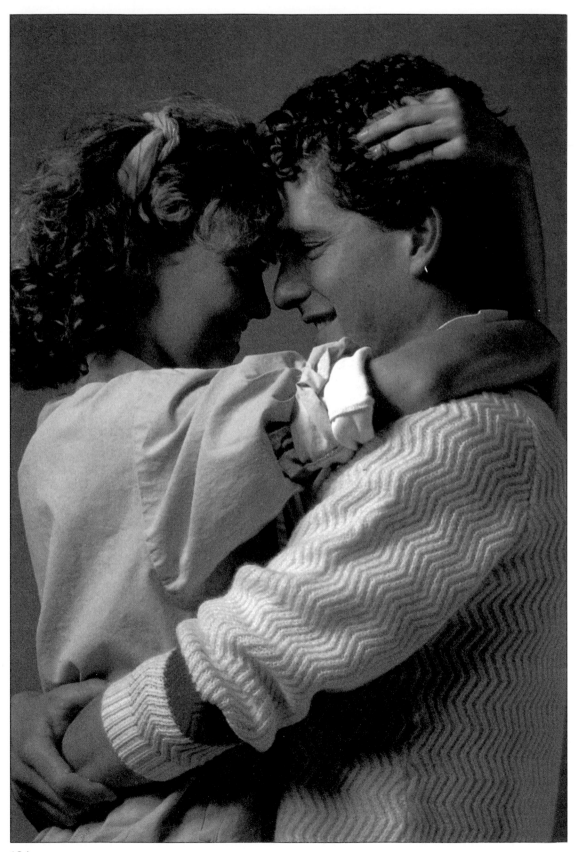

YOUR
SEXUALITY

A rewarding sex life is one of the ingredients of a continuing sense of well-being. While everyone has the potential for a healthy and fulfilling sex life, developing and maintaining it is not always easy. Problems arise for a variety of reasons, including a lack of understanding about sexuality and sexual response, feelings of guilt about desires and behavior, insecurity about technique, illness, ignorance about contraception, and stresses from other aspects of life that spill over into relationships. When things go wrong in a relationship, people often do not know what to do.

It is important to understand that sexual attitudes, activity, and experience evolve with the years, along with changes in physical and emotional development. This chapter examines the development of sexuality during childhood and adolescence, when attitudes are formed, and follows the years through to midlife and menopause. It includes essential information on sexual functions, contraception, health screening, and problems that might impair sexual satisfaction. It shows how, with knowledge and understanding, care and effort, you can achieve happy and fulfilling sexual relationships, and thus improve the quality of your life.

Sexual feelings are inherited or instinctive, but sexual behavior is something that has to be learned. From the age of three or four, children are aware of sex differences. They are interested in, and enjoy touching, their own and each other's bodies. Since the male sexual organ is easily accessible, boys tend to become familiar with sexual feelings earlier than girls.

The onset of puberty marks the beginning of a period of great upheaval and can be a trying time for everyone. The self-consciousness and self-centeredness of adolescence are intensified by the inner conflict created by a child struggling to assert independence while he or she is still very aware of the need for emotional and financial support from parents. In addition, "late developers" may be particularly worried about the delayed onset of physical maturity. The attitudes formed toward sex and relationships at this time, however tentative, have profound repercussions later. Although it is sometimes hard for parents to be sympathetic, adolescents need to be treated with understanding in order to achieve a healthy sexuality and to ease the transition to adulthood.

Sexual development spans almost a decade—from the age of 10 to 18—for both sexes, but tends to begin and end earlier in girls than in boys.

Physical changes: girls

Female puberty begins about two years before the onset of menstruation, when the pituitary gland at the base of the brain begins to secrete hormones. These stimulate the ovaries to release estrogen, the female hormone that triggers the growth of secondary sexual characteristics.

The breasts begin to develop first. The areola, the pigmented area around the nipple, enlarges. As the breasts gradually grow, fat develops in them, producing the rounded contour. It takes about two and a half years for the breasts to become fully formed, and it is quite common for one breast to begin to develop before the other.

Straight, unpigmented hair begins to grow sparsely in the pubic area, gradually becoming darker, coarser, curlier, and more profuse throughout puberty. Underarm hair begins to appear about the time of menarche, or the first menstrual period. The pelvis widens, and fat is deposited over the abdomen and hips.

The most significant landmark in a girl's sexual development is menarche. Stimulated by the pituitary gland, the ovaries release estrogen and progesterone, the two hormones that control the menstrual cycle. Menstruation usually starts at 13, but can begin at 10 or be delayed until 17 or 18.

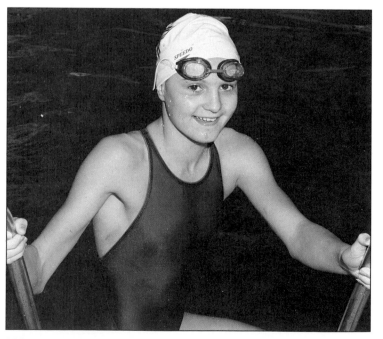

Many girl athletes reach their peak of performance during adolescence. This maximum seems to coincide with, or follow soon after, the last growth spurt, which brings them to their adult height. For all girls, sports should be encouraged and not regarded as in any way unfeminine.

A girl usually is not fully mature and able to conceive until a few months after menarche, when ripe eggs are released and the ovaries have enlarged to sustain the monthly emission of eggs. At this stage the uterus has enlarged sufficiently to accommodate a fetus, and vaginal fluid can be secreted to facilitate sexual intercourse.

Some girls welcome menarche as the arrival of womanhood; others may be subconsciously afraid of the responsibilities, particularly the sexual implications, of adulthood and seek to cling onto childhood.

The rate of development for girls is enormously variable. Throughout childhood, girls are, on the average, half an inch shorter than boys. However, their growth spurt starts sooner, at around the age of 11, so that by 13 girls are about one inch taller than boys on average. Their bones grow and mature quickly, so a year later most girls have finished growing, while boys are just beginning their growth spurt.

Physical changes: boys

Male puberty usually starts at around 12. The pituitary gland begins to secrete gonadotrophins, which stimulate the testes to produce androgens and, later, sperm. After about a year, the testes release the male hormone, testosterone, which triggers the growth and development of secondary sexual characteristics.

Fine hair begins to appear around the base of the penis, and gradually becomes denser, coarser, and curlier. About two years later, hair begins to grow in the armpits and a fine down sprouts on the upper lip and chin, eventually becoming a coarse moustache and beard that make shaving necessary. Hair grows on the chest and sometimes on the back. The skin and hair become more oily and body odor develops.

For boys, the greatest source of concern about the physical changes they are undergoing is the maturing of the genitals. The skin of the scrotum changes in color and texture. At the same time the testes enlarge and begin to produce sperm, and the penis gradually grows toward its full size and becomes more erectile. It is usual for boys to experience nocturnal discharge of semen, and they are capable of fathering a child as soon as the sperm are fully formed. In some cases, boys also develop slightly enlarged breast tissue under the nipples, but it is a temporary condition.

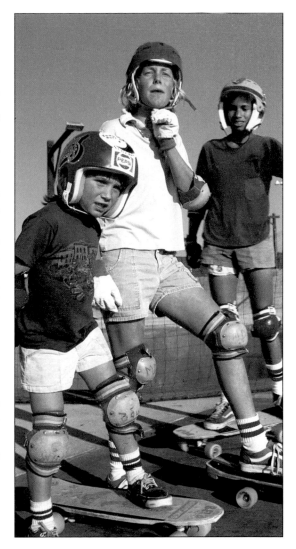

These 14-year-old boys illustrate the variable rate of sexual development: only the one in the center has begun his growth spurt.

The rate of sexual development in boys is highly variable. The growth spurt might begin at 13, but is more usually delayed until 16, and full height may be reached between 18 and 21. The hands and feet begin to grow first, then the arms and legs, and finally the torso. After the bones have grown to full length, the muscles begin to strengthen and the figure broadens. Meanwhile, the facial features become more pronounced and the voice breaks due to a thickening of vocal cords and enlarging of the voice box cartilage.

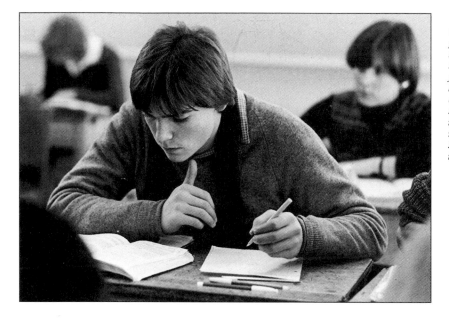

The teenage years are often dogged by academic pressures. For some boys, study is an excuse not to socialize and can lead to feeling uneasy with girls in later life. Others are distracted from work by sexual thoughts and may ignore their schoolwork. A reasonable balance between study and a social life is important.

Mental and emotional changes

While coping with the physical changes, adolescents have also to grapple with social pressures and search for an adult identity. This can be an exciting time when individuals take pleasure in their new appearance and explore new ways of expressing themselves. Not surprisingly, the psychological stresses imposed by so many changes can also lead to sudden, dramatic mood swings and emotional insecurity.

The most common way of dealing with accumulating insecurities is to conform to the peer group. Within this circle of friends, adolescents may discuss various aspects of physical development and sex, and experiment with new modes of behavior. Inevitably, conflicts arise between adolescents striving for independence and parents and other adults anxious to retain control. The revolt against authority manifests itself in many ways. Experimenting with smoking, alcohol, drugs, extreme politics, wild music and clothes, and various forms of antisocial behavior are

---

What to tell young people

Sex education is taught in most schools, but many questions remain unanswered because of the sheer embarrassment of asking them.

● Tell your daughter about menstruation when you think she is old enough to understand so that menstrual periods will not come as a shock to her. Remember that a girl may start to menstruate by the time she is 10.

● Make sure your children are familiar with the basics of male and female anatomy and reproduction so they will not be misled by misinformed friends.

● Make sure they are properly informed about the various methods of contraception.

● Remind them gently of the implications of sexual intercourse, including getting pregnant or fathering a child, and the risks of contracting a sexually transmitted disease.

● Encourage them to feel responsible for their bodies and to discuss sex and the emotional side of relationships openly with you; it can help them to form their sexual code and standards.

● Do not scorn or ignore the subject of masturbation but place it in the context of normal sexual drives.

common expressions of rebellion, with which parents may find it difficult to cope.

Discovering sexuality

In adolescence the sex drive increases and masturbation is common in both sexes. Young adolescents also frequently develop crushes on members of their own sex. Sexual fantasies and masturbation can result in feelings of guilt. Adolescents should understand that both of these are normal, not a perversion nor a threat to health or mental stability.

Curiosity and awakening sexual instincts lead to an increasing interest in the opposite sex. Adolescents need to work out a sexual identity that conforms to their wishes and the prevailing moral climate. Experimentation invites the risk of rejection, confusion, and ridicule, which can result in great anguish and color subsequent encounters.

Although the majority of parents and teachers would deny that they sex-type children, most boys and girls identify with their own sex from infancy. They seem to enjoy games in which they imitate the behavior of adults of their own sex with whom they are most familiar. For example, most little children play "mommy and daddy" and "doctor and nurse" games. As they get older, of course, they see and are influenced by adults in a wider range of activities.

Changing social attitudes and the prohibition of sexual discrimination have resulted in people having jobs and engaging in domestic activities that were once restricted to members of the opposite sex. However, this does not mean that traditional sexual stereotyping has disappeared. For example, even in movies, television series, and magazines that portray career women and tender, loving men, these women are often still depicted as sex objects ultimately ruled by their emotions, whereas the men are shown as being in control of their emotions and the situation, and sexually dominant. It is not uncommon for young people to use such fictional characters as role models. They may emulate them in manner and dress, and expect life to imitate fiction too.

Devising a personal sexual code often demands more maturity than most teenagers possess. Some girls deny their sexuality and become obsessed with "neutral" interests, such as sports; others express their frustration by mooning over pop stars or becoming sexually promiscuous at a young age, often through the pressure of the peer group and anxiety and confusion about sex. Some boys hide their strong sexual feeling for girls behind an affectation of disinterest.

The way in which adolescents respond to their sexual awareness and needs depends not only on the peer group, but also on the attitudes expressed at home. If parental signals are negative, adolescents might associate sex with guilt, which can lead to problems in adult life. When parents are positive and understanding, it can help adolescents develop a healthy sexuality.

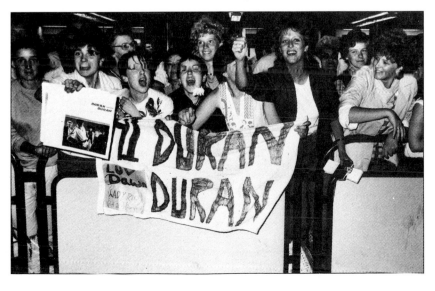

Idolizing the stars at a pop concert can provide teenage girls with the chance to release their sexual frustrations. Such occasions are also an opportunity to escape from the parental lifestyle and to dress in the style currently favored by a girl's peer group.

Sex and the forming of relationships are essential to well-being in both men and women. The diffferences in attitudes and approach depend on the nature of sexuality in the mature male and the mature female.

The male sex organs

The penis, the most obvious of the male sexual organs, consists of a shaft of spongy, erectile tissue. Its sensitive tip, the glans, is covered by a fold of skin, the foreskin, which is surgically removed in circumcized males. The testes, which are contained in the scrotum, produce the male sex hormone, testosterone, and sperm cells. The sperm pass from the testes into the epididymis, where they mature. They are then carried by a tube, the vas deferens, through the prostate gland and into the ejaculatory duct, which joins the urethra, the tube from the bladder to the penis. In the mature male, sperm production is a continuous process. The sperm are either ejaculated or reabsorbed into the system when no ejaculation takes place.

During intercourse, masturbation, or other sexual stimulation, the sex organs undergo change that occurs in a series of phases. In the arousal phase, there is a rush of blood to the penis, making it erect. The skin becomes more sensitive and responsive to stimuli, breathing deepens and quickens, and the heart rate increases.

In the plateau phase the penis reaches its maximum size and the testes enlarge. Drops of seminal fluid (which contains sperm and could lead to pregnancy) might appear on the head of the penis.

During the third phase, orgasm, the sperm are mixed with fluids secreted by the seminal vesicles and prostate gland to form semen, which is forced out of the penis by a series of rhythmic contractions. In the resolution phase the system returns to its nonaroused state.

The female sex organs

The external part of the female sexual system consists of the highly sensitive, erectile clitoris, which is covered by a small flap of skin, and the vulva, which consists of inner and outer lips—the labia minora and labia majora, respectively. Within the body lie the vagina, a muscular passage leading to the cervix (the neck of the uterus), and the uterus. The hymen is a thin membrane just inside the vagina, which can be ruptured by vigorous exercise or sexual intercourse.

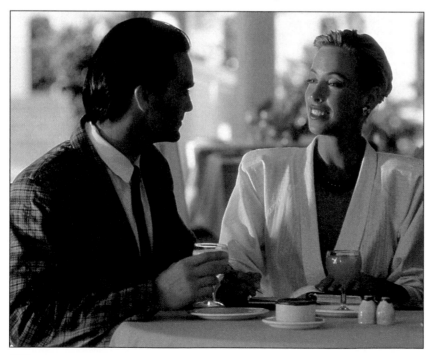

The way men and women look at each other and their physical attitudes – their body language – are sexual stimuli.

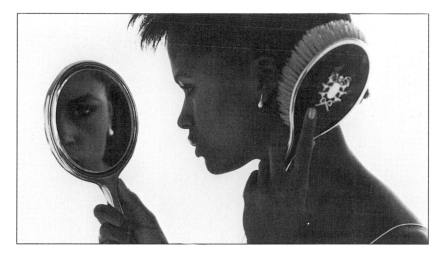

Most people try to look their best to attract other people to them and to reflect their self-image.

As with males, there are four phases in the female orgasmic cycle. In the arousal phase a reflex action causes both the internal and external sex organs to fill with blood. The vagina expands in length and width, and the vaginal walls produce a lubricant that facilitates intercourse. The breasts might enlarge and the nipples become erect. The skin, particularly in the erogenous zones (areas sensitive to sexual stimulation), becomes more sensitive. Breathing deepens and quickens, heart rate increases, and a flush might appear on the cheeks and breasts.

In the plateau phase the vagina entrance narrows to grip the penis. The clitoris becomes fully erect and draws back into its hood. If a woman is sufficiently aroused and is receiving clitoral stimulation, she might experience orgasm. For a man, ejaculation and orgasm are simultaneous events.

In the resolution phase the sexual organs return to their normal state as the blood that swells them drains away. Breathing slows and the flush disappears.

Sexual display and arousal

Most sexual relationships are motivated to some extent by the libido, or sex drive. But how men and women go about attracting each other and what makes them sexually aroused are largely the results of cultural influences, learned associations, and also of individual preferences and needs.

In most societies men have been, and continue to be, conditioned to be independent, assertive, competitive, and sexual. The role of women in Western societies, however, is changing. In the past women were brought up to be passive, dependent, receptive, and far less sexually direct than men, although there have always been exceptions to this rule. It is gradually being more widely accepted that women also can be independent, assertive, and competitive in their careers and their personal relationships.

Both sexes try to attract sexual partners by highlighting their positive attributes. They are sensitive to mental, visual, and tactile sexual cues and stimuli—a look, a touch, a smell. A man may maintain a fairly constant level of arousal because of the continuous production of testosterone, while a woman's level of arousal is influenced by her menstrual cycle; each woman has points in her cycle when she is more easily aroused.

Dispelling the myths

Sexual arousal can be inhibited by stress, feelings of guilt, or worries resulting from a lack of sex education or experience. Some men, for example, worry about the size of their penis because they believe that a woman's satisfaction is in direct proportion to it, and some women worry that their vagina is too small. In fact, penis or vagina size is irrelevant to satisfaction. Some people also believe that men know intuitively how to satisfy women. But sexual behavior is learned, and since everyone has different sexual needs and tastes, communication between partners is essential for mutual satisfaction. Thus the relationship within which you experience sex is important.

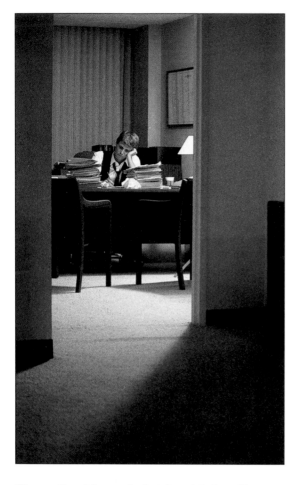

The continual demands of a job can interfere with developing and maintaining a healthy social life, and some people may use it as an excuse to avoid forming relationships.

Relationships

The type of relationships people seek are, like sexual attitudes, governed not only by their needs and desires but also by the moral code of the society in which they live. In the recent past the accepted stereotyped behavior for a young man was to have a number of short-term relationships—"sow his wild oats"—until he had established a foothold in his career. Then, it was assumed, he would marry, become a father, and be the support of the household. Similarly, the stereotyped ideal for a young woman was to marry, have two or three children, and be a supportive wife and mother.

The introduction of the contraceptive pill in the 1960's is credited with being largely responsible for the revolution in these attitudes and the emergence of the "permissive society." For a time the release from fear of an unwanted pregnancy meant that women, like men, could and did have short-term relationships, and people experimented with communal living. Now the fear of herpes and AIDS has changed attitudes yet again. People are tending to be more discriminating in their choice of sexual partners, and placing more emphasis on building lasting relationships.

However, some changes that began in the 1960's and 1970's remain and have a growing impact on society. Many women now establish themselves in a career, sometimes combining it with marriage and children. Although marriage is still the ideal for many people, a large number are choosing to marry later and have fewer children, while others are remaining single, either living alone or in a relationship outside marriage. These facts, plus the high divorce rate, mean that family lifestyle in North America has become considerably more diverse.

Homosexuality

Homosexuals are people who are sexually attracted to members of their own sex. Many people develop a crush on someone of their own sex during early adolescence, and may even have homosexual experiences at some time in life, but this is often a passing phase and does not mean that they are homosexual. For some people, however, it remains the preferred style for mature relationships. Although homosexuality is now increasingly accepted, many myths and prejudices still remain.

Homosexual men are not necessarily effeminate in appearance or manners, nor are lesbian women necessarily mannish, although some individuals may conform to this pattern, just as some heterosexuals conform to feminine and masculine stereotypes. Homosexual people are not necessarily promiscuous and many maintain stable, long-lasting relationships.

Some homosexuals marry and have children before they are aware of their true orientation, and some men and women find that they are bisexual, that is, attracted to people of both sexes. In spite of changing social attitudes, homosexuals and bisexuals might still experience difficulty in coming to terms with their sexuality, and the support of family and friends can be very helpful.

The romantic ideal of marriage still exists and many women still consider themselves failures if they remain single.

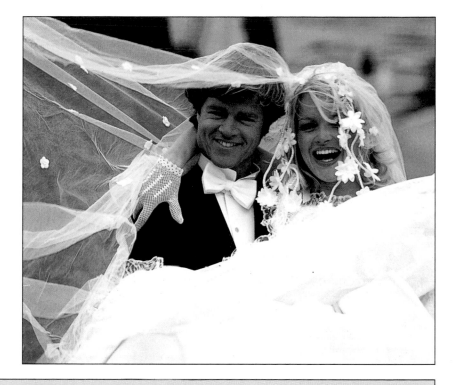

Sexually transmitted diseases

Anyone who is sexually active can get a venereal disease, so it is important to take precautions to reduce the risks: use condoms or spermicidal vaginal jelly or foam before intercourse, and urinate and wash the genitals with soap and water before and after sexual activity. If you have, or suspect you have, a sexually transmitted disease, go at once to your doctor or a public health clinic, tell your partner immediately, and do not resume sexual relations until the doctor says you may.

Acquired Immune Deficiency Syndrome

AIDS is caused by a virus or viruses that destroy a person's immune system so that the body cannot defend itself against other infections. As far as is known, the virus is transmitted in semen, vaginal fluids, and in infected blood. The incubation period can vary from three months to six years, and there is no cure yet.

Candidiasis

Previously called monilia and also known as thrush, candidiasis is an infection of the vagina caused by a yeast-like fungus. Women may have no symptoms or may have itching or burning in the vagina and a creamy white discharge. Men who contract the disease from women often get a rash on the penis. Candidiasis is usually treated with creams and vaginal suppositories, and is curable.

Genital herpes

Herpes is caused by a virus and produces painful sores on and around the genitals. The sores heal in about two or three weeks but can recur. Antiviral drugs are used with some effect to prevent recurrences but there is no cure yet.

Gonorrhea

Gonorrhea is caused by the bacterium *Neisseria gonorrhoae*. In men the symptoms usually are a burning sensation when urinating and a yellowish discharge; the majority of women have no symptoms. The disease can be cured with antibiotics.

Nonspecific urethritis

NSU is very common and is not always sexually transmitted. There are more than 70 causes of NSU, including the herpes virus, trichomonas, chlamydia, and the candida fungus. The symptoms are similar to those of gonorrhea: an inflamed urethra, a burning sensation when urinating, and a discharge. Various antibiotics are used to cure NSU.

Syphilis

Syphilis is caused by the bacterium *Treponema pallidum* and occurs in three stages. In the first stage there is a sore at the point of infection. The second stage produces a flulike illness and rash about a month or two later. The third stage can result in blindness, paralysis, and death. Syphilis can be diagnosed by a blood test and cured with antibiotics.

IMPROVING YOUR SEX LIFE

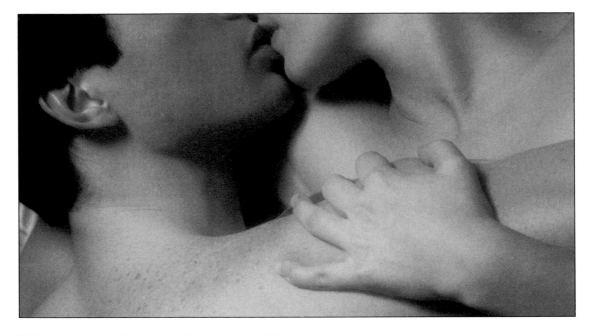

When sex is no longer a pleasure for either partner, it can become a source of tension that spills over into other areas of life. Today there is no need for couples to "just live with it." You can revitalize a stale sex life and overcome any difficulties you may experience.

Self-help
A sexual relationship can lapse into a routine or be so limited that it leaves one or both partners dissatisfied. This does not happen overnight; it is a result of two people getting so used to each other that they fail to appreciate the subtleties of their needs and desires and the fact that these can change over time. Sex then ceases to be a special experience and instead becomes a ritual like brushing your teeth or, for some, a chore.

Putting pleasure back into sex involves a shake-up of attitude, both toward sex and toward your partner. Each member of the partnership must again see the other as an individual, whose personal qualities were once a source of attraction. You should not take your partner or the sex act for granted. This means starting over and re-establishing lines of communication.

When sex becomes a problem, it is important for partners to be frank and honest with each other. Try to express dissatisfaction in a nonhurtful way as a shared problem, not your

If making love has become sporadic or boring, then it is time for a change of attitude. Use your imagination to discover more about your partner and to find new ways of making love. Discuss any problems or grievances openly and honestly.

partner's fault, and consider ways of remaking a sexually successful relationship. A simple airing of frustrations, stresses, and dissatisfactions, combined with a discussion of positive aspects of the relationship, can do a great deal to bring a couple closer, and to emphasize that only joint effort will bring sexual happiness.

Do not regard it as a personal failure if you cannot think of ways to improve your relationship but rather as an incentive to resolve a situation that has developed into a problem. Books can help with specific difficulties and give hints for improvement. Your family doctor or gynecologist might be willing to answer questions and provide counseling, or might recommend marriage guidance or sex therapy.

Although most of the sex aids on the market have little practical value and are often expensive, some can loosen inhibitions or add a charge or some humor to lovemaking.

Sexual problems
A great many people experience some sexual problems at some time. Many of these problems

194

are occasional, for instance when a man has had too much alcohol and cannot achieve an erection, or a woman has had a tense day and cannot become aroused. More enduring sexual problems can be a serious source of guilt, worry, and introspection if you do not do anything about them.

Most sexual problems arise from a subtle and complex mixture of psychological causes, attitudes, upbringing, and tension in daily life or in relationships. Problems experienced by both sexes include a lack of interest in sex, the inability to become aroused, and painful intercourse.

The most common problems in men are erectile dysfunction, or impotence, which is characterized by the inability to achieve or sustain an erection; premature ejaculation; retarded ejaculation; and ejaculatory incompetence, that is, the inability to release semen into the vagina.

In women the most common problems are vaginismus, spasms or clamping of the vaginal muscles that prevent penetration, and difficulty in achieving orgasm.

Nonconsummation that is due to impotence or vaginismus often occurs as a result of intense fear on the part of either or both partners. In some cases, however, nonconsummation might simply be the result of a lack of knowledge.

A few sexual problems have medical causes. An overtight foreskin, for example, can make intercourse painful, while an undescended testicle might cause embarrassment; both can be treated surgically. Some illnesses, such as diabetes, heart, lung, or kidney disease, and previous prostate surgery, can cause impotence. Some drugs, notably those prescribed for depression and high blood pressure, and tranquilizers, can affect sexual response, particularly in men.

During the midlife transition men often experience a drop in sexual desire and performance. In women, vaginal soreness after childbirth, reduced lubrication in the vagina as a result of menopause, and gynecological problems, such as ovarian cysts and vaginal infections, can make intercourse uncomfortable or painful.

Obtaining help

If doctors, marriage counselors, or sex therapists themselves cannot help you, they might be able to suggest other therapies available. With perseverance and a positive attitude most couples can overcome their problems.

No contraceptive has yet been found to be 100 percent reliable, suitable, practical, and without side effects or possible health risks. However, there are many contraceptive methods available, and it is more than likely that you will be able to find at least one that suits you. Single people need to accept the responsibility for contraception as their own, but couples can share it.

A tremendous breakthrough was made with the oral contraceptive pill, but since the mid-1960's the question of its safety has given rise to much controversy. Since no birth control method is ideal, extreme remedies, such as male and female sterilization, have gained popularity and relieve the burden of birth control, particularly for couples over the age of about 35 who are satisfied that they have completed their families.

The contraceptive pill
The pill is one of the most reliable and reversible methods of birth control, and its release onto the market in 1960 transformed the sexual behavior of millions of women. There are two main types: the combined pill, which uses two synthetic hormones, progestogen and estrogen, to stop ovulation; and the mini-pill, a progestogen-only pill, which alters cervical secretions to impede the sperm's journey to the uterus. Although the pill is still the first choice as a contraceptive for the majority of women, a succession of "pill scares" has led to some caution.

Just how safe is the pill? Early on, the high estrogen levels in the combined pill were found to contribute to blood clotting, which in turn can cause thrombosis (blood clots) and circulatory problems. Since this made women more vulnerable to heart disease and strokes (although they are still five times less vulnerable than men of the same age), the estrogen levels were lowered. If they are too low, however, breakthrough bleeding (bleeding between menstrual periods) occurs and the pill might be ineffective in preventing pregnancy.

Opinion is now divided about the safest strategy to use. Some doctors say that with the low-estrogen formulas, women run only a small risk of thrombosis. Others recommend that all women over 35, and those over 30 who smoke, should stop using the combined pill and switch to a progestogen-only pill. In view of such disagreement, it would appear that for ultimate safety a woman in her twenties should have her blood pressure and blood cholesterol monitored frequently, stop smoking, and discuss with her gynecologist the advisability of discontinuing the combined pill and using an alternative method of birth control (see pages 198–199) at around the age of 30 or 35.

The "scares" of the early 1980's centered on research that appeared to establish a causal relationship between the pill and breast and cervical cancer. However, the results of the various studies contradicted each other and it is clear that more research is needed before the pill can definitely be linked as a causal agent in cancer of the breast, cervix, ovary, or uterus. Some scientists believe that, until more time has passed, it will not be possible to make an exact assessment of the real long-term effects of the pill. Meanwhile, women who have chosen or are considering the pill as a method of contraception should take into account that there might be some health risks.

Barrier methods
The three types of contraceptive that block the entry of sperm into the uterus are the condom, the diaphragm, and the sponge. Although these methods are not as convenient, may not be as effective, and do not allow the same spontaneity in sexual relations as the pill, they have other advantages.

A condom is a thin rubber sheath worn over the penis during intercourse, which prevents sperm from entering the woman's body. It is available over the counter and not only enables the man to take responsibility for contraception, but also provides the best protection against AIDS and other sexually transmitted diseases (see page 193). However, there is a risk that a condom can tear or slip off during use.

A diaphragm is a circular rubber device that is worn over the cervix. A woman must be measured for a diaphragm by a doctor, who will check that it fits properly and may also instruct her on using it. To offer any protection against conception, the diaphragm must be inserted so that it completely covers the cervix. To ensure maximum effectiveness, it should be used with a spermicide (see pages 198–199). It is reusable, but should be checked for holes each time it is inserted.

The sponge is made of polyurethane foam and

STERILIZATION

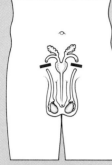

Male sterilization

Male sterilization involves cutting and tying each vas deferens to block the path of sperm from the testes. The operation, under local anesthetic, usually takes about 15–20 minutes, but contraceptive precautions are needed for the next 3–6 months, until all stored sperm is ejaculated.

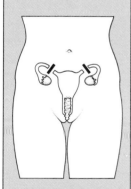

Female sterilization

This is performed by cutting, clamping, or tying the Fallopian tubes. Operations to remove the ovaries or uterus also result in sterilization. These operations are usually conducted under a general anesthetic and take effect immediately.

contains a spermicide. The foam blocks and absorbs sperm, and releases a spermicide. Because the sponge fits loosely over the cervix, insertion is easier, one size fits everyone, and it is available over the counter. Each sponge can be used only once. This method carries some risk of toxic shock syndrome (see page 205). To reduce this risk, do not use the sponge during a menstrual period, nor leave one sponge in the body for more than 30 hours.

Sterilization

For those who do not wish to have any more children, sterilization provides a permanent solution to the problem of contraception. The decision to be sterilized should not be taken lightly, however there is an increasing chance of reversing the procedure. In men, each tube (the vas deferens) that carries sperm from the testes to the penis is cut in the scrotum and then closed off at the ends. A vasectomy will not inhibit sex drive nor the secretion of male hormones, but contraceptives must be used for up to six months or until laboratory tests show that the seminal fluid is sperm-free.

The most common operation for women is performed on the Fallopian tubes, which carry eggs from the ovaries to the uterus. The tubes are cut, clamped, or pulled through a tight plastic ring. In rare cases the tubes can rejoin, sperm can travel through a clamp, or an ectopic pregnancy, in which a fertilized egg is trapped in a Fallopian tube, could occur. Periods will continue as normal after the operation, and menopause occurs at the natural time.

If the ovaries are damaged or diseased, the operation to remove them also results in sterilization and might precipitate the menopause. The third method is hysterectomy, the removal of the uterus, which is usually considered only if a woman has other gynecological problems that could be treated most effectively this way.

Sterilization, which takes effect immediately in women, should not affect a woman's weight or sex drive and might even improve sex once the fear of pregnancy is removed. Nevertheless, counseling is advisable before any decision is made, and sterilization should never be performed at the same time as an abortion because the emotional turmoil of pregnancy termination might force a hasty decision.

Contraceptives of the future

Contraceptive developments in the future remain uncertain, since current research into birth control is confined to refinements of old methods. The most revolutionary foreseeable change is a vaccine that would make the female body reject sperm, but this is unlikely to be perfected until the 21st century.

The male pill needs to contend with the problem of halting the ever-moving production line of sperm and of male resistance to the idea.

Other modern methods yet to be evaluated include a nasal contraceptive spray that suppresses ovulation, spermicide-releasing vaginal rings, and a diaphragm that needs no spermicide.

With so many birth control methods available, most people can find at least one type of contraceptive to suit their age and circumstances.

The chart lists the main contraceptive methods with an analysis of their effectiveness, safety, and convenience. Additional information can be obtained from your doctor or from the Planned Parenthood Association, which you will find listed in your telephone directory.

Remember that if neither partner uses a contra-

Method	How it works	Advantages
Combined pill	Synthetic progestogen and estrogen hormones mimic those produced during pregnancy. Since no message is sent out for an egg to be released, no ovulation takes place. Pills are taken for 21 days, followed by 7 days of dummy pills or 7 pill-free days.	Easy and convenient to use. Regularizes periods. Can reduce menstrual bleeding, period pain, and premenstrual tension. Does not inhibit lovemaking. Might protect against cancer of the ovaries and the uterus.
Mini-pill	A progestogen-only pill, taken every day. It thickens mucus in the cervical canal, inhibiting sperm entrance and implantation of the egg in the uterus.	Easy and convenient. Safe for older women. Less risk of heart problems. Suitable while breast-feeding.
Condom, or "rubber" (women should use a spermicide).	Worn over the penis during intercourse to block the sperm.	Easy to use. Allows the man to take responsibility for birth control. Helps prevent passing of sexual disease.
Intrauterine device (IUD)	A device made of plastic. How it prevents a fertilized egg from implanting or developing in the uterus is unknown.	Effective immediately (unless you are already pregnant). Especially suitable for those over 35 and those who have completed their families. Does not interfere with lovemaking.
Diaphragm with spermicide	A saucer-shaped device of rubber or rubber and plastic is inserted into the vagina so that it covers the cervix. Spermicide must be inserted no more than 2 hours before intercourse. Diaphragm and spermicide together prevent the sperm meeting the egg.	No side effects, no health risks. Might protect against cervical cancer. Can be used at any age.
Spermicides	Spermicidal foams, creams, jellies, and suppositories contain nonoxynol-g and, as their name implies, kill sperm.	Can be used at any age. Used at every sexual contact can protect against some sexually transmitted diseases.
Sponge	A soft, circular, polyurethane foam sponge containing spermicide is inserted in the vagina to cover the cervix up to 24 hours before intercourse. Must be left in place for 6 hours after intercourse.	Effective for 24 hours and for repeated intercourse within that time. One size fits all. No fitting required.
Injectable	Synthetic hormone progestogen is injected into a muscle, and slowly released into the body, where it stops ovulation.	Depending on type, one injection is effective for 8 to 12 weeks. Does not inhibit lovemaking.
Rhythm method	The calendar method entails working out the pattern of menstrual cycles to predict safe days. The temperature method indicates a slight drop in temperature just before ovulation, and is considered unreliable on its own. The Billings, or mucus, method relies on detecting changes in cervical mucus near ovulation. The combination, or symptothermal, method involves temperature recording, and noting changes in cervical mucus and other symptoms of ovulation, such as backache and depression.	No side effects except sexual frustration. Partners share the responsibility.
Coitus interruptus (withdrawal)	The penis is withdrawn from the vagina before ejaculation.	No side effects except possible frustration. Allows the man to take responsibility for birth control.

ceptive, pregnancy can occur without female orgasm, sometimes without full penetration, and even if the woman douches after sex. Also, breast-feeding does not protect a woman against becoming pregnant. It is always better to be safe than to take the risk of an unplanned conception.

Although there are risks and failures attached to the use of contraceptives, it should be emphasized that, with careful use, most of them work safely most of the time.

Disadvantages	Comments	Reliability
Possible initial side effects of nausea, headache, sore breasts, water retention, between-period bleeding, depression, and loss of libido. Possible risk of thrombosis; possible link with breast and cervical cancer.	Not recommended for smokers over 35, those with a family history of heart disease or strokes, and some diabetics. Safest have low progestogen/estrogen formulation. Additional precautions are needed to counteract vomiting or diarrhea, with some drugs, and if a pill is taken more than 12 hours late. Regular blood pressure checks, cervical smears, and monthly breast examinations advised, as for any other woman.	98–99 percent
Same initial problems as combined pill. Higher risk of ectopic pregnancy. Most effective 4 hours after taking. Can cause between-period bleeding and irregular periods. Possible link with cervical cancer.	More suitable for women over 35 who wish to stay on the pill. Must be taken at the same time every day; if more than 3 hours late, extra precautions and checks needed, as for combined pill.	97–98 percent
Interrupts lovemaking. Can slip off or tear. Can impair sensitivity.	Must be held in place until withdrawal is complete. Never reuse. Lubricate with a specially formulated jelly.	95–97 percent *with careful use*
Can be expelled from the body. Must be replaced every year. Possibility of pelvic infection, which might cause sterility. Chance of ectopic pregnancy.	Unsuitable for women with heavy periods. Must be removed before starting a family.	95–98 percent
Might inhibit lovemaking. If worn too long, can cause toxic shock syndrome. (See also spermicides.)	Must be inserted and fitted correctly so that the cervix is covered. Must be left for at least 6 hours after last intercourse, then washed, dried, powdered, and stored in a cool place. Must not be used by women with pelvic disorders. Check for small holes and renew every year, after a birth, miscarriage, or termination, or a loss or gain of 14 pounds in weight.	80–95 percent *with careful use*
Creams, jellies, and foams can be messy, and more must be added if intercourse occurs more than 2 hours after insertion or on a second occasion. Suppositories effective for 1 hour, 10 minutes after insertion. Can cause irritation in men and women.	Require careful timing.	82–95 percent *with careful use*
Should not be used during a period. Some people might be allergic to the spermicide.	Must not be left in place for more than a total of 30 hours.	80–90 percent *with careful use*
Periods usually become irregular. Return of regular periods and fertility might be delayed up to a year after the last injection.	Must be prescribed by a doctor. Mainly for women for whom other methods are unsuitable. Link with cervical cancer not known.	Over 99 percent
Demands constant checking. Calendar method is unsuitable if the cycle is irregular. Unsuitable during times of change. Temperature method can be unreliable. Billings method is difficult to learn.	The only method approved by the Roman Catholic Church. Comparatively unreliable.	Calendar method— 53 percent Temperature method— 66 percent Billings method— 80 percent Combination method— 85 percent *with careful use*
Difficult to time exactly; some sperm can enter vagina before withdrawal is complete.	Inefficient and unsatisfactory for many. Used successfully in some cases, but requires a cooperative man.	75–80 percent

RELATIONSHIPS UNDER PRESSURE

No marriage or long-standing relationship can ever hope to be perfect all the time; nor can a couple's sex life. You may have started out with great expectations and a grand passion but the pressures of life inevitably intrude. It is possible, however, to identify problem areas and in doing so to look at ways in which to effectively revitalize relationships.

All in the family—children

The family is a demanding unit that at times can be delightful, at other times, distressing. At best it can enrich life, at worst it can enslave its members. From the moment the first child is born to the day the last child leaves home, the lives of parents are limited by the demands and the needs of their offspring.

The arrival of children often precipitates a dramatic shift in roles and relationships. Despite the current vogue for shared parenthood, most mothers are still the caretakers of their children. A sexual split between partners might begin with the exhaustion of childbirth and the physical and emotional demands of the new bond between a mother and her baby.

As time goes on, children's demands on both partners, but particularly on the mother, begin to grow, and a parent can be pulled in conflicting directions. Commonsense dictates that care and attention be given to the most vulnerable party, usually the child, but a man or woman might not be any less in need of attention than a child. Many children learn to play off one parent against the other, reinforcing the emotional split between them, and a parent might use a child as a weapon in a troubled relationship.

The presence of children also reduces privacy. Lovemaking becomes constrained by late nights and locked doors, particularly when the family is living at close quarters. Although adults do not need to, many hide all aspects of their sexuality and displays of affection from their children. As a result, young people, as they grow older and start to be sexually aware, may view their parents' lovemaking with skepticism or disgust.

To alleviate some of the pressures inherent in their relationship, parents need to share the work load honestly, allowing enough time and energy for a fulfilling emotional and sexual life. Parents have to learn to be selfish enough to insist on being partners too. This might mean making a

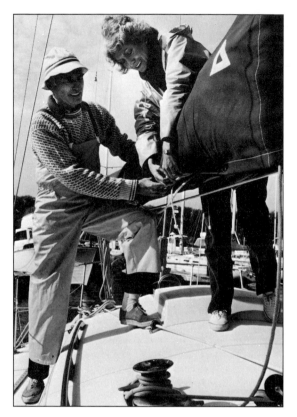

An activity-oriented vacation away from all the aggravations of everyday life might be just the tonic your relationship needs, since stress and tiredness are the twin enemies of libido. Choose the type of vacation that you will both fully enjoy.

concerted and deliberate effort to set aside the demands of parenthood from time to time. Couples might find it helpful to set aside an evening each week on which to go out together or to take occasional trips without the children.

All in the family—parents

When an aging, single parent moves in, it can impose unexpected strains on any family. Even the most thoughtful and sensitive couple cannot foresee how roles and relationships will be revised. There might be settling-in problems, especially if the parent comes from a different city or town and is used to an independent life, routine, and longstanding friends.

Conflicts and guilt inevitably result when one partner slips back into a childhood role, allowing the parent to drive a wedge between man and

Identifying problems

When a relationship suffers, so will sex.

● Nagging, pushing, shouting, and sulking are symptomatic of underlying problems; arguing about trivia provides an excuse to attack each other.

● The problem may seem to be money, work, the children, elderly parents, or sex, but it could just be lack of communication.

● Taking the trouble to find out what bothers a partner is never a waste of time.

Revitalizing a relationship

● Try to talk—it should have a good, if not dramatic, effect.

● Try to remember why you first loved, respected, admired, and enjoyed each other.

● Recognize that you have both changed and look for new reasons to love, respect, and enjoy each other now.

● Examine your joint goals.

● Reveal your thoughts and feelings and recognize each other's frustrations and aspirations.

● Make up your quarrels—it is the most loving thing you can do.

woman, or stands back while the grandparent takes over the role of bringing up the children or gives advice from the sidelines. In such a tense situation, particularly if physical space is also limited, relaxed lovemaking might cease.

For the couple's loving and sexual relationship to survive, each partner must exercise great patience, make strenuous efforts to adapt to the new situation, and work hard to smooth over divided loyalties.

The world of work

Work puts enormous pressure on a couple's relationship because of its inherently stressful nature, its energy-sapping qualities, and the amount of time it claims. Too tense, too tired, and too busy for sex, was once the cry of male partners, but it is now echoed by many working women. Furthermore, with breadwinning increasingly shared, conflicts arise about the division of family responsibilities. There might also be jealousy about financial contributions, success, independence, and absence from home. It is all too easy for a couple pursuing their personal ambitions to become two separate, exhausted adults who happen to live under the same roof and share the same bed.

The only way to revive a "work-sick" sex life is to revise priorities and to compromise; to care about work without allowing it to supersede the needs of the relationship. Work is best done and left outside the bedroom door.

Extramarital affairs

Casual sex outside marriage usually has serious effects on both partners. Some people feel the need for sexual variety, the thrill of secrecy, and extra emotional support, and a few relationships thrive on such sexual uncertainty.

Many relationships, however, simply cannot survive the strain of extramarital affairs. For many people, infidelity goes against their moral upbringing, dispels their trust, shatters their security, arouses feelings of guilt, and repels them. Even if the marriage survives, there will often be residual distrust and fear that the partner could be unfaithful again. The outcome depends on the strength of a couple's commitment to each other, the limits of tolerance and love, and the belief each has in the value and the lasting worth of the bond.

Should you keep your relationship alive?

All relationships have their ups and downs, and the divorce rates indicate that in many cases the downs are greater. Ask yourself the following questions; your answers will indicate whether or not you think your relationship is still a source of joy and comfort. Then consider how you could improve it (see pages 194–195, 296–297).

● Do I care about my partner?

● Have we lost our appeal for each other?

● Would I go out of my way to support my partner?

● Do we have common interests?

● If my partner left me, how would I feel?

● Is my partner my best friend?

● Do we respect each other?

● Do I feel disillusioned with our relationship?

● Can we overcome the sources of irritation?

● Have we grown together or apart?

● Would I feel happier if we separated?

● How do I feel when I look back on our life together?

● Should we stay together (for the moment at least) for the sake of the children?

PREMENSTRUAL SYNDROME

An average of five out of every 10 women may suffer some physical and emotional distress during the two-week interval between ovulation and menstruation. Dubbed the premenstrual syndrome (PMS), or premenstrual tension (PMT), the condition is now recognized and treated medically.

Physical symptoms of PMS include:
Bloated abdomen and fingers.
Swollen, tender breasts.
Weight gain: sometimes up to $6\frac{1}{2}$ pounds.
Headaches, often on one side.
Aching back, legs, shoulders, knees, and ankles.
● Craving for sweet, high-carbohydrate foods.
Pimples, boils, spontaneous bruises, clumsiness, dizziness, or faintness.
● Exacerbation of asthma, epilepsy, migraine, conjunctivitis, and contact lens irritation.

Among the emotional symptoms of PMS are:
● Tension, anxiety, depression, tearfulness, forgetfulness, lack of concentration, irritability, and inability to make decisions.
● Violent mood swings.
Lethargy.
● Some loss of confidence and disinterest in sex, work, and social life.

Theories and treatments

No single cause for PMS has yet been identified. A number of theories, however, have been proposed and have led to successful treatment.

Sometimes more than one treatment must be tried, but with trial and error, a great measure of relief can usually be found. It is important that any treatment is approved by your doctor.

One theory is that PMS is caused by an imbalance of the hormones estrogen and progesterone. Estrogen levels normally rise until ovulation occurs, then fall, but research has shown that in 40 percent of PMS sufferers estrogen levels remain high in the second half of the menstrual cycle while progesterone levels are abnormally low. The treatment consists of doses of progesterone, which reduce fluid retention, breast tenderness, headaches, spontaneous bruising, and nausea, and also relieve many of the emotional symptoms, such as anxiety and depression.

Another theory is that women with PMS suffer from low levels of pyridoxine (vitamin B_6), which works on many parts of the body, including the brain and the pituitary gland—the menstrual trigger—and on the body's response to stress. This deficiency lowers the output of progesterone and estrogen. Doctors who advocate this theory treat PMS with vitamin B_6 tablets from three

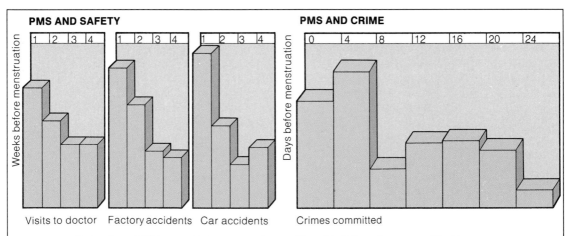

PMS AND SAFETY

Weeks before menstruation

Visits to doctor   Factory accidents   Car accidents

Women suffering from PMS have a higher proportion of car and factory accidents, and visit their doctors more often, during the two weeks before the onset of menstruation. Suicides also peak at this time, when emotional control is at its lowest ebb. Loss of efficiency during PMS can upset a promising career.

PMS AND CRIME

Days before menstruation

Crimes committed

Almost half the crimes committed by women occur during the 8 days before the onset of menstruation. Violence by women toward their children and husbands is more common during PMS than at other times, a point that has become the center of controversial legal debate in the courts.

days before the symptoms start, up to menstruation. It has been effective in relieving depression and headaches in some women. An alternative theory, however, is that stress is, in fact, the cause not the effect of hormonal imbalance.

There is strong support for the theory that an excess of prostaglandin hormones cause nausea, moodiness, and water retention. Treatments with anti-prostaglandin drugs have achieved good results.

A recent theory is that PMS is caused by a deficiency of essential fatty acids, particularly gammalinolenic acid. The seed oil of the evening primrose, *Oenothera biennis*, is a natural remedy used by the American Indians. PMS sufferers for whom other treatments have failed have found the oil to be successful in relieving their symptoms. Ask your doctor about it.

Other treatments include synthetic diuretics, which help to relieve water retention; tranquilizers; antidepressants; and treatment with the pill. These last three, however, have made symptoms worse in some cases.

A plan of action

Many women have found relief through self-help. Use a chart such as the one below to establish your personal pattern of symptoms, and then treat yourself as follows:

● Try to plan your life so that you do not put yourself under strain premenstrually.

● Reduce water retention by reducing your intake of sodium (see pages 64–65).

● Don't worry about the temporary weight gain; you will lose retained water naturally during the menstrual period.

● Keep food cravings in check; weight gained by eating large quantities of chocolate or other sweet foods will not be so temporary.

● Lift your mood by planning to go to a concert, a play, or the movies.

● Take up yoga, relaxation, or meditation to relieve tension.

● Take extra care if you are prone to accidents, dizziness, or fainting.

● Do some aerobic exercise, such as running or swimming.

● Alert your family and friends so that they are more understanding.

● Develop an awareness of the symptoms and try to exert more self-control.

If you believe you are suffering from PMS and have been unable to find relief with self-help measures, consult a doctor about medical treatment. You should not try to treat yourself with vitamins or drugs, which can have serious side effects.

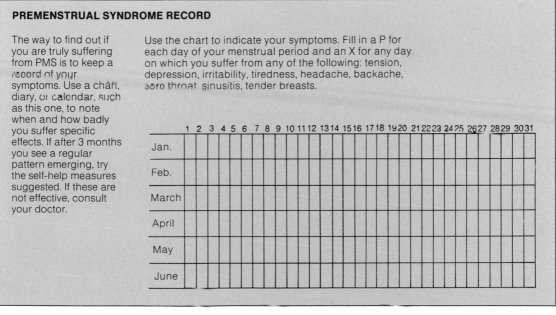

PREMENSTRUAL SYNDROME RECORD

The way to find out if you are truly suffering from PMS is to keep a record of your symptoms. Use a chart, diary, or calendar, such as this one, to note when and how badly you suffer specific effects. If after 3 months you see a regular pattern emerging, try the self-help measures suggested. If these are not effective, consult your doctor.

Use the chart to indicate your symptoms. Fill in a P for each day of your menstrual period and an X for any day on which you suffer from any of the following: tension, depression, irritability, tiredness, headache, backache, sore throat, sinusitis, tender breasts.

	1 2 3 4 5 6 7 8 9 10 11 12 13 14 15 16 17 18 19 20 21 22 23 24 25 26 27 28 29 30 31
Jan.	
Feb.	
March	
April	
May	
June	

Despite the current trend toward fitness and well-being, many women still do not take enough care of their bodies. Far too often they assume that good health means an absence of disease or that female complaints are the necessary burden of their sex. These assumptions are incorrect, often dangerously so. Cervical cancer, which can be symptom-free in its early stages, has a death toll in Western countries of about one in 5,000 women. Pelvic infections, if left untreated, can be the cause of permanent sterility.

The range of tests

Some women shy away from gynecological examination. Every woman should make regular screening part of her health program, since cervical (Pap) smears and breast examinations are crucial to early detection of disease.

All women are advised to have a full gynecological examination at least once a year. Women should have their breasts examined by a doctor or specially trained nurse every year, especially if they are taking the pill or are over 35. Pap smears are usually advised once a year. Women on the pill should have their blood pressure monitored regularly. These tests take only a few minutes and they might make the difference between life and death.

The gynecologist begins a full examination by taking your medical, personal, and gynecological history. It is helpful if you have handy details of previous tests and problems, dates of your last few periods, any premenstrual symptoms that you experience, and any other facts you think might be relevant, including your method of contraception.

The gynecologist examines your breasts and, if necessary, refers you for mammography (X-ray) and gives instruction in breast examination (see pages 206–207), all with the purpose of detecting abnormalities that can give early indication of breast cancer.

He will examine your pelvic region for any signs of disease, abnormal growths, or damage or infection in the uterus, cervix, or vagina.

Next he will take a Pap smear (also called cervical smear or cytotest)—a routine of all gynecological examinations. The procedure entails lightly scraping off some of the cells of the lining of the cervix (neck of the uterus). The sample is sent to the laboratory to be examined for

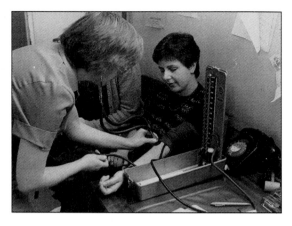

Blood pressure measurements are an integral part of female medical screening. They are particularly important for women who are on the pill, since the hormones this contraceptive contains might lead to high blood pressure.

possible malignancy. Women who have taken, or whose mothers took, the steroid DES or whose Pap results are abnormal will have a colposcopy, a painless examination of the cervix with the aid of a specially designed microscope. Cervical precancer, if detected in its earliest stages before it becomes invasive (it can take up to 10 years to develop), can be treated simply and with complete success. If it is left untreated, cervical cancer can be fatal.

Women who have abnormal discharges are tested for vaginal and cervical infections by taking a sample for laboratory culture. In this way, common infections such as candidiasis or trichomoniasis and any venereal diseases that might show can be diagnosed and treated (see pages 192–193).

Additional tests for blood pressure, anemia, urinary infections, diabetes, and rubella, which can damage a fetus or cause miscarriage or stillbirth (see pages 214–215), will also be taken where appropriate. After the examination, when the doctor discusses his findings, remember to ask any questions you might have; it is useful to make a list of such questions.

Menstrual problems

Women's menstrual periods vary enormously, but the average monthly loss of blood is only two fluid ounces. Irregular, painful, heavy periods are not unusual, but you should get a proper diagnosis from your doctor or gynecologist.

CERVICAL SMEAR TEST

Annual cervical smear, or Pap, tests are essential, since cervical cancer can be prevented if cellular changes are detected before they become widespread, or invasive.

A Pap test consists of a scrape of tissue taken from the cervix (neck of the uterus). The cells are stained and viewed under a microscope.

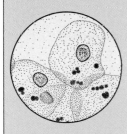

Healthy cells are large with small, dark nuclei.

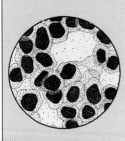

Cancer cells from the cervix are small with large, dark nuclei almost filling them.

The worst symptoms of menstrual problems can be alleviated through self-help or medical treatment. Irregular bleeding (metrorrhagia) can be caused by emotional upsets as well as physical disease or the onset of menopause, and can be light or heavy. If treatment of the cause is not successful, hormones can be given until the cycle is regular again.

Absent periods (amenorrhea) not caused by pregnancy might be due to emotional upsets, anorexia nervosa, stopping the contraceptive pill, or even too much exercise. Painful periods (dysmenorrhea) can be primary (spasmodic acute cramps, common in women before their first pregnancy) or secondary (congestive, dull aching, and heaviness, usually coupled with the premenstrual syndrome and spanning the later years up to menopause). Severely painful periods arising from medical causes are treated with drugs and sometimes with surgery.

Self-help treatments, including painkillers, curling up with knees on the chest, or with a hot water bottle, can relieve period pain. Exercise such as swimming, dancing, or jogging, both before and during a period, is also effective. Medical treatment is available if self-help measures are unsuccessful.

Extremely heavy periods (menorrhagia) are common in the early menstrual years, but should be investigated by your doctor. Any sudden change to heavier periods might be symptomatic of a serious complaint, so report it to your doctor.

Toxic shock syndrome (TSS) can occur if a tampon is left in the body for too long during a period or inadvertently left in at the end of a period. The symptoms typical of it are headache, nausea, stomach pain, vomiting, diarrhea, dizziness and faintness. If you suspect you have TSS, see a doctor immediately.

Investigations of menstrual problems

Menstrual problems that do not respond to self-help treatments often demand more thorough medical investigation. One of the commonest of these is the D and C, which stands for dilation (of the cervix) and curettage (of the uterus). In a D and C the uterine lining is scraped under general anesthetic and a sample of tissue taken for examination. Often the scraping alone is sufficient to solve the problem; if not, drug treatments might be required.

Checklist

● Have you had a full gynecological examination in the last year?

● Have you had a professional breast examination in the last year?

● Have you had a Pap smear in the last year?

If you answer "no" to any of the above, make an appointment now.

● Have you recently noticed a sudden change in your periods?

● Have you noticed a recent change in your breasts?

● Do you think you may have a disease or disorder?

If you answer "yes" to any of the above, see your doctor as soon as possible.

It is a cruel fact that breast cancer affects one in every 10 women, and that it is probably still the single most common cause of death in women between 40 and 44.

Although breast cancer cannot be prevented, there is a good chance of a cure if it is detected in its earliest stages. This is why it is essential for women to make a habit of examining their breasts every month and to have regular medical checkups. Remember that 20 percent of all cancer deaths are due to breast cancer.

Breasts undergo subtle and normal changes throughout a woman's life. The rise and fall in the levels of the female hormones, estrogen, progesterone, and prolactin, contribute to breast changes during the menstrual cycle, during pregnancy, when breast-feeding a baby, and at the time of menopause. The contraceptive pill can also cause changes. Every woman needs to distinguish these normal changes from new lumps. Most are benign; only one in 10 will be cancerous.

Who is at risk?
The cause of breast cancer is not yet known, although according to some researchers the contraceptive pill might be a contributing factor, possibly by delaying the first pregnancy. The Western way of life is another contributory factor. Those most at risk are women over 35 years old, childless women, those who had their first child after the age of 30, those with previous benign breast problems, and those closely related to someone who has had breast cancer.

Self-examination
All women should examine their breasts every month from puberty onward. Do it immediately after each period (because the breast might feel tender and lumpy in the week before menstruation) or, after menopause, on the first day of the month.

The crucial signs to watch out for when you examine your breasts are: a lump in the breast or local lumpy areas; unusual increase in the size of one breast; one breast unusually lower than the other; puckering or dimpling of the breast skin; turning in of the nipple; fluid emerging from one nipple only, especially if it is bloodstained; a rash on the nipple; swelling of the upper arm; enlargement of the lymph glands in the armpit.

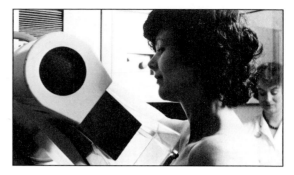

Mammography can detect signs of breast cancers before they become noticeable through physical examination. Early detection improves the chances of making a full recovery.

If you notice any abnormality, see your doctor immediately. Breast disorders, such as chronic mastitis, cysts, and benign tumors are fairly common but their symptoms might mimic cancer.

In chronic mastitis, the breast feels swollen, lumpy, and painful, particularly before and during menstruation. This condition is most common in women between 30 and 50 but can occur at any age. Cysts, small sacs in the breast tissue that become filled with liquid, are most common in women in their mid-thirties and forties. Cysts can cause pain, discomfort, and a discharge from the nipple, and might need to be removed surgically or aspirated. Often, innocent lumps in the breast are clumps of fibrous tissue that can swell and cause pain. They are usually permanent and might require surgical removal.

Breast screening
Regular screening entails examination of the breasts by a doctor, often together with a breast X-ray, known as a mammogram, which reveals any malignancy as an irregular opaque patch on the resulting image. This procedure can detect about 92 percent of cancers. Although not always comfortable, mammography is not painful. It should, however, be avoided if you are, or might be, pregnant.

An additional diagnostic test is a needle biopsy, which involves inserting a needle into the lump. If liquid is aspirated and the lump disappears, the problem is due to a cyst. If the lump is solid, a few cells can be drawn into the needle. Laboratory tests will subsequently distinguish between malignant and benign disease.

HOW TO EXAMINE YOUR BREASTS

The aim of self-examination is to get to know your breasts and to be able to detect any abnormal changes in them that warrant further medical examination. Most growths are benign but all changes in the breast tissue should be investigated at once. Only by detecting abnormalities early can cancer be fully cured.

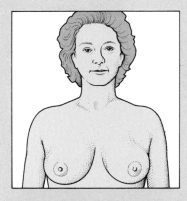

Sit in front of the mirror stripped to the waist. Sit completely straight, then carefully study your breasts. Look for any marked change in size and see if one breast has recently become lower than the other. Look at the skin for any puckering, dimpling, rashes, or changes in texture. Has the nipple drawn back or turned in since your last examination? Look inside your bra for any signs of discharge.

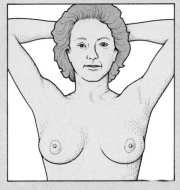

Lift the breasts to examine them underneath. Raise your hands above your head and see if there is any swelling or skin puckering on the upper breast or around the armpit. Turn from side to side and check again.

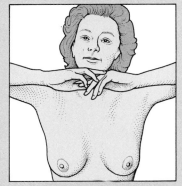

Lower your arms and raise them to chin level. Have both nipples moved upward to the same extent? Lean forward and examine each breast for unusual changes in outline, dimpling, or retraction of the nipple. Press your palms together and look for any changes.

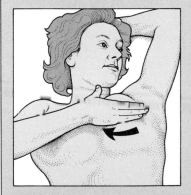

Lie down in a relaxed, comfortable position, either on a bed with a folded towel under your left shoulder blade, or in the bath. Put your left hand under your head. Examine your left breast with your right hand. Use the front part of the flat of your hand and keep your fingers straight and close together.

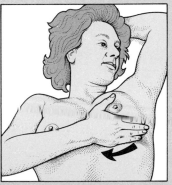

Slide your hand above and below the nipple, from the armpit to the center of the body. Using a circular motion press gently to feel for lumps. Lower your arm and feel for lumps again.

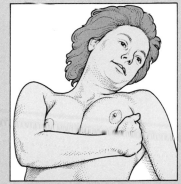

Pass your hand from the bottom of the breast, across the nipple, and upward to the armpit. Slide your hand sideways and diagonally across the breast and over the nipple, making sure you have felt all parts of the breast. Feel for any lumps in the armpit or the top of the collarbone. Now examine the right breast with your left hand.

Menopause marks the end of a woman's reproductive life. It can be a difficult time for many women, since it involves not only adjusting to the psychological fact of losing fertility but also coping with physical symptoms caused by hormonal changes, which can be unpleasant. In the past, the "change of life" was dreaded as the beginning of a steady decline. Now, however, women view menopause more positively, and with self-help and medical care, they can expect an easier passage to a new and fulfilling life.

What is menopause?

Menopause is a stage in life that lasts a year or two. It is not an illness. The cessation of regular menstrual periods characterizes menopause. The ovaries become resistant to instructions from the pituitary and stop maturing the eggs that have been present in them since birth. Since the stock of eggs has been depleted over 30 to 40 years, progressively fewer eggs are released. This interrupts the cyclic production of the hormone progesterone, which in turn prevents the release of sufficient hormones from the pituitary to trigger the growth and shedding of the uterine lining (menstruation).

The end of menstruation can occur at any time between the ages of 36 and 56, though the median age seems to be 48. There is no truth in the old wives' tale of early puberty/late menopause and late puberty/early menopause. Sometimes menstruation stops abruptly. More commonly, however, a few months of irregular bleeding are followed by normal losses, then a few more months of irregular bleeding until bleeding ceases altogether. A year without bleeding in a woman under 50, or six months in a woman over 50 can usually be taken as the end of menstruation. Contraceptive precautions must be used during the entire menopause since there is still a slight chance of pregnancy occurring.

Menstruation stops if a woman's womb is removed before she reaches menopause. This operation, called a hysterectomy, is carried out in about 19 percent of females 15 years and older. Most hysterectomies are performed to treat gynecological problems, including pain. If the ovaries are left in place, they will continue to secrete female hormones until the natural menopausal changes take place. If the ovaries are removed, estrogen replacement therapy is usually prescribed.

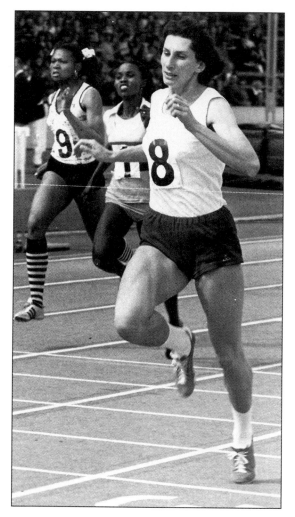

Gold medal winner *Irena Szewinska, the Polish 400m runner, approaching midlife, and still competing successfully against girls 20 years her junior.*

Problems of menopause

Women suffer menopausal problems to different degrees. The major physical symptoms are hot flashes and sweats and loss of lubrication in the vagina, which are believed to be caused by low estrogen levels.

Hot flashes can occur frequently or infrequently either during the day or night. A feeling of intense heat lasting several seconds or minutes suddenly spreads over the upper part or whole body and sometimes causes a reaction similar to blushing as well as sweating. Night sweats often

Hormone replacement therapy (HRT): the facts

● Suitable only for women with a clean bill of health.

● Those found suitable are given estrogen and/or progesterone in pill form, by implant, or injection.

● Estrogen creams can be applied locally for dry vagina or dry nasal mucous membrane.

● HRT helps to relieve hot flashes, night sweats, dry vagina, and osteoporosis.

● Treatment is given for three years or longer, and is also used to counteract the effects of aging.

● Some studies suggest that HRT might lead to cancer of the breast and uterus, heart disease, and gallstones, but these might merely be signs of aging.

cause insomnia, a reason in itself for exhaustion, irritability, and depression during waking hours. Some women never have them, others have them for years, but most experience them spasmodically for a few months.

One of the most troublesome symptoms for sexually active women is loss of lubrication of the vagina caused by reduced estrogen levels. The lining of the vagina also becomes thinner, which may make intercourse uncomfortable. It may also make a woman vulnerable to vaginal and urethral infections, which can cause bleeding and ulceration of the vaginal walls. The resulting disinclination for sex can fit in well with the aging male partner's loss of sexual interest or capacity, or can become a source of friction between two people whose sexual desires no longer happen to coincide.

Women might also complain of other symptoms, including irritating dryness of the nasal mucous membrane, headache, palpitations, dizziness, weight gain, abdominal pains, nausea, vomiting, swollen ankles, and loss of memory and concentration. As yet there is no established link between menopause and these symptoms, and according to one study only 20 percent of women suffer them severely enough to cause any disruption of life. Symptoms should not be endured— they can be treated, so seek expert advice from your doctor or gynecologist.

Reassessing your lifestyle

Emotionally, menopause is a highly charged time and some women find it difficult to separate physical from emotional symptoms. The end of childbearing can be traumatic for those who equate worth with motherhood, particularly if menopause coincides with the time when children start to leave home. Many women believe that menopause signals the end of their sex lives; most find this time of reassessment painful and disquieting. The stress of midlife problems can lead to depression as a woman struggles to achieve a new role and meaning in life. If severe, this needs expert treatment (see pages 278–279).

Yet the "change" can be a change for the good. Positive rethinking is crucial to "life after youth." With the burdens of menstruation and fear of an unwanted pregnancy lifted, women should search for new interests, work, and continue to enjoy a full sex life.

Checklist

Seek medical attention if you are suffering from any of the following:

● Hot flashes

● Night sweats

● Nasal dryness

● Vaginal dryness

● Irregular vaginal bleeding

● Headaches

● Palpitations

● Dizziness

● Abdominal pains

● Nausea

● Swollen ankles

If the menopause is upsetting you emotionally:

● Speak to a close friend or therapist.

● Explain it to your partner, friends, and children.

● See your doctor.

● Exercise regularly.

● Eat sensibly.

● Find a new interest or hobby.

● Pay attention to your appearance to keep up your morale.

● Think positively about your future.

MALE HEALTH SCREENING

The midlife transition strikes many men hard. Although there are no sudden hormonal changes as in women, men can feel abnormally stressed— a feeling that often results in some dramatic alteration of behavior.

Awareness of the implications of the midlife transition makes it easier to cope and to develop a more positive attitude. For midlife is not the end to a man's sex life, particularly if he pays careful attention to his health.

Health screening for men

Sexual health is an integral part of whole body health. If a man does not feel well in himself, is constantly overtired or under pressure, is suffering the effects of drink excesses or drugs, or is prey to a debilitating illness, his sexual needs and performance will decline. Although every man should make routine health screening part of his health program before he reaches middle age, it is more important during middle age since there is an increased risk of cancer, strokes, and heart, lung, and liver disease.

A comprehensive screening that should be able to detect diseases and disorders will include tests for blood pressure, and heart and lung function; analyze the blood for fat content and liver, kidney, and metabolic disease; and test the urine for diabetes. Since such tests build up a comprehensive picture of a man's health, the doctor can suggest alterations in lifestyle and habits. Cutting out smoking, reducing drinking, eating a healthier diet, and making time for more exercise, vacations, and outside interests will all contribute to improved fitness, which will be reflected in a more vital sex life.

Within this context, there are only a few conditions that actually inhibit a man's sexual performance and comfort. Aside from physical defects, which require surgical treatment, the main problems include urinary infections, enlargement of the prostate gland, sexually transmitted diseases, drugs, and alcohol. Any infections demand immediate treatment and abstinence from sex until they have cleared up. Antidepressant drugs, often prescribed to combat the emotional problems, frequently diminish a man's sexual desire, which can increase his anxiety, and deepen his depression.

A partner must be reassuring to avoid a complete breakdown in sexual relations, and men might gain closeness and pleasure from sexual contacts other than intercourse. Alcohol, with its depressant qualities, is often the reason for incapacity. After a number of failures, a man might become psychologically impotent, thus exacerbating his physical failure. Less alcohol and a realization of its effect will do a great deal to restore a man's potency.

The midlife transition

Middle age has a curious way of stealing up and catching you unaware. For a man suddenly confronted with this undeniable reality, the physical facts of aging can be traumatic. As a result, many men develop uncharacteristic vanities and attempt to recapture their youthful appearance to little effect.

Many men feel pressured into a reappraisal of their lives, and those who are already insecure, anxious, and defensive might become distressed about the future, their financial status, their career, domestic problems, health, and much more. All this self-obsession leads to the typical midlife symptoms: tension, depression, irritability, resentment, and a concern for the male image. Such turmoil can create problems for a man's partner, who might herself be undergoing a similar rethinking of her life, as well as coping with the physical symptoms of menopause.

Some men are known to experience physical symptoms such as hot flashes, insomnia, palpitations, loss of memory and so on, similar to those experienced by women during menopause, although there is no evidence of a diminished hormone output in men of this age group.

Many men regard the gradually diminishing sexual powers of the middle years as an affront and as a threat to their masculinity. The solution for some is to seek out younger women, who they hope will restore their virility and self-image; some achieve temporary or long-term satisfaction in this way, others do not.

Improving relationships

Reduced sexual interest within a marriage can be upsetting for both partners, and the woman might feel she no longer inspires affection or desire. She then suppresses her own desires until the man also feels rejected, and the resulting tension spills over into other areas of the relationship.

It is important for a man to realize that his

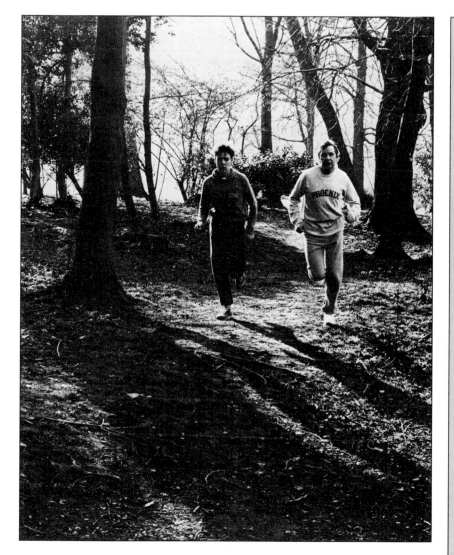

Regular exercise can do much to revitalize a man's middle years. It will not only give him more physical and mental energy but will also help to counteract the effects of stress. At a time when teenage children are beginning to grow away from their parents, a shared activity such as running can help promote the development of a caring, adult relationship between a father and his sons or daughters.

When your sex life suffers:

● Try reducing your alcohol intake to improve potency.

● Have a urinary test if you suspect an infection.

● Lose some weight to improve general fitness and vitality.

● Do more exercise to increase energy.

● Consult your doctor for a change of drugs or other advice.

● Have a complete health screening.

● Take a vacation with the woman you love.

● Try having sex in the mornings and on weekends, not on week nights when you are tired after the working day.

sexual prowess and desire will decline as he ages. This is a fact of mature sexual life. There will be a gradual curtailment of libido, a lengthening of the time taken to achieve an erection, and a decline in orgasmic potential. If the physical quality of sex wanes with aging, the emotional pleasure and intimacy can still remain. It is, therefore, essential that couples take time to reopen lines of communication and reassure each other about their continuing affection, attraction, and sexual abilities (see pages 194–195).

Middle age should not be an end. There are many years ahead, and there is no reason why sex should not be an integral part of them.

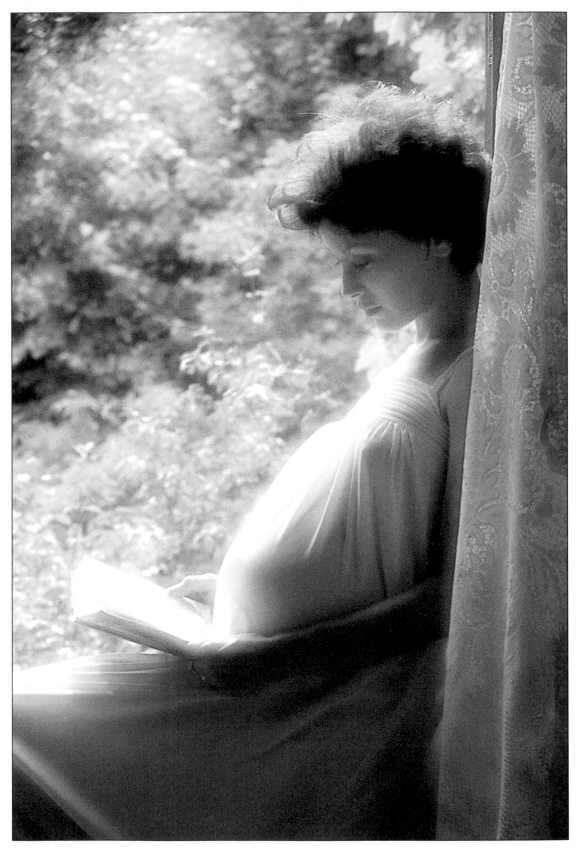

PREGNANCY AND BIRTH

The discovery that a baby is expected is one of life's most exciting moments. During the next few months, especially if it is a first baby, both parents-to-be will experience a wealth of new feelings, from exhilaration to fear.

Over the last half century, increasing self-awareness and concern for healthy living have produced an enormous change in attitudes toward pregnancy and birth. No longer are women confined, literally, during their pregnancy; many work outside the home until ten weeks before the birth. Diet and exercise, and giving up cigarettes and alcohol, are now considered as important a part of prenatal care as medical checks. There is the growing movement toward encouraging prospective parents to look at, and if necessary reform, their lifestyles even before a baby is conceived.

Medical science, working toward safer births and improved health of mothers and babies, has made enormous strides. It has also presented the expectant mother with many more choices. For example, she can decide on the position she prefers for labor, and whether or not to have an anesthetic.

From the mine of information and advice that exists on pregnancy, this chapter focuses on the essentials, to provide parents with the basic information they need about fitness and well-being during pregnancy, labor, birth, and after delivery. In most cases, a healthy mother means a healthy baby and a healthier start to life.

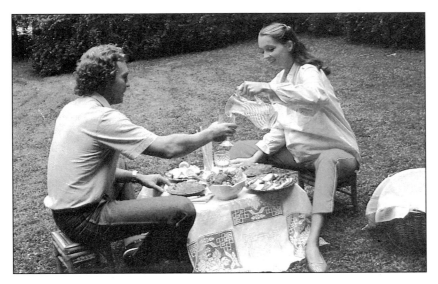

Both partners should be
nutrition-conscious when
they are planning to have a
baby. Do not eat high-protein
foods to the exclusion of
carbohydrates. Choose fresh
foods and avoid foods
preserved in sugar.

*Unrefined foods contain
more desirable nutrients.
Proteins, vitamins, and
minerals, such as calcium
and iron, are needed for
body building, the prevention
of illness, and avoiding
problems during pregnancy
such as iron-deficiency
anemia.*

Pregnancy is a time in a woman's life when it is important for her to be as fit as possible. Increasingly, doctors are also stressing the significance of health care and fitness during the months prior to conception for both the potential parents. If you are already pregnant, then do not worry about what you should or should not have been doing up to now. Whatever stage you are at, it is not too late to begin working toward a healthier lifestyle for the rest of your pregnancy, and it is important that you do not feel guilty about events that are already in the past.

Preconception care

A healthy way of life adopted before conception might lessen the risks to the growing baby during the crucial early weeks of development, when a woman might be unaware that she is pregnant. The baby's spinal cord develops between $4\frac{1}{2}$ and $6\frac{1}{2}$ weeks, the arms during the same period, the legs between $5\frac{1}{2}$ and $7\frac{1}{2}$ weeks, and by the eighth week of pregnancy, the fetal heart is beating.

If you are planning a baby, then first you must stop contraception. If you are taking the pill, you should switch to a barrier method, such as the diaphragm or condom (see pages 198–199) for at least three months to allow time for the natural pattern of hormone production and egg release to be re-established. And remember that it takes one in eight couples longer than a year to conceive.

If you and/or your partner smoke, try to stop, or at least cut down. Reduce your alcohol consump-

tion as well—even an occasional overindulgence is not a good idea. Diet is also very important. Your doctor might prescribe iron and folic acid supplements. Pay attention to your weight before conception. While being overweight is not ideal, crash dieting can impair fertility. You should not go on a reducing diet once you are pregnant, but you can make sure that you are within the desired weight range for your height and build before you conceive (see pages 72–75).

There are several other matters that call for medical guidance. Ask your doctor to check that you are immune to German measles (rubella). If you need immunization, continue to practice birth control for at least three months afterward, for while the vaccine is taking effect, it might damage a growing fetus.

If you work with children or in a hospital, beware of infections, especially any viral infections, such as rubella or mumps, to which you may not be immune. Discuss with your doctor any noxious chemicals that you or your partner might have contact with or be exposed to at work. The possible effects on the unborn child of many chemicals is unknown, but if you work with such substances, explore the possibility of transferring to another department for the duration of your pregnancy. Avoid any unnecessary X-ray examinations during pregnancy.

Talk to your doctor about any medications you are taking, including creams, sprays, and cough mixtures. Some antibiotics and steroids are

The menstrual cycle is governed by hormones and operates so that an ovum, or egg, is released from the ovary approximately once every 28 days, a process known as ovulation. The cycle also ensures that the uterus is prepared to receive and nurture the egg if it is fertilized by a sperm. If fertilization does not occur, then the uterine lining is shed as the menstrual period. If the ovum is fertilized, continued hormone production ensures that menstruation does not take place.

THE MENSTRUAL CYCLE

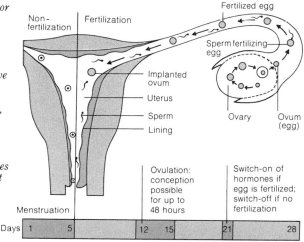

Smoking and alcohol

Nicotine, carbon monoxide, and alcohol are poisonous substances that damage the placenta, thus reducing the amount of oxygen and food reaching the baby. This raises the fetal heart rate, leading to fetal distress.

Congenital problems also result from deficiencies of vitamins, minerals, and calories at an early stage of fetal development.

A woman who smokes during pregnancy has a 00 percent greater chance of miscarrying or losing the baby through complications at birth. The baby is also more likely to be premature, have a low birth weight, and run a greater risk of infection.

Drinking can affect the development of the fetus, causing fetal alcohol syndrome—malformation of the heart, limbs, and face.

potentially harmful to a fetus. Ask the doctor's advice about taking aspirin or aspirin substitutes. For safety's sake, it is advisable to do without any medications if you can. Of course, drugs of addiction or habituation are definitely harmful to the baby.

If you take medication for a chronic condition, such as diabetes or epilepsy, consult your physician before you attempt to conceive. Your doctor might suggest altering your medication and you might need time to adjust to the new dosage.

Remember to tell your dentist too that you are planning to have a baby before he prescribes any drugs or gives you an anesthetic.

If you are concerned about handicaps and diseases passed on in the family of either potential parent, ask your doctor if he can recommend a genetic advisory center. Otherwise, contact any large hospital in your area. A genetic counselor will be able to advise you and your partner of the risk of your baby being affected.

Many genetic abnormalities cannot be tested for before conception. Down's syndrome, or "mongolism," for example, is caused by an extra chromosome, so the fetus has 47 instead of 46 chromosomes. The chances of giving birth to a baby with Down's syndrome increase with the mother's age: at 35 the risk is 1 in 300, at 40 it is 1 in 100, and by 46 it is 1 in 40. Spina bifida, in which the spinal cord develops abnormally, is not related to the age of the mother. Both can be detected during pregnancy (see pages 218–219).

Preconception checklist

Before you try to get pregnant:

● Stop contraception: if on the pill, switch to a barrier method for 3 months first.

● Stop smoking: if you cannot, a maximum 5 cigarettes a day is a reasonable target.

● Reduce consumption of alcohol: 2 glasses of white wine a week is a good target.

● Eat a balanced and nutritious diet.

● Check with your doctor about rubella and other viral infections.

Sports

If you have never exercised or played a sport, then pregnancy is not the time to take up vigorous activity. A brisk walk every day is excellent exercise, and swimming is one of the best forms of all-around exercise. Start an exercise program specifically tailored for pregnant women (see pages 224–229). Some women if they are already fit, successfully continue playing tennis or other sports until well into their pregnancies.

Infertility

Despite preconceptual care, one in 10 couples is thought to suffer from infertility, with the causes lying roughly 60 percent in women and 40 percent in men.

Causes: Most female infertility results from either ovulation dysfunction—problems with the growth and release of the egg—or problems with the reproductive organs, such as blocked Fallopian tubes, or scar tissue around the ovaries, uterus, and tubes. Other causes of infertility involve the uterus, which must be in good condition to allow for implantation and proper growth of the fertilized egg; and the cervix, which has to produce a good-quality mucus to provide a proper environment for the sperm.

A man is considered infertile if he has a low sperm count (oligospermia) or defective sperm. The causes are many and varied, and include hormonal disorders, chromosome abnormalities, disorders in the body's immune system, a varicose vein in the testicle (varicocele), undescended testicles, infections, disease of the prostate gland or seminal vesicles, defects in the penis, and blocked transport ducts. In some men no cause can be found for a low sperm count.

Both partners might have one or more fertility problems. It is also common for both partners to be only slightly infertile, or subfertile. Each one matched with a more fertile partner might produce children, but together they are infertile. Sometimes a couple fails to achieve pregnancy simply because they use lubricants, which can immobilize sperm, or because they have intercourse prior to ovulation.

Tests: Both partners need to be examined. A woman's ovulation can be checked by measuring body temperature and by blood tests. Simple surgical investigations will detect blockages of the Fallopian tubes or scar tissue binding the reproductive organs.

Semen analysis, the main way to ascertain a male's fertility, is carried out on a sample of seminal fluid. It shows the quantity and quality of sperm and the volume and quality of the fluid.

Treatments: Depending on the cause of infertility, a woman might be treated with fertility drugs to promote ovulation, or have surgery to remove any blockages or adhesions in her reproductive organs. If her Fallopian tubes are irreparable, she might be suitable for *in vitro* fertilization, which offers only a 5 to 10 percent chance of success.

A man with a low sperm count might be advised to wear loose underwear and avoid exposure to excessive heat. If necessary, he can be treated with fertility drugs, and have surgery to correct blockages and varicose veins.

Artificial insemination with the partner's sperm is also a possibility.

Miscarriage

Miscarriage, or spontaneous abortion, occurs in 15 to 20 percent of pregnancies, most often before week 12. After week 28, it is called premature labor. Abnormal development of the fertilized egg due to a chromosome abnormality is the most common reason. Other causes include hypertension, kidney disease, hormonal imbalance, certain drugs, malformed uterus, fibroid tumors, and weak cervix.

Some miscarriages are accompanied by minor cramps, and some are completely painless. A woman should consult her doctor about any vaginal bleeding during pregnancy. A missed abortion is the term used when an embryo dies and is retained in the uterus. Many of the signs of pregnancy disappear, but menstruation does not return. The pregnancy will eventually abort spontaneously, but a D and C, short for dilation and curettage (see page 205), is usually performed as soon as the condition is diagnosed.

After a miscarriage, a woman will have a D and C to ensure that all the products of the conception have been removed from the uterus to reduce the risk of heavy bleeding and possible infection.

A miscarriage is difficult for both partners to cope with emotionally, particularly because there is no tangible evidence of loss. It is important not to blame yourselves or each other. Remember too that grieving is both a normal and necessary part of accepting what has happened.

A woman's chance of a normal pregnancy is not affected by having one or more miscarriages, unless there is a recurring cause. If you have had a miscarriage, discuss with your doctor the best time to try to conceive again. This will depend partly on the stage of the pregnancy at which you miscarried and partly on your feelings about trying again.

Once you suspect you are pregnant, you will want confirmation as soon as possible. A missed period may well be the first indication, but there are other symptoms that could give you a clue. Your breasts might feel tender and swollen; you might urinate more frequently; you might feel tired and listless for no apparent reason; you might experience nausea, find certain food and drinks distasteful, or lose your desire for alcohol and cigarettes. The feeling of being pregnant is so distinctive that many women in their second and subsequent pregnancies know within a matter of days that they have conceived.

Pregnancy testing

You can use a home pregnancy test available from drugstores or ask your doctor or gynecologist to have a test done. Most testing requires a urine sample. If you are pregnant, it will contain the tell-tale hormone, human chorionic gonadotrophin (HCG). A urine test is reliable six weeks after the start of your last period. A blood test will confirm pregnancy earlier. Alternative means of obtaining a pregnancy test include family planning clinics, health centers, and pregnancy advice services.

Once your pregnancy is confirmed, your doctor will calculate when the baby is due. Pregnancy lasts, on the average, 266 days from conception, but since few women know exactly when they conceive, 280 days are added to the date of the first day of the last menstrual period, to give an estimated delivery date. This, in fact, adds up to nine months and seven days, but a full-term baby could arrive two weeks before or two weeks after the estimated delivery date.

Because this is such an important time in your life, be certain to choose a doctor with whom you feel comfortable discussing your concerns. Your doctor will make arrangements for your prenatal care once your pregnancy is confirmed. He will arrange a schedule in order to monitor your health and that of the developing fetus. Initially these visits will be on a monthly basis, becoming more frequent during the weeks immediately preceding the birth. You might have to visit the hospital for special tests (such as ultrasound or amniocentesis, see pages 218–219). Alternatively, depending on where you live and your doctor, you might consider a home birth with a doctor and midwife.

Prenatal checks

During your first visit to the doctor after your pregnancy is confirmed, he will ask for many details of your personal medical history and that of your partner. He will also enquire about your work and lifestyle, and that of your partner, to pinpoint any danger areas. Remember that this is your opportunity to ask questions, too.

From then on, your visits to the doctor should be every month until the twenty-eighth week of pregnancy, after which they will be every two weeks until the final month, during which you should see him every week. Regular prenatal visits are essential. The results from tests carried out at your first visit are the yardstick against which all subsequent findings are compared. Any fluctuations in readings that might be significant to the health of either mother or baby need to be carefully monitored at all stages of pregnancy to reduce risks as much as possible.

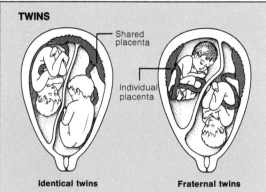

TWINS

Shared placenta

Individual placenta

Identical twins   **Fraternal twins**

Identical twins are formed when one egg splits into two. Nonidentical, or fraternal, twins occur when two eggs are fertilized at the same time. A woman whose mother had fraternal twins is almost twice as likely to have twins as a woman with no twins in her family. You are more likely to have twins if you are between the ages 35 and 40, and if you already have children (especially twins).

The position of the uterus can be the earliest clue to twins. With a singleton, the doctor can feel a firm lump behind the pubic bone by the twelfth week of pregnancy; with twins this might be evident by the eighth week. If the doctor thinks you might be carrying twins, an ultrasound scan will confirm or deny his suspicions any time after the eighth week.

You are more likely to become anemic if you are carrying twins, and your doctor might prescribe more than usual quantities of iron and folic acid tablets to counteract this. The difficulties or problems associated with pregnancy increase more quickly in a multiple pregnancy, but twins go to full term (40 weeks) only occasionally.

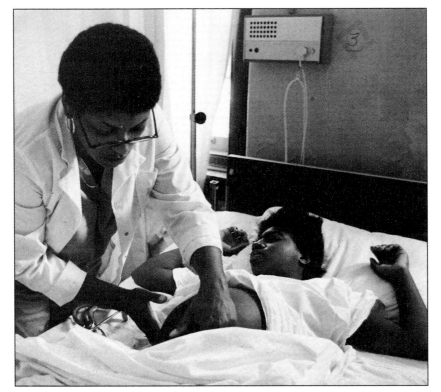

By feeling, or palpating, the abdomen, a doctor can detect the position of the baby.

Routine tests

Routine tests on urine and blood enable checks on several aspects of your health. The urine sample will reveal any kidney infections (many of which would otherwise go unnoticed but cause complications during pregnancy) and diabetes. The urine protein level is also tested, since later in pregnancy its rise can indicate pre-eclampsia, a medical problem that puts the baby at risk because it interferes with the proper functioning of the placenta.

A blood test will reveal your blood type. If you are Rhesus negative and your baby inherits a Rhesus positive blood type from his father, you can build up antibodies that can harm subsequent babies. This problem is easily dealt with by giving the mother an injection of anti-D globulin after the birth of the first child. Tests on the blood will also show whether you are anemic, immune to rubella, or have a disease harmful to you and the baby, such as syphilis.

Blood pressure measurement is part of the prenatal routine. Blood pressure tends to increase in 20 to 25 percent of pregnancies and can indicate serious problems that need careful medical monitoring to protect the baby.

At each prenatal visit the doctor will feel the abdomen to locate the top of the uterus and the position of the baby. This gives a clue to the stage of your pregnancy, although only an ultrasound examination (see opposite) will give an accurate estimate of this. Initially you will have a vaginal examination to enable the doctor to feel the uterus and check for pelvic abnormalities.

Self-help routines

The establishment of a routine of prenatal care goes hand in hand with your self-care, once you know that you are pregnant. The commonsense practices recommended in preconceptual care, such as giving up smoking and drinking, are now essential to maintain maximum fitness and health during pregnancy. The correct diet and exercise, as well as regular check-ups, will give your baby the best chance of a healthy start in life. They will also prepare you in the best possible way for the physical and psychological impact of the months before and immediately after the birth.

THE GROWTH OF THE BABY

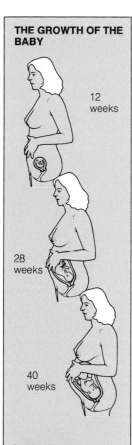

12 weeks

28 weeks

40 weeks

At 12 weeks the baby is about 2 inches long and all major organs have formed. By 28 weeks the baby is often head-down, ready for delivery. It would have a slim chance of survival if born now. At full term (40 weeks), the abdomen may appear to get smaller as the baby's head enters the pelvis.

Special tests

As well as routine prenatal checks, your doctor may advise certain special tests. If these tests reveal a fetal deformity, parents may decide to terminate the pregnancy. Tests for serum alpha fetoprotein (AFP) are routine in many hospitals. AFP enters the mother's bloodstream if the baby is suffering from an abnormality such as spina bifida. It can also indicate multiple pregnancy. AFP tests are usually carried out at about the sixteenth or seventeenth week of pregnancy and are routine if the mother has already given birth to a child with spina bifida or if either parent has a family history of the abnormality.

Amniocentesis to detect Down's syndrome involves the insertion of a needle into the uterus. A small amount of the amniotic fluid that surrounds the growing baby is obtained, and its cells studied for chromosomal and other defects. At the moment, this test cannot be carried out until the sixteenth week, although it may soon be possible much earlier. It carries with it the risk of spontaneous abortion of approximately 1 in 300. It is usually offered to women aged 35 and over; at 35 there is a 1 in 300 chance of having a baby with Down's syndrome.

Ultrasound safety
Ultrasound gives instant results with no risk of miscarriage.

Between the 12th and 16th weeks of pregnancy, a scan can estimate the gestational age of the baby by measuring it. At this stage, a scan will reveal twins or other prospective multiple births and some abnormalities.

Between 30 and 36 weeks, a scan can assess fetal maturity and thus confirm the delivery date. At this stage a scan will also reveal the position of the baby, which might have implications for the delivery. The position and condition of the placenta can also affect the passage of the baby down the birth canal.

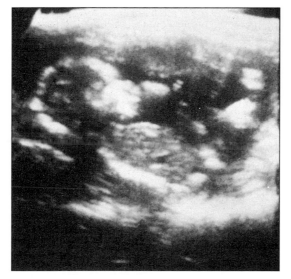

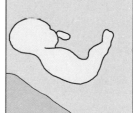

This simple interpretation of the ultrasound scan (at left) shows the development of the unborn baby to be normal for 18 weeks. The head and body are clearly visible, and one leg, with a well-formed foot, can also be distinguished.

An ultrasound scan involves bouncing ultrasonic sound waves off certain body tissues to reveal an image of the baby on a screen. The image is often fuzzy and unclear, and can be interpreted only by someone with a trained eye. The operator will point out the baby's limbs and head, certain organs, such as the heart and stomach, and the placenta. Most prospective parents find the experience both exciting and reassuring.

STAYING FIT IN PREGNANCY

Make staying fit and healthy throughout pregnancy your goal. Right from the early stages, it is important to learn about and practice a healthy lifestyle. You are now concerned with the health and well-being of two people: you and your baby. Pregnancy is an individual experience and each woman reacts differently. Real and rapid changes will occur, and it is a time to pay particular attention to the messages that your body sends you.

More and more women work outside the home during pregnancy, and they also continue to work closer to the time of birth than their mothers did. However, it is wise to know and respect your limitations at this time. Try to rearrange your hours of work so that you do not travel at the height of the rush hour, and avoid strain and tiredness. Try to rest for an hour with your feet up when you get home. If you are not going out to work, make sure that a period of relaxation becomes part of your daily routine.

The nine months of pregnancy are customarily divided into trimesters, or three-month periods. Each has an individual character that you can generally predict, but do not become alarmed if your pregnancy does not exactly match the expectations. Your doctor is the best person to answer any questions that you might have regarding your baby's development.

The first trimester
Because of the hormonal changes taking place during the first three months, you might experience increased fatigue, nausea, and heightened emotional sensitivity. The demands on your body are greater now, so plan some time to rest and try not to get overtired. To combat nausea, eat small portions of plain, easily digestible foods rather than large meals, and avoid greasy, salty, and sugar-laden foods. Antinausea medication should be taken only on your physician's advice.

Get proper nutrition in the form of a well-balanced diet (see pages 52–93), and definitely do not begin any type of weight loss program during your pregnancy. By the same token, under no circumstances should you "eat for two" at this time. Although weight gain is personal and does vary widely, 25 to 30 pounds is a reasonable amount of weight to gain during the next nine months. As a rough guide, you will put on a quarter of your total weight gain between about weeks 12 and 20, half between weeks 20 and 30, and the remaining quarter after that. Many women stop gaining weight following about the 36th week, and some start to lose weight in the days before the birth. Remember that it is notoriously hard to lose excess weight after the birth, so try to keep your weight in check without dieting. It is also recommended that you completely eliminate cigarettes and drugs, and eliminate or reduce to a minimum your consumption of caffeine and alcohol.

Hormonal changes can slow bowel movements and cause constipation. Drinking plenty of water and eating high-fiber foods, such as fruits and vegetables, whole-wheat bread, and cereal, will help this condition. A constant need to urinate might prove an inconvenience, so be certain you have easy access to a restroom. Possible vaginal discharge can lead to irritation and an increased susceptibility to vaginal infections. All-cotton underwear is a good idea, and wearing white will

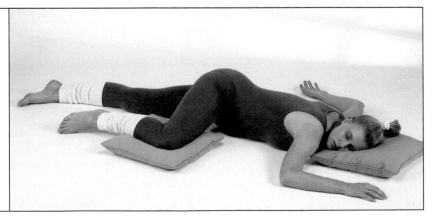

RELAXING
Lying on your side, with all parts of your body supported, is a good position in which to relax. You might also find this a comfortable position to adopt during the early part of labor.

help you to detect a discharge. If you experience vaginal bleeding, treat this as serious and consult your doctor.

The second trimester
After the 12th or 14th week you might develop the "bloom" of pregnancy, with shining hair, a clear skin, and a general glow of well-being. Any initial fatigue and nausea should have abated, and you will have renewed energy. Regular exercise will be a very important factor in your health during and after your pregnancy. It is not the time to embark on any type of new, rigorous activity, but continuing a familiar program or sport is beneficial. An exercise program for pregnant women begins on page 222. Aside from the physical benefits of a fitness routine, you will have increased pep and energy, and looking better enhances your self-image.

As the baby grows and you begin to feel its movement, you will experience a shift in your balance and posture. Your waistline will begin to disappear, so wear comfortable and loose-fitting clothing, preferably made of natural fibers that can "breathe." You have 40 to 60 percent more blood in your body by now, which can lead to leg cramps and varicose veins. Exercises that tone leg muscles help to pump blood more efficiently and will compensate for circulatory changes. The varicose veins usually disappear after pregnancy.

Take a positive approach to these middle months by keeping up a meticulous routine of personal hygiene. This includes having your teeth checked by your dentist, since you could experience trouble with your teeth and gums. When you brush your teeth, the gums might bleed

easily and become inflamed. Your teeth might also suffer from calcium depletion as the baby's bones are built, so be sure to include calcium-rich foods, such as dairy products and leafy green vegetables, in your diet.

You may wish to start massaging your breasts and nipples to prepare for feeding. This might be especially necessary if you have flat or inverted nipples. Draw them out with your fingers or wear a plastic nipple shell inside your bra. Your breasts will be heavier throughout pregnancy, so a well-fitting, or specially designed, maternity bra is essential for comfort and support.

The third trimester
During the last trimester, as the baby completes its growth, you might feel more tired and experience a change in your breathing pattern. Deep-breathing techniques will help you to feel more energized and will ensure proper oxygen supply to the baby. Remember to eat properly and get extra rest. Do not put unnecessary demands on your body. Avoid lifting, long periods standing up, and crowded situations. Plan ahead to make sure you can be comfortable.

Your partner
While you are experiencing the varied joys of pregnancy, it is important to share events and feelings with your partner. There is no reason why normal sexual activity cannot continue during this time, although your doctor will advise you if you need to exercise caution during the first trimester and final weeks before delivery. Modify and experiment with sexual positions that ensure your comfort as the baby grows.

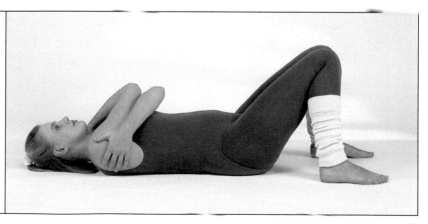

CONSTRUCTIVE REST
Lie on your back, with your knees bent and resting together. Cross your arms on your chest and gently hug your shoulders.

Close attention to your health and well-being during the months of your pregnancy will pay off in dividends of easier labor, delivery of your baby, and postnatal recovery. If your pregnancy is normal and uncomplicated, you can exercise. A strong and flexible body works more efficiently and tires less easily. Exercises can be relaxing and enjoyable. They should be done regularly, and setting a specific time will help you to remember to do them every day. As with any exercise program, wait at least one hour after eating to begin activity, wear comfortable and nonbinding clothing, and avoid extremes in temperature.

The exercises and positions that you see in these and the next four pages can be done throughout your pregnancy. Modify them to accommodate your new size as your baby grows. Remember to be sensitive to the changes in your body, and discontinue any exercise that causes you pain or discomfort.

Points to keep in mind when planning your fitness program are good posture and muscle tone to prevent back pain, pectoral strength to prevent sagging shoulders, and strong leg, back, and arm muscles to compensate for the shift in your center of gravity. Cardiovascular exercises, such as walking, bicycling, and swimming, are excellent for increasing your level of aerobic fitness. But understand that vigorous exercise raises the body temperature and heart rate. Be sure to monitor your pulse rate during these activities and do not exceed a safe level. Check with your doctor. Joggers who wish to continue their sport should generally limit workouts to 20 minutes in order to prevent overheating.

Pelvic exercises are important. You should be particularly aware of the muscles of the pelvic floor that control the vaginal and anal openings. Practice the pelvic tilt exercise shown here. It will teach you to maintain proper posture and alignment while sitting, standing, and walking. The head roll and shoulder circle exercises will help you to relieve upper back and neck tension, and should be done frequently during the day.

Pay close attention to how you move while performing daily activities. When you are lifting, always bend your knees and keep objects (or small children) close to you. Use your strong thigh muscles for support. Practicing the "cat" position and twist will teach you how to stretch and relax your back muscles and maintain flexibility.

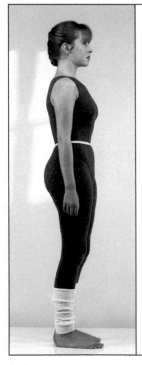

POSTURE
Good posture is important. Use your abdominal muscles to straighten your spine. Tuck your bottom in and keep your shoulders down.

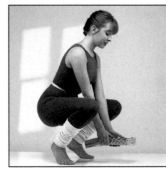

LIFTING
When you are lifting, always bend your knees to avoid back strain. This is especially important if you already have small children.

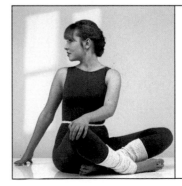

SIDE TWIST
Sit cross-legged on the floor, with your back erect. Grasp your right knee with your left hand, and twist your shoulder and neck so that you are looking over your shoulder. Repeat 5 times on each side.

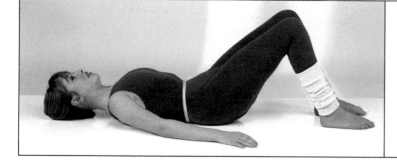

PELVIC TILT
Lie on your back, with your knees bent. Tense your inner thighs and groin area. Then press in your abdomen as your pelvis tilts up. Tighten your buttock muscles to hold and set the position.
Repeat 5 times.

CAT POSITION

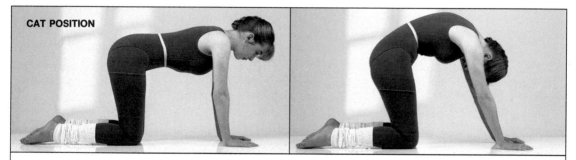

1. On your hands and knees, arms straight and stomach in, make your back as flat as a table as you inhale.

2. Exhale and pull your head down, pressing your stomach in and rounding your back. Lift your tailbone and return to flat back position. Repeat 5 times.

HEAD ROLLS
1.

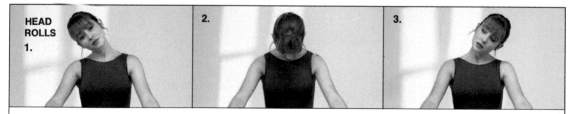

1. Sit cross-legged on the floor. Bend your right ear toward your shoulder.

2. Continue down and through to the opposite side. Inhale as the head goes back, exhale as it goes forward.

3. Reverse direction. Repeat 5 times in each direction.

SHOULDER ROLLS
1.

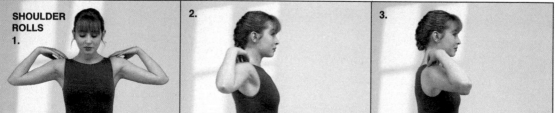
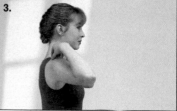

1. Sit cross-legged on the floor, or sit on a chair. Put your hands on your shoulders.

2. With your fingertips on your shoulders, draw backward circles in the air with your elbows.

3. Don't hunch your shoulders— keep a long space between your ear and shoulder. Repeat 5 times.

Because of the hormones produced during pregnancy, you might find it easier than ever before to do stretches. During this time it is important not to overestimate your flexibility, which could strain joints and cause problems later. Focus your attention on graceful movements (perhaps to music) that are in harmony with your body in terms of its constantly changing shape and weight. Perform your exercises slowly and carefully to gain maximum benefit.

You might begin to experience swelling in your legs and ankles due to water retention and increased weight. To encourage better circulation, avoid sitting cross-legged, do the ankle circles as shown in the hamstring stretch exercise opposite, and wear low-heeled shoes.

Now that the important abdominal muscles are less available, increase the strength of your arms, legs and back to support you. The curl-up and side stretch are designed to stretch and strengthen the muscles around the rib cage and waist. Chair sitting against the wall helps to lengthen and relax lower back muscles while it firms your thighs. You will find that the cat stretch is a great stress-reliever.

Plan a regular exercise routine that fits into your lifestyle. Twenty minutes each day is all you need to perform the exercises shown here. Try to do at least five repetitions, and remember to breathe fully, exhaling on the effort.

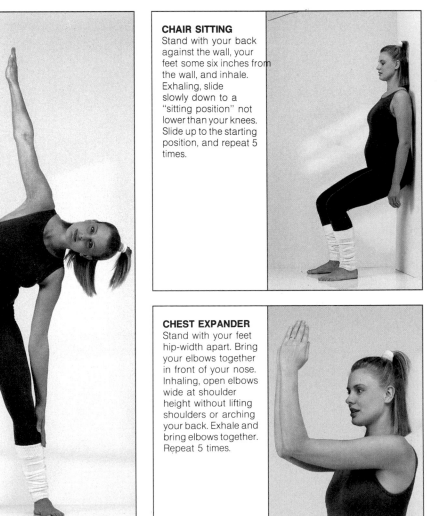

STANDING SIDE STRETCH
Stand with feet apart, arms out to the sides. Keep your hips to the front, lift your upper body from the hips and lean to the left. Slide your hand down your leg as far as you can, raising your right arm. Stretch the hands away from each other. Slowly increase the extent to which you can lower your left arm. Repeat 5 times each side.

CHAIR SITTING
Stand with your back against the wall, your feet some six inches from the wall, and inhale. Exhaling, slide slowly down to a "sitting position" not lower than your knees. Slide up to the starting position, and repeat 5 times.

CHEST EXPANDER
Stand with your feet hip-width apart. Bring your elbows together in front of your nose. Inhaling, open elbows wide at shoulder height without lifting shoulders or arching your back. Exhale and bring elbows together. Repeat 5 times.

BREATHING

It is important to breathe properly so you will have more pep and energy. Aim to breathe 4–6 times a minute; it will help to count to 5 as you exhale. Practice breathing as follows: **1.** Breathe in deeply; feel your ribs expand, and imagine the breath going all the way down into your stomach as your diaphragm contracts. **2.** Breathe out, making a hissing sound to emphasize your exhalation. This reduces stress.

Next breathe just from the chest. Then practice shallow panting, which is used for strenuous exercise and at the peak of contractions. Keep your mouth slightly open and rest your tongue on the floor of your mouth. During labor, exhale while muscles are contracting and inhale when muscles are relaxed.

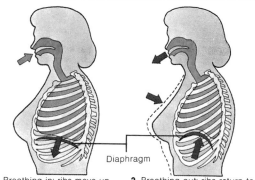

Diaphragm

1. Breathing in: ribs move up and out; diaphragm contracts.

2. Breathing out: ribs return to rest position; diaphragm releases.

HAMSTRING STRETCH

Lie on your back with your knees bent. Raise one leg in the air with the knee slightly bent, and rotate your ankle 5 times in each direction. Repeat on the other side.

CURL-UP

Lie on your back with your knees bent, hands resting on thighs, and inhale. As you exhale, reach toward your knees, lifting your head and shoulders off the floor. Inhale as you roll back. Repeat 5 times.

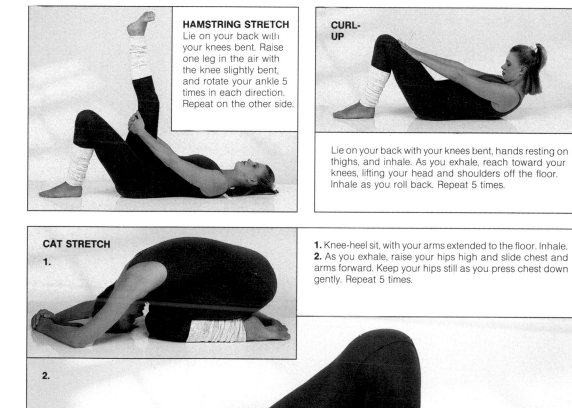

CAT STRETCH

1.

2.

1. Knee-heel sit, with your arms extended to the floor. Inhale.
2. As you exhale, raise your hips high and slide chest and arms forward. Keep your hips still as you press chest down gently. Repeat 5 times.

During the final months leading to delivery continue your fitness program. Protect your joints (hips, knees, ankles) and the extra weight they bear by paying special attention to body alignment. If you experience any difficulty sleeping as a result of your growing belly, try lying on your side with a pillow between your knees. Use the constructive rest position on page 221 to relax your back frequently throughout the day.

The following exercises will help to prepare you for delivery. Add them to your regular routine. The sitting side stretch, standing leg extension, hip circles, and deep twist will stretch and lengthen the muscles in your thighs and pelvis. Use the reach-through exercise for relaxing the upper and middle back. Foot pedaling will tone your calf muscles and encourage good circulation.

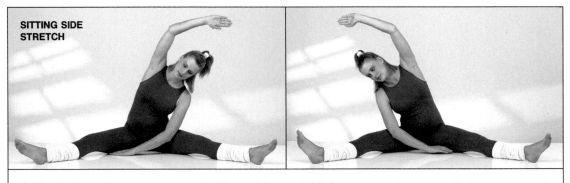

SITTING SIDE STRETCH

1. Sit on the floor with your legs wide apart. With your left palm flat on the floor and your right arm raised, inhale. As you exhale, bend to the side and hold to a slow count of 5.

2. Inhale as you return to center, and exhale as you repeat to the other side. Repeat 5 times to each side.

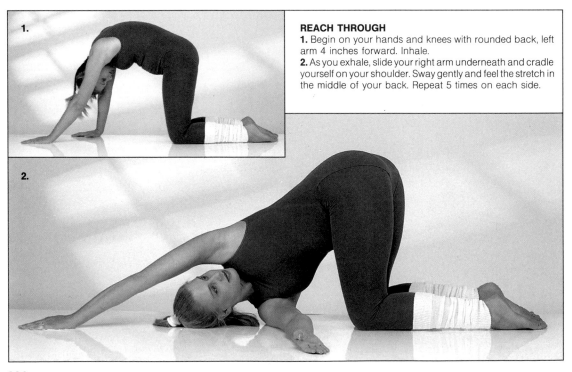

REACH THROUGH
1. Begin on your hands and knees with rounded back, left arm 4 inches forward. Inhale.
2. As you exhale, slide your right arm underneath and cradle yourself on your shoulder. Sway gently and feel the stretch in the middle of your back. Repeat 5 times on each side.

FOOT PEDALING

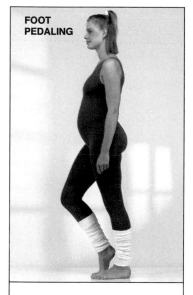

Stand with one leg straight, foot flat on the floor, and the other knee bent with your heel off the floor. Breathe rhythmically and shift your weight from one foot to the other in a pedaling motion.

HIP CIRCLES

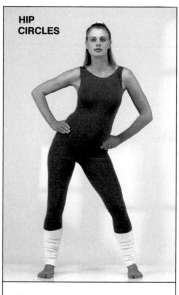

Stand with your legs wide apart, knees bent, and hands on hips. Imagine scraping the inside of a bowl with your hips as you describe a large circle. Repeat 5 times in each direction.

STANDING LEG EXTENSION

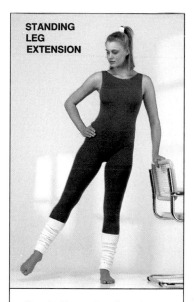

Stand with your hands resting on the back of a chair or table. Inhale. As you exhale, slowly lift one leg, keeping hips stable. Repeat 5 times on each side.

DEEP TWIST

1. Stand with your feet wide apart, hands on the inside of the knees, thumbs pressing out. Inhale.
2. As you exhale, press your left shoulder down as you look over your right shoulder. Inhale and return to center. Exhale and repeat on the opposite side. Repeat 5 times on each side.

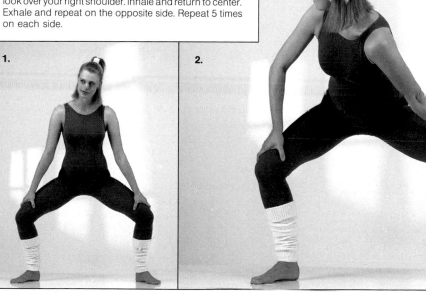

1.

2.

GIVING BIRTH

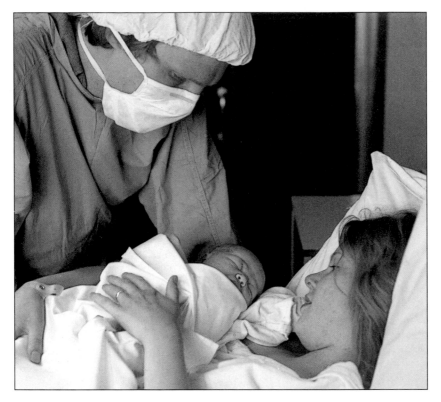

The baby is presented to the mother as soon after birth as possible. Some doctors recommend doing this before the cord is cut. Such close contact is thought to help in the formation of the bond between mother and baby.

Adopting routines of relaxation and breathing will help you during labor and birth. Many women worry that in labor they will forget all they have learned beforehand, but this is where your partner comes into his own. Fathers are now widely accepted as an invaluable source of support during labor, but a close relative or friend may accompany you if you wish. If your partner is unable to attend prenatal classes, repeat any instructions to him when you get home, and practice together.

Signs of labor

Strong, regular contractions may herald the first stage of labor, which is to dilate the cervix, but their intensity and frequency can vary. They usually start at the rate of six to seven per hour. When the cervix (the neck of the uterus) is fully dilated, the second stage of labor begins, and it ends in the birth. The third stage is the delivery of the placenta.

It is best to move around at home during the first stage of labor for as long as you can, but remember that second and subsequent labors are often shorter than the first. You should think about going to the hospital when the contractions are coming at about 10-minute intervals and lasting for 20 to 40 seconds. You should go to the hospital in any case if the fluid-retaining membranes around the baby break, which can happen before you get contractions. Labor might be preceded by a "show," as the mucus plug from the neck of the uterus is passed out. This alone is not a sufficient reason to go to the hospital.

Relax during the build-up of a contraction and breathe as regularly as you can. Try to conserve energy by remaining calm, and try to stay upright. Positions you might find comfortable are squatting, supporting yourself in front with your arms; sitting the wrong way around on a chair, leaning forward on a pillow; or sitting the right way around, leaning on your partner. In these positions he can massage your back to assist relaxation and pain relief. In the hospital, keep mobile if your doctor allows you to.

The method of childbirth you choose will depend on your preference and your medical history, and will be modified by hospital facilities

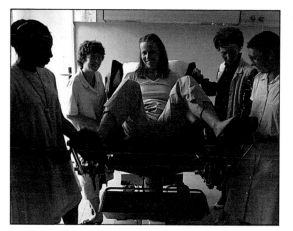

A modern version of the old-fashioned birthing chair is now favored by some obstetricians. Giving birth in an upright position means that labor is assisted, rather than hindered, by the force of gravity. To encourage an atmosphere of calm, hospitals are also installing birthing rooms, in which a couple can make themselves reasonably comfortable during labor.

and attitudes. Supporters of "natural" birth believe that a woman should be free to determine the conduct of her own labor and should not automatically be confined to bed to give birth in a recumbent position. They reject the increasing use of drugs and fetal monitoring in favor of more natural methods, although these are not necessarily safer.

Whatever your preferred method of childbirth, you might find that your medical history or the progress of your labor demands medical intervention. The baby's heartbeat will be monitored to detect any signs of distress; for example, if you have suffered from high blood pressure. If the doctor suspects a risk to the baby, he may advise you to have the birth induced through the administration of hormones or by rupturing of the fluid sac around the baby.

Induction of your labor will probably be recommended if you have experienced weight loss recently, if the doctor suspects that the baby might be at risk from the inadequate functioning of the placenta, if there is a marked reduction in the baby's movements, or if the baby is overdue. A Caesarean delivery (cutting through the abdominal wall) will be necessary if the placenta is blocking the neck of the uterus (placenta previa); if the baby is in an awkward position, for example, bottom down (breech); if your baby is too large for your pelvis; or if you are suffering from the venereal disease herpes.

Painkillers

During labor and birth, you might feel the need for painkillers and should not feel guilty about this. A mixture of gas and air can be breathed in through a face mask. This has the instant effect of making you feel lightheaded and can be used to help you over the worst of each contraction. It has no side effects. Demerol, administered in the form of an injection, takes about 20 minutes to work and lasts about 2 hours. This drug is normally safe, but might make you feel sick and can hamper the baby's breathing if it is administered too late in labor.

You might also be offered an epidural, which is an anesthetic injection into the spinal cord that numbs all sensation in your lower abdomen and birth canal. An epidural depends upon the availability of a trained anesthetist, and it necessitates a medically controlled labor and birth. If you have an epidural, you will have to lie on your side throughout; you may need an intravenous (IV) drip, and the baby's progress will be monitored throughout labor.

A few women suffer a blinding headache after an epidural, and the baby's ability to suck can be temporarily affected. However, an epidural can be a boon in a long labor and can also be used for a Caesarean so that you can see the baby being born. If you do not like the idea of drugs, you might prefer acupuncture or hypnosis as a means of pain relief (see pages 318–319, 330–331).

Whatever happens, do not attempt to stick to your original preferences come what may, and remember that the hospital staff are there to help you. At all times during labor and birth, feel free to ask what options are open to you and to discuss the reasons for the obstetrician's recommendations and their implications.

For about 10 days after the birth of your baby, you will need special care and attention, whether the birth was at home or in hospital. During this early postnatal period, you will have routine checks on your blood pressure and temperature, and examination of your uterus and any stitches.

Vaginal bleeding continues for up to two weeks. It might turn into a white discharge, which can last for six weeks. If the blood remains bright red and the flow is heavy, if there are clots in it, or you are aware of an offensive smell, report it to your doctor as soon as possible.

If you have been stitched for a cut or tear, adding two cups of table salt to your bath is immensely soothing. Constipation is a common complaint after the birth. Do not expect a bowel movement for a few days. A high-fiber diet and plenty of liquids should help. If you experience painful contractions from your uterus, breathe through them as you did in labor.

Feeding your baby

Most women are able to breast-feed their babies if they so desire. You should not feel guilty if this is not your choice, or if your milk supply is inadequate. Sometimes large amounts of milk are produced from the time the milk comes into the breasts two or three days after the birth, but breast-feeding often takes about a week to become established. It might also take the baby a while to get used to sucking. If your nipples are sore, let the air get to them or apply a commercial cream. If you do not breast-feed, you can express milk from the breasts to relieve the discomfort.

Once you start to supplement breast-feedings with a bottle or cup, your milk supply will probably start to dry up. It is important to pay meticulous attention to hygiene when bottle-feeding and to follow the manufacturer's instructions exactly.

Feeding your baby

The advantages of breast-feeding are:
- Colostrum, produced in the first few days, and breast milk contain antibodies against gastrointestinal and respiratory infections.

- The baby is less likely to get fat or develop diaper rash.

- Breast milk is always available, suitable for the baby, sterile, and at the right temperature.

- Supply meets demand, and flow varies according to the baby's degree of hunger.

- Physical contact encourages bonding.

NOTE: Cigarette smoking suppresses milk production; oral contraceptives may be passed on in breast milk.

The advantages of bottle-feeding are:
- People other than the mother can feed the baby.

- It is easier to keep a definite track of exactly how much the baby is eating at each feeding.

- The baby is not affected by drugs the mother is taking or her diet.

- The milk flow is not affected by any negative aspects of the mother's state of mind.

- Bottle-feeding is less tiring to the mother.

Check your progress
Weight: Unless you were overweight before the birth, you should not have difficulty losing weight afterward if you eat a healthy diet (see page 54 ff). Breast-feeding aids weight loss.

Diet: Do not go on a reducing diet if you are breast-feeding. Your food requirements will not differ from those during pregnancy, but you may supplement your milk and whole-grain intake. You will need 500 calories a day more than a nonpregnant woman to produce enough milk. Drink plenty of liquids (other than milk).

Exercise: Start gentle exercises as soon as you wish, but do not begin the exercise program given on pages 232–233 until 2 weeks after the birth.

SLEEP PATTERNS

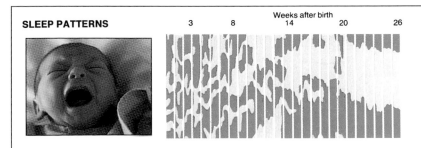

Weeks after birth
3   8   14   20   26

A baby is not instinctively aware of the pattern of night and day. In the first few weeks after birth there is a shifting pattern of sleep (*blue*) and waking (*pink*). A 25-hour rhythm between 5 and 25 weeks. Shortly afterward, this reduces to a 24-hour rhythm, with most hours of sleep at night.

Emotional reactions

With the birth of a baby, especially if it is your first, you embark upon a new phase of your life—one that will be both challenging and rewarding. However, the days and even weeks after birth can be a time of conflicting emotions for a mother, and can prove confusing or distressing for a new father, who might be experiencing a wealth of hitherto unfamiliar and disturbing feelings.

After the initial joy of the birth, you might come down to earth with a bump: many women experience the "baby blues" on about the fourth day after the birth. This mood does not usually persist, but you might feel in low spirits for a while and cry a lot for no apparent reason.

Postnatal depression that lasts after the first week or so affects some four percent of women to some degree, although relatively few seek help. Symptoms can include chronic lethargy, back-ache, headache, poor appetite, loss of interest in sex, sleeplessness, tearfulness, and irrational fears about the baby's health. Do not be afraid to consult your doctor about the problem, but also help yourself by making sure you get some rest for each part of the day, by not neglecting your diet, by enlisting your husband's support, and by doing regular aerobic exercise of some kind.

Getting into routine

Your daily routine will be dictated by your baby's needs. Sleeping and feeding patterns established in the early days can change suddenly and inexplicably, and a baby who was initially contented might suddenly cry a lot and be difficult to placate. The problems become easier to solve as the baby gradually settles down to a more regular pattern of eating and sleeping, as you are able to sleep more, and as you begin to be able to distinguish between the cries that mean hunger, pain, frustration, and so on.

Sex may well be the last thing on your mind at this time. Your stitches might only just have healed, and sleepless nights may mean you have barely enough strength to cope with your baby's needs, let alone your own or those of your partner. There is no time limit upon the resumption of lovemaking, but penetration is not advisable until you are sure that any stitches have healed and until all vaginal discharge has ceased.

At about six weeks after the birth, you will have to see your obstetrician or gynecologist for a postnatal check-up. This will involve an internal examination of the condition of your uterus to see if it has returned to its normal size, possibly a Pap smear (see pages 204–205), and a check that all has healed well. Your breasts and abdomen will also be checked to make sure that they are normal.

If you are returning to work, it is probably best from the baby's point of view if you do so at between three and six months, and in any case not before you are well healed and rested. It is essential, of course, that you make arrangements for the baby to be looked after. Do not feel guilty about either returning to work or not working. Your decision is bound to be a complex one, based on your financial, emotional, and intellectual needs. Only you can decide what is the right balance for you.

POSTNATAL CARE/2

Wait at least two weeks after your baby is born to begin your postnatal exercise program. However, you can start your pelvic floor exercises (squeezing the vaginal and anal muscles) as soon as you feel able. These will help healing and start toning your muscles. Seek the advice of your doctor on when it is safe for you to begin getting back into shape. As always, a regular fitness program will help to enhance your self-image as you gain the strength that you need for your new responsibilities. Remember, it is important to be good to yourself and set aside time each day to address your own personal needs.

This program emphasizes regaining abdominal strength, and toning and firming body parts that tend to lose tone during pregnancy. The exercises described in the prenatal routine are also suitable after delivery. Expand your program by planning more aerobic exercise to combat fatigue and to burn calories. Consider long walks in nice weather with your baby as a good way to begin. Refer to the section on aerobics to plan your program (see pages 106–123).

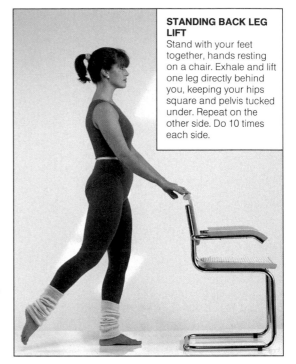

STANDING BACK LEG LIFT
Stand with your feet together, hands resting on a chair. Exhale and lift one leg directly behind you, keeping your hips square and pelvis tucked under. Repeat on the other side. Do 10 times each side.

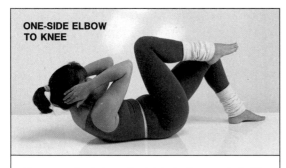

ONE-SIDE ELBOW TO KNEE

Lie on your back, knees bent. Inhale. As you exhale, lift your head and shoulders off the floor, touching right elbow to right knee. Repeat 5 times on each side.

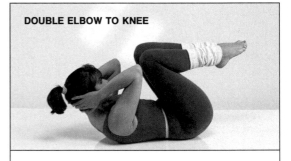

DOUBLE ELBOW TO KNEE

Lie on your back, hands behind head, knees bent into your chest. Inhale. As you exhale, lift to touch both elbows to knees. Repeat 10 times.

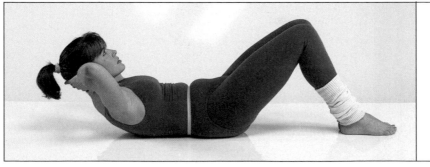

CRUNCHES
Lie on your back with your hands behind your head, knees bent, feet flat. Inhale. As you exhale, tuck your chin into your chest and curl your upper body forward until your shoulder blades clear the floor. Repeat 10 times.

CURL BACK
1.

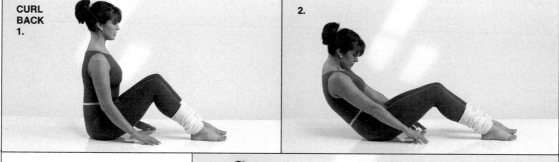

2.

3.

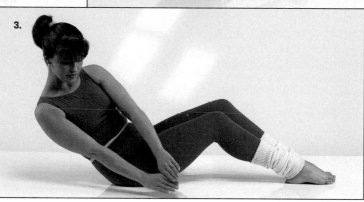

1. Sit with feet together, knees bent, feet flat. Inhale.
2. As you exhale, slowly roll back toward the floor, stopping before your lower back touches it. Do not let your feet lift off the floor. Hold for a slow count of 5, then pull forward to the starting position. Repeat 5 times.
3. Follow instructions above but roll back on the diagonal. Repeat 5 times on each side.

TRICEP TIGHTENER
1. Bring your elbows in tight to your body.
2. As you exhale, extend your arms back and up as high as you can without lifting your shoulders or slumping your chest. Inhale as you bend your arms in and forward. Repeat 10 times.

1.

2.

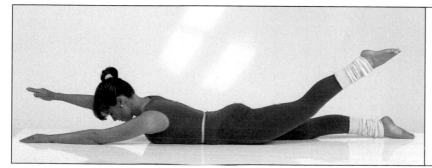

OPPOSITE LEG AND ARM LIFT
Lie on your stomach, keeping your waist pulled in off the floor. As you exhale, slowly raise one arm and the opposite leg. Repeat 4 times each side, alternating sides.

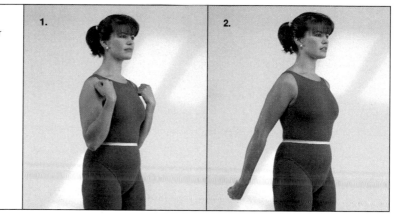

EXERCISES TO DO WITH BABY

Your baby's health and fitness routine can start right from the beginning. The physical relationship that the parent has with the baby will be important in developing strength and flexibility. A gentle touch can soothe the restless sleeper; rock him slowly and tap his buttocks lightly. After the first month, your baby will enjoy some massage, especially to ease cramps. Stroke the baby's limbs and trunk, working away from the heart. Use only the weight of your hand and take care not to exert pressure. Touch very gently when you massage the abdomen, and make sure that your hands are warm.

Always support the weight of the baby's head with your hand and remind others to do so as well. Prevent the baby's head from lolling back before strong neck muscles develop. Resist the temptation to swing the baby by his arms; what looks like fun can cause a dislocation of the shoulder joint. In general, be supportive but not over-anxious; let the baby progress at his own rate regarding standing, crawling, and walking.

Flexing and stretching your baby's feet, arms, and legs will be a fun way to stimulate strong muscle development and motor skills. Mobiles and brightly colored toys will encourage the baby to reach and will sharpen his visual perception. Always let your baby's natural movements be your cue in making exercise selections.

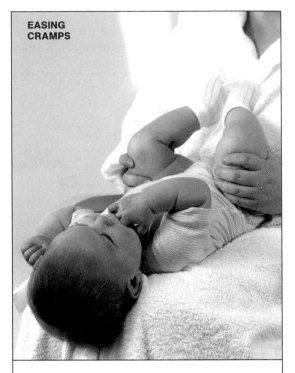

EASING CRAMPS

Place the baby face up on your legs, with his head toward your knees and his legs folded against your stomach. Bending the baby's legs will relax his abdominal muscles.

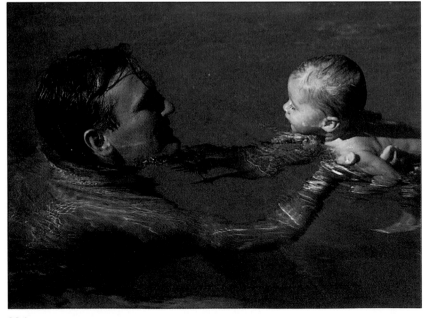

Resuming leisure activities as soon after the baby's birth as you can will help you to define the family unit. Try to find ways that you can include your baby in what you are doing. Swimming, for example, is not only good exercise for both parents, but also is an activity that a baby can enjoy.

MASSAGE

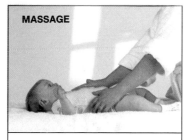

Use gentle pressure of your hand in outward strokes over the whole body. This will result in total relaxation of the arms, legs, neck, and back. Work slowly, regularly, and very gently. Try massage after the baby's bath.

BABY ESCAPES

Place the baby on his stomach over a rolled pillow. Place a favorite toy on the opposite side to lure the baby toward it. Gently hold him back at the knees or ankles while he tries to "escape" to his toy. Don't allow the baby to become frustrated; let him accomplish his escape after a few attempts.

BABY CRUNCHES

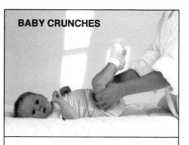

Press the baby's knees gently toward his abdomen to encourage contraction of the abdominal muscles. When the baby breathes out, release the pressure on the knees. Take care not to press for more than 2–3 seconds. Repeat 5 times.

ANKLE ROTATIONS

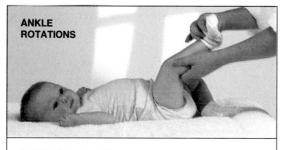

Hold the baby's calf loosely in one hand while gently rotating his foot in each direction. With the flat of your hand, lightly press the sole of his foot to flex and point positions.

LEG PRESS

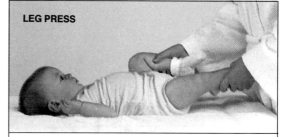

Gently press the baby's knees toward his stomach. Alternate pressure and release of your hands will encourage a bicycling motion that will help the baby to strengthen and stretch his leg muscles.

BABY PUSH-OFFS

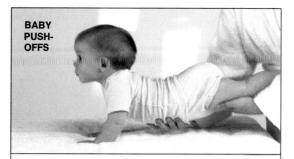

For the 3- to 6-month-old. Hold the baby with one hand under his chest and one hand at his knees. Lean his body forward until his hands press flat on your knees or other surface and he supports himself. When he makes an effort to push away, lean him away briefly, and then repeat.

LEG STRETCHES

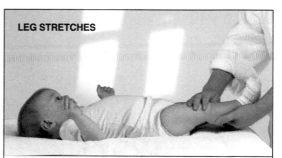

With the baby flat on his back, legs together, place one of your hands under his calves, the other on his knees. Gently stretch his legs out straight. Take care to stay within the baby's natural range of movement—if you try to stretch his legs too far, the baby will arch his back, which might strain it.

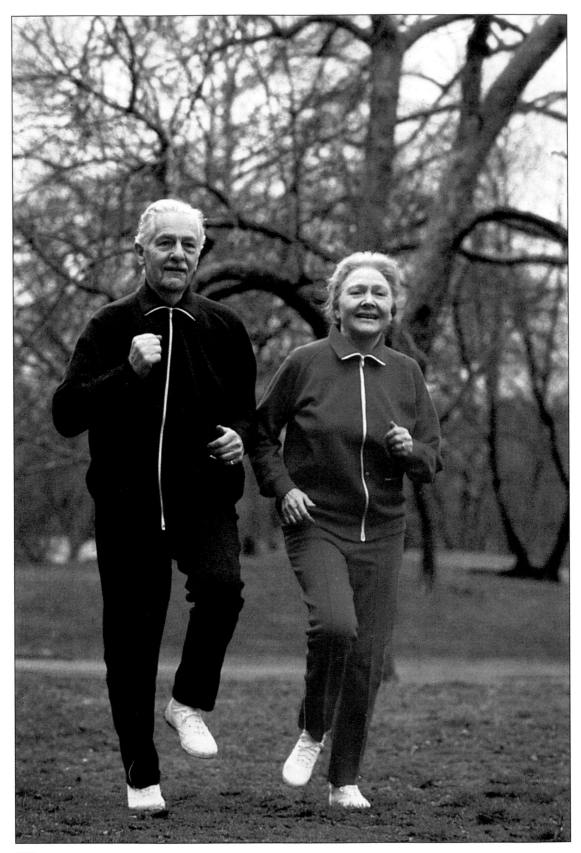

FEELING GOOD, STAYING YOUNG

Older citizens are receiving more and more attention as their numbers increase. There is ample evidence that older people—those over the age of 65—are more numerous, more fit, and have more to offer than at any time in the past. Today many well-known politicians, businessmen, entertainers, and artists are continuing to work and to contribute to society well beyond the usual age of retirement.

On the eve of his seventieth birthday, the French cellist Paul Tortellier claimed he owed his youthful appearance and vigor to his belief that everyone should aim to die young but delay doing so for as long as possible. The longevity of some creative artists might well be due to the fact that they never "retire," but keep up those activities that to them are a part of their being, not just a job. It certainly makes sense to try to follow their example, and to recognize that retiring from employment does not mean retiring from life. In fact, this time should be thought of as a bonus, and as an opportunity for a renaissance.

Looking forward to the future with enthusiasm, and being confident of your potential to grow, keeps the vital spark within you alight. The challenge is to keep mentally and physically stimulated. Perhaps the most telling sign of success in retirement is wondering when you ever had time to go to work.

AGING AND ATTITUDE

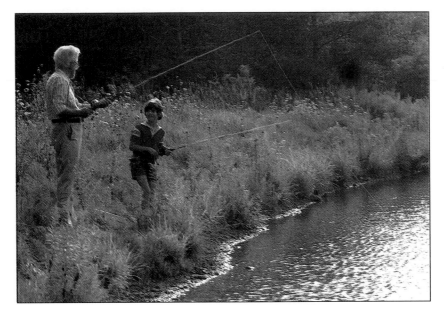

Young and old can often bridge the generation gap with consummate ease. Grandfather and grandson find no difficulty in communicating, or in sharing pursuits and pastimes such as fishing. It should be possible to extend this sharing and caring attitude to the elderly across all sectors of society, both inside and outside the family, so that the aged are not isolated or written off as a burden to society.

From the time you are born, your behavior and your attitudes are influenced to a greater or lesser degree by the rules and attitudes of the society in which you live. As you grow older, you may feel that you live in an age and a society that is obsessed with youth, in which old age is associated with chronic disease, and being old is "unfashionable," unattractive, and at times even frightening.

A place in society
Television, newspapers, and magazines endorse this blinkered view by constantly celebrating the vigor, beauty, success, and sexual prowess of youth, and by portraying the elderly as pathetic and neglected. You might, unknowingly, contribute to this attitude and provoke indifference on the part of younger generations by not making an effort to get to know and understand them, or by not managing your affairs as best you can. Furthermore, as you get older, your view of other people's aging tends to be negative and does a disservice to both the young and the old. First, it creates a self-fulfilling prophecy, a stereotype; and, second, it does not correspond to the reality of aging, which is more positive and satisfying than many people expect.

The traditional roles of the elderly have been greatly undermined in Western industrialized nations. In nonindustrialized societies, elderly people often continue to be active members of their communities, which in turn benefit from their skills and abilities. Yet in the West you are frequently considered obsolete as soon as you retire. You become officially unproductive—a burden to society—something most old people are at pains not to be. Far from being venerated, the "village elders" can become the community's cast-offs, euphemistically dismissed as "senior citizens." And although you have many more constructive and rewarding years in store, the fund of knowledge, experience, and wisdom you have accumulated with age may be largely ignored.

Responses to the elderly
The view that old age is a rehearsal for death permeates all levels of society. In day-to-day life, some people's responses to the elderly are shaped by the firm belief that if you are old, you must be decrepit. Consequently, you may find as you get older that you are being managed, bullied, treated like a child, or protected to an extent that severely cramps your style.

Such attitudes often conceal people's unresolved fears of growing old, particularly among those who don't have an extended family and rarely come into contact with the elderly. Take an honest look at the way you treat older people. The box at the top of the opposite page covers many widely held views about the elderly. Like most

How do you treat the elderly?

If your answers to the questions below reveal a negative attitude, consider whether these actions make sense in relation to you or to older people that you know well. When you treat people as stereotypes, you lose opportunities for close relationships. Young and old share the basic human needs for warmth, understanding, support, dignity, and companionship.

Do you:
- Avoid elderly people?
- Believe they can't make reasonable decisions?
- Show impatience?
- Overprotect them by withholding information about health or other matters?
- Talk over their heads?
- Make allowances for their age and mobility?
- Seek their advice?
- React enthusiastically to their plans?
- Involve them in your activities?

The aging process

Physiological changes occur with age, but their rate and extent follow no set timetable and vary from person to person. The effects of aging include the following:

Skin and hair
A gradual loss of elastic tissue (and of fat beneath the skin) causes the skin to sag and wrinkle. Changes occur in skin pigmentation and hair loses color. Weakened blood capillaries often cause the skin to bruise more easily, and changes in blood vessels, genetic factors, and exposure to the sun can produce brown spots on the hands.

Skeleton and muscles
Height decreases with age because of shrinking of the disks between the vertebrae. Loss of elasticity in the connective tissue causes the joints to stiffen and enlarge. The bones become more brittle (osteoporosis), and muscles lose some of their bulk and tone.

Heart and circulation
Arteries harden and thicken inside. This means the blood circulates less freely. There is some reduction in the supply of oxygen to the tissues, and a poor response to any sudden demand for an increased burst of energy.

The heart, which becomes less efficient with age, has to work even harder to pump blood through the narrowed arterial pathways, and this might cause the blood pressure to rise.

Lungs
The tissues of the lungs lose elasticity with age so that maximum breathing is reduced, although it is still efficient.

Abdominal organs
The capacity of the abdominal organs is less, and the kidneys are slower to filter impurities from the blood.

Brain and nervous system
The brain shrinks with age, but this does not seem to affect intellectual powers. Short-term memory, however, fails. The main threat to the brain is shortage of oxygen due to the impaired blood supply. The reaction time of the nerves increases, making responses slower.

Senses
Some sensory loss is to be expected. The two most common effects are a reduced ability to focus on nearby objects and a degree of hearing loss (particularly for the higher tones). Taste, smell, and touch are diminished to some degree, and the mechanisms of balance become less acute. Older people might also become less aware of temperature changes, and so dress inadequately for cold conditions.

generalizations about a group of people, these views don't depict the total reality. For example, one stereotype of aging is that old people complain increasingly about their health. In fact, studies have shown that generally the elderly tend to under-report symptoms of chronic conditions. Also, the older population tends to be more, rather than less, diversified in social, health, economic, and other characteristics than the young. The greater variety of goals, values, preferences, and capacities of the old compared to the young population means that generalizations apply to some, not most, individuals.

A positive attitude

As you grow older, it is important to recognize, and come to terms with, the unavoidable physical effects of aging. At the same time, beware of negative expectations about aging, as they might limit your own ability to find satisfaction in the later years.

In aging, as throughout your life, it is very important to keep active and stay interested in the world around you, and to find supportive and challenging contexts in which to promote continued personal growth and obtain fulfillment. For this reason many people consider planning for retirement to be a life-long pursuit. Fortunately, most older people maintain independent and active lives in the community.

The elderly population of the developed world is at an all-time high, and indications are that more people alive today will survive to a ripe old age than ever before. Since the elderly now represent an increasingly influential and vocal segment of the community, governments are finally being forced to look at them in a different way.

The "graying" of nations

Three major factors have brought about the progressive "graying" of industrialized nations: a falling birth-rate, a drop in the infant mortality rate, and increased life expectancy.

One of the most dramatic examples of this aging trend is in Japan, where, following the post-war baby boom, the fertility rate went into steep decline. When, in recent times, a head count was taken on Japan's Respect for the Aged Day, the over 65's (11,320,000 people) were found to account for 9.5 percent of the population.

This is a relatively low proportion compared to the United States' 11 percent or Britain's 14 percent. Yet by the year 2000, as the chart opposite shows, Japan will have a greater percentage of elderly people than both these countries. And by the year 2025, an estimated 21.3 percent of the Japanese population will be over 65—the highest proportion in any advanced nation. By this same year, West Germany will be populated by 20 percent of old people, Britain and France by 18.6 percent, and the United States by 15.8 percent.

Geriatric experts stress that the health problems of the elderly should not be viewed too pessimistically. There are in fact millions of old people who have never had a stroke, who have never fallen and broken a bone, who do not suffer from incontinence, and who are not confined to their homes or beds. In fact, between 85 and 90 percent of elderly people have few health problems, and lead active lives.

In the early 1980's, the World Assembly on Aging put forward the idea that the fit elderly could, if mobilized, be a productive resource. However, no government has yet firmly acted on such a possibility, perhaps because of the prevalence of widespread high unemployment.

Significantly, Japan, with its prosperity, low unemployment, and tradition of working into old age, has raised the retirement age from 55 to 60, and workers reaching formal retirement are fre-

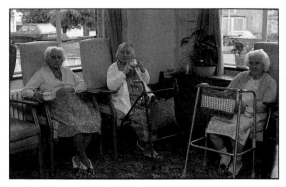

The fate of thousands of elderly people is to spend their days in sedentary occupations. Enlightened approaches to the care and needs of the elderly recognize that such a restricted way of life is unfulfilling and often unnecessary. The elderly have much to offer, and should be motivated and encouraged to use their time and energy to the full.

quently re-employed by their companies, albeit at a lower level. The US has abolished the mandatory retirement age except in a few professions, in which it is 70. Some other countries are, however, considering voluntary retirement for people in their fifties.

The concept of formal retirement arose in the days when average life expectancy was perhaps 20 to 30 years less than it is today. Now that more people in the developed world can expect to live well into their seventies, the need for a retirement age of around 60 is probably an anachronism.

The claims of the elderly

In many ways, the elderly have never had it so good. Many receive annuities from their company pension plans or from Social Security. In addition, those in need may receive help with housing and medical expenses. But money is not enough.

Many old people, no longer content to remain a passive lobby, are beginning to press their own claims. In the United States today, for instance, the elderly are much more active in politics and more vocal about political issues than are their contemporaries elsewhere.

At the moment, then, it is sheer pressure of numbers that is forcing governments to start taking notice. But if the American initiative were to be taken up internationally, elderly people could be organized into an active political force. Then perhaps they would again be recognized as a vital part of society.

THE GROWTH OF THE ELDERLY POPULATION

Key
P = Total population
EP = Elderly population

Elderly as % of population

% of elderly living in institutions

Elderly as % of population in the year 2000

Country

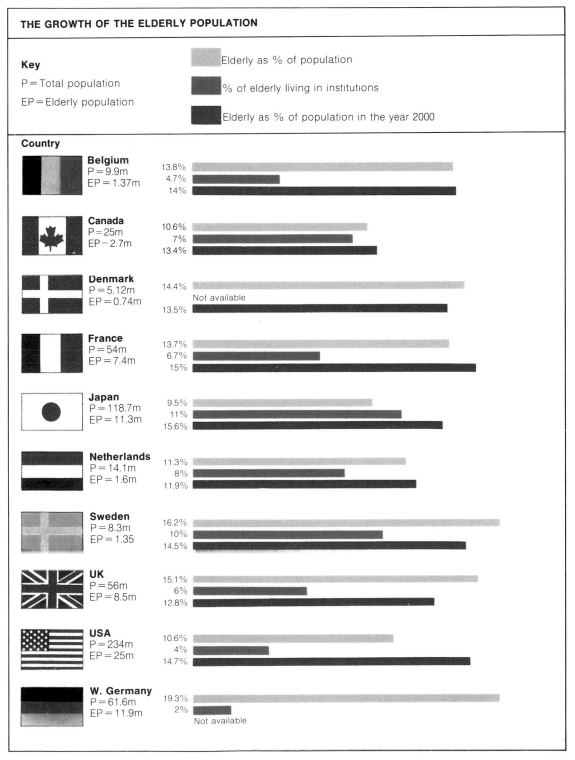

Belgium
P = 9.9m
EP = 1.37m
- 13.8%
- 4.7%
- 14%

Canada
P = 25m
EP - 2.7m
- 10.6%
- 7%
- 13.4%

Denmark
P = 5.12m
EP = 0.74m
- 14.4%
- Not available
- 13.5%

France
P = 54m
EP = 7.4m
- 13.7%
- 6.7%
- 15%

Japan
P = 118.7m
EP = 11.3m
- 9.5%
- 11%
- 15.6%

Netherlands
P = 14.1m
EP = 1.6m
- 11.3%
- 8%
- 11.9%

Sweden
P = 8.3m
EP = 1.35
- 16.2%
- 10%
- 14.5%

UK
P = 56m
EP = 8.5m
- 15.1%
- 6%
- 12.8%

USA
P = 234m
EP = 25m
- 10.6%
- 4%
- 14.7%

W. Germany
P = 61.6m
EP = 11.9m
- 19.3%
- 2%
- Not available

Retirement is an important transition in the life cycle. Like marriage, the birth of children, and the time of the empty nest, it affects both mental and physical well-being. At the same time it offers an opportunity to discover new ways of achieving personal satisfaction. Millions of people today are finding these leisure years as rewarding as their working years.

Planning ahead for the bonus years

Many aspects of retirement can be anticipated and prepared for, and thoughtful advance planning will ensure that the transition is made as easily as possible. Difficulties encountered in adjusting to retirement are usually related to the extent to which personal identity and meaning in life have come from activities and relationships at work. Retirement can be most satisfying if you keep up old interests as well as develop new ones. If you replace job-related interests when you retire, you are less likely to feel a sense of loss. For example, a schoolteacher whose satisfaction in life came from participating in the education of children might find volunteer work—as well as a sense of continuity—at a day-care center or a children's library.

However, the chief executive officer of a company who has derived great satisfaction from his high-ranking position might have more difficulty satisfying his need for status in retirement; but he, too, can succeed. For example, as an officer of his neighborhood or tenants' association he might exercise leadership and enjoy the recognition of an elected position.

New interests and activities do not just happen. Experience shows that the key to successful retirement is facing up to it—and well ahead of time. Today, when retirement can extend to two decades or more, you need to review your life and relationships long before the gold watch is due in order to make the most of these bonus years.

This is the message of the many organizations set up to help older employees facing retirement. The American Association of Retired Persons (AARP), the largest such organization in the country, found that, with proper foresight and planning, many problems could be averted. To help people who are approaching retirement age plan for the future, AARP provides printed materials, films, and videos for retirement planning seminars, and

even a guidebook for seminar leaders. In the seminar you are introduced to some of the challenges and opportunities of retirement. Topics include health, safety, and changes in physical capacity across the lifespan; housing and location; the pros and cons of staying in your present home or moving to a retirement community; structure and use of time; financial planning and legal affairs. Seminar participants can become members of AARP and receive publications and prescribed drugs at a discount by mail.

It is essential to remember that the materials and information provided by a retirement preparation seminar only suggest possible options. The crucial next step is individualized planning, which takes into account your personal goals.

Since the 1970's the majority of Americans have retired from full-time work before the age of 65, but only a small minority have had any kind of preparation for it, and then often only at the last minute. This leaves the mass of working people to develop some sort of positive philosophy on their own. At 50 most people find their family responsibilities easing, and this is when you should start to lay the groundwork for your future comfort, happiness, and security if you haven't done so already.

Money matters

Finance is a high priority, since it can take years to save an adequate nest egg. Over the 10 years leading up to retirement, you should fulfill the following objectives.

You should consider whether it is to your advantage to clear existing debts, bank loans, installment plan balances, or mortgages. Anticipate and carry out major undertakings, such as reroofing the house or financing a move, while you are still on a full salary. If possible, begin to accumulate savings and arrange an investment income to supplement Social Security and private pension.

If you are not a financial wizard, seek the help of a bank manager, accountant, or investment adviser, who will find the best returns for your cash. Remember, however, that any plan will need to be reviewed at intervals.

Five years before you retire, you should formulate some ideas of where and how you want to live. One of the most common and miserable pitfalls of retirement to be avoided is moving to a

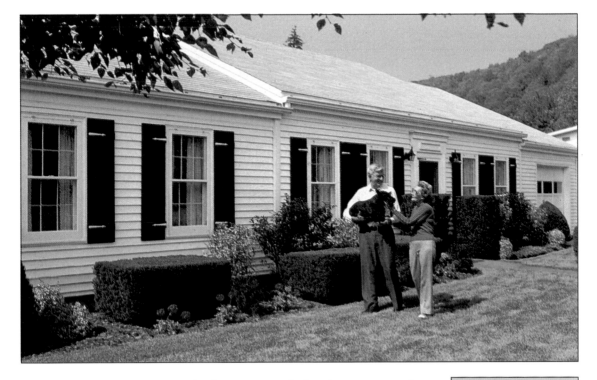

Don't get carried away by romantic locations when it comes to considering where you will live when you retire. Familiar faces and places can be reassuring when your working life changes. A smaller, more convenient house in your present locality might be the best answer.

completely strange or isolated area, remote from family and friends. In this way, you double the problems of adjustment, leaving both work and your familiar surroundings behind.

However, if you want to move, this is the time to decide on your retirement setting. Over the coming years, spend the occasional vacation or spare weekend scouting the area you are interested in. Check out its public transportation, hospital, and library—facilities that will become increasingly important to you in later years. These expeditions may also lead to some new social contacts. Bear in mind that investigating is not a commitment.

As you get the feel of the area, you will discover what kind of property comes into your price range. Single-story houses are popular with older people, although they can be just as expensive as two-story houses of comparable capacity. A house with stairs might become difficult to manage in later years; or you might feel that an apartment without a garden would prove too limiting, and so on. Whatever your choice, plan your move well before retirement, since you may have to wait until the housing you desire becomes available, and so that the cost of moving can be borne on a full-time salary.

Ten steps to retirement

● Find out about your pension.

● Clear financial debts.

● Reassess your investments.

● Get an appraisal on your house.

● Check that your insurance policies are adequate.

● Decide where to live.

● Survey social amenities in the area you plan to move to.

● Explore possibilities for part-time work.

● Make a will.

● Develop your leisure interests.

RETIREMENT COMMUNITIES

Planned retirement communities are designed to provide a safe, crime-free environment. They are an attractive option to living alone. Some provide only housing, while others include social, recreational, and medical services. Many also provide housekeeping, meals, and transportation. In some cases you pay for each service as you need it, and in others you pay an initial lump sum plus monthly carrying charges that entitle you to comprehensive care.

Who lives there?

Many such communities were once restricted to people aged 60 and above, but today a growing number of so-called adult communities are open to people over the age of 50. This wider age range means a greater mix of people and range of activities. If you are considering a retirement community, think about the sort of social and recreational interaction you would want. Would restrictions on children under 18 be a blessing—a freedom from noise and crying babies? Or would you miss the opportunities to watch young children at play or to hear their laughter? In general, communities in which half or more of the residents are of the same age tend to have higher rates of participation and interaction than those in which there is a bigger difference in the age of the residents.

All communities are shaped by the people who live in them, so take some time to meet prospective new neighbors, find out about their interests, and hear their views and concerns.

Checking credentials

Sponsors of some of the very early retirement communities did not manage their finances well, and commitments to provide health-care services, apartment and grounds maintenance, and security were often unfulfilled. As a result of these experiences, most states have now established regulations and monitoring safeguards for these communities.

One step in evaluating the credentials of a sponsor and the reputation of a retirement community is to check with your state or local department for the aging, health department, or social services department. These agencies may also be able to answer questions about other aspects of retirement living; their number is in the telephone book.

Locations

New communities are coming onto the market throughout the country. An increasing number of people are electing to stay where friends and family, resources and services, the climate and the cost of living are familiar. Moreover, many retirees who moved to "traditional" retirement states such as Florida, Arizona, and California are returning to their home states for these same reasons.

Types of housing

Most retirement communities will provide you with an independent apartment unit. Cottages and townhouses may also be available. In choosing a residence, look for design features, such as nonslip floors, that make it easy for you to carry out daily living activities. Use the checklist opposite to help you.

Financial considerations

While all types of housing units are available among the array of retirement communities, you will find that financial arrangements and the availability of health care vary. The most common types of communities are listed below.

● **Life-care communities:** These are total-care facilities that provide housing and comprehensive health-care services. You make an initial lump-sum payment to cover all these costs and usually pay a small monthly fee for grounds maintenance and real estate taxes. The emphasis in these communities is on long-term economic security and health-care service.

● **Continuing-care communities:** These are like life care in the range of services available, but they require a co-payment (that is, you must pay a share of your medical costs). The method of calculating the resident's contribution varies according to his age, state of health and financial resources, and must be considered carefully.

● **Retirement housing:** A third type of community provides housing and residential services such as housekeeping, meals, and transportation to shopping and activities, but you have to arrange for your own general health care. A 24-hour emergency call system is usually built in to each housing unit.

Retirement housing checklist

How many of the following design features, based on an AARP checklist, does your current or prospective retirement home have? Score 1 point for each feature it has.

1. All the rooms are on the same level, with no thresholds or walking hazards.

2. The floors are nonslip surfaces, such as wall-to-wall carpets, or unglazed ceramic tiles.

3. The doors are at least 30 inches wide and open easily from both sides.

4. The windows open and close easily.

5. The halls are between 36 and 48 inches wide.

6. Automatic heating maintains every room at a minimum of 70°F.

7. Air conditioning maintains a cool environment in a hot climate.

8. High-intensity light is available where needed.

9. There are night lights in the bedroom and bathroom.

10. Electrical outlets are 28 to 30 inches from the floor.

11. There are sufficient closets and storage facilities so that nothing needs to be stored on the floor.

12. The bathroom is near the bedroom.

13. The bathtub is low with a flat, nonskid bottom and a place to sit on the side.

14. The shower has an adjustable showerhead and a nonskid floor.

15. Grab bars are firmly anchored at the bathtub and toilet.

16. Kitchen counters, range, and sink are continuous.

17. The refrigerator has an easily accessible food compartment.

18. The overhead cabinets are no more than 12 inches deep, with top shelves no more than 72 inches from the floor.

Add up your score. If you score 16–18, the facilities are excellent; 13–15, facilities are suitable; 12 or less, some changes probably are necessary—take steps now to make your environment more suitable.

Where should you go?

Be sure to consider:

● Proximity to friends, family, and commercial and recreational facilities.

● Access to high-quality medical services.

● Age of the community population, and of the housing units and facilities.

● Access to public transportation.

● Features such as well-lit public areas, locked entry doors, and security patrols, as well as on-site health clubs, activities, and housekeeping services.

● The type of emergency call system and how it is monitored.

● What the fees cover, and what remedies you may have if you find the services unsatisfactory. Seek financial advice before making a commitment.

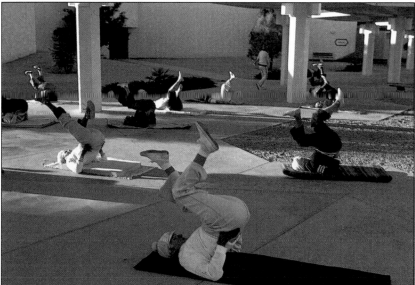

Some retirement communities offer a wide range of indoor and outdoor activities. These give you opportunities to keep fit, learn new skills, and meet people.

Your retirement plan should begin to take final shape five years, and certainly no later than two years, before the anticipated date on which you will retire. This is not a simple question of filling the 2,000 hours a year normally spent at a job, but of formulating a comprehensive and practical retirement philosophy, designed to ensure a rounded existence.

At this stage, having already tackled the long-term issues of money and housing, you should be resolving practical details of how you want to live. Do you want to embark on a second career or to look forward to at last having time for leisure interests?

Surprisingly, perhaps, most people want to continue to work. About 30 percent of retired Americans would like to be working, at least part-time, and no fewer than 75 percent of those still in employment would like to go on to some kind of paid, part-time work. As average life expectancy increases, and the elderly continue to enjoy better health, many more individuals choose to remain in the labor force. In addition, the prevailing economic climate may encourage people to continue at work or seek part-time employment.

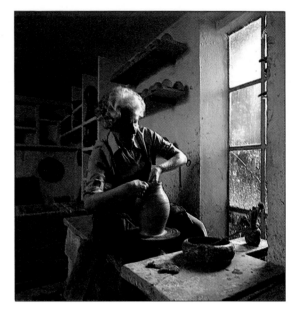

Retirement offers a wonderful opportunity to develop new skills. Taking a course in pottery, for example, might also allow you to earn some money by selling the objects you produce.

Seeking employment
Research has repeatedly shown that work in retirement improves health, morale, and life expectancy. But since it is not always easy to find, it is essential to explore job possibilities well before you retire.

The most fruitful approach to job-hunting is probably through your own personal grapevine. As retirement approaches, let your contacts know that you will soon be on the job market, if only for a part-time commitment that will fit in with your new lifestyle.

Volunteer work
Older people are often willing and supremely able to do volunteer work. Their wisdom and experience is of great value to volunteer organizations, the work less stressful than it is in paid employment, and there is no age discrimination. Volunteer work can take the form of informal assistance to friends, neighbors, or relatives, or an organized service, such as helping out in a hospital, or working for a charitable organization. Like the ideal job, in which work matches the preferences and abilities of the employee, volunteer jobs need

to provide opportunities for learning, growth, and self-expression. Participants should feel they are of use to a community.

More than two-thirds of elderly volunteers in the United States work in programs that provide services to the elderly. The services of these volunteers enrich their own lives as well as the lives of those they serve. Structured programs include:

● **The Senior Companion Program:** One-to-one relationships between the well and the frail elderly are established to reduce isolation.

● **The Service Corp of Retired Executives** (SCORE): Retirees aid small businesses and community organizations by providing financial and managerial advice.

● **The Retired Senior Volunteer Program** (RSVP): Retirees are linked to service programs such as day-care centers, nursing homes, libraries, courts, schools, and museums. This federally-funded program also provides transportation and lunch reimbursement to the volunteer.

At last there is time to try your hand at something you have long wished to attempt, and there is much to gain, both socially and intellectually.

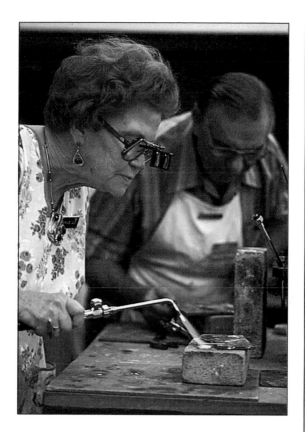

Tips on work

● Ask around among friends for employment.

● Consult employment agencies for part-time or consultancy work.

● Consider becoming a foster grandparent.

● Sign up for courses or classes at your local college or high school.

● Resume or take up a potentially lucrative hobby or craft.

● Go to your local hospital or church to discuss the possibility of some kind of volunteer work.

● **Tax Aid** and **Volunteer Income Tax Assistance** (VITA): Retirees are trained to act as tax preparers for senior center members. Retirees can also participate in inter-generational programs, applying the experience and skills they have acquired to problems faced by youngsters and younger adults.

When making inquiries about any kind of work, it helps to have a timetable in mind that will leave you time for other things. Now, more than ever, is the time to balance work with leisure, creating a healthy lifestyle for this new phase of your life. Retired people can enjoy sports as much as the young. Any glimmer of talent for writing or painting, for example, can also be developed with practice and guidance. Academic and technical courses for mature students are also available at local high schools or colleges.

Whatever you choose, remember that continued mental and physical stimulation are the two essential keys to feeling good and staying young as you grow old gracefully.

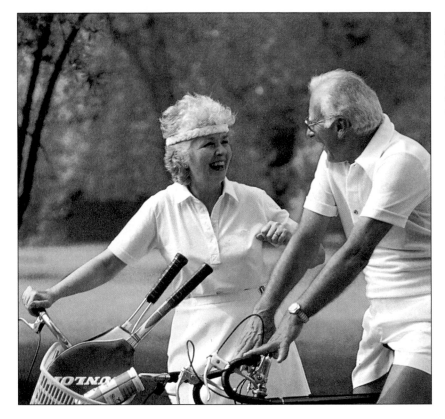

Social contacts in the retirement years are often easily fostered by mutual interest in a game such as tennis. The companionship, competition, and stimulation such contacts provide are essential to the sense of well-being.

Retirement can provoke a crisis of identity every bit as real as the traumas of adolescence or the midlife crisis. Some newly retired people enjoy a feeling of euphoria and look forward to enjoying their leisure; others are seized by a compulsion for feverish activity, such as springcleaning, home improvements, or gardening. Yet many others—men especially—suffer a keen sense of deprivation, even depression. When the farewell speeches are over, a feeling of bereavement sets in, which affects not only the retiring person but also those around him.

Relationships

All marriages suffer the ripples, if not the full impact, of retirement shock. If both partners are prepared for this and have a positive philosophy for these years of leisure, the shock is more readily absorbed. Women, generally, are less reticent than their male partners about the need for reappraisal, and the transition comes more naturally to women who have devoted their lives to the home. However, such women must also get used to sharing the house all day long with their partner.

Couples need to plan their new life together. It is a good idea to attend a pre-retirement course together and to draw up a list of goals still to be achieved. A couple's domestic routine may have to be readjusted and chores shared more equitably. This should be a time of fulfillment for both partners, not an embittered siege.

Friendships

Now, more than ever, is the time to maintain old, and cultivate new, friendships outside the home. Working life may have obscured a general lack of social contacts, and when business friendships fizzle out after retirement, as many inevitably do, life is at serious risk of becoming dreary. Women are often better at maintaining social momentum, but both partners should concentrate on renewing and cementing old friendships as well as remaining open to, and actively seeking, new ones. Friendships can be based on shared interests, experiences, and memories, and on the evidence

Aging can be a happy experience if loneliness does not become a problem. It is up to you to seek out others whose company you enjoy.

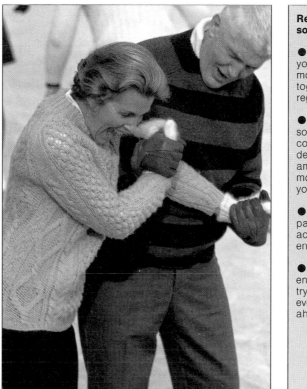

Reorganizing your social life

● Make a list of people you would like to see more often, and get together more regularly.

● Are there routine social or family commitments that demand unnecessary amounts of time, money, or effort? Can you change them?

● Decide which of your partner's social activities you most enjoy and try to join in.

● Keep an engagement diary, and try to plan some social events for the weeks ahead.

of many late marriages, new romantic attachments are certainly not out of the question at this stage of life.

Single people living on their own are most at risk of becoming lonely in these later years. It is especially important for older singles to learn the art of self-sufficiency and be diligent in keeping up with friends and making new contacts.

Younger generations

It helps to gather a good mix of ages around you, as many people wisely do long before they retire. Getting involved with people of all ages will make your transition to retirement easier and your retirement years more varied and enjoyable.

In socializing with members of other generations—whether they are your children, neighbors, or friends—it is important to realize that younger people are not automatically healthier, wealthier, and more carefree than you. They, too, have problems; they, too, get lonely. Many young people appreciate being able to call on the wisdom of age in a crisis.

Sex after 60

Sexual relations can be pleasurable and gratifying in your later years. The main problem is the shadow cast by certain unfounded beliefs—that sex in the later years is somehow distasteful, or that older people are "past it." True, there is some decrease in libido (although less in those who remain sexually active), but men do not automatically become impotent at 60, nor do women lose interest in sex after menopause. Unless indicated medically, there is no need for intercourse to cease in old age. If you have always had a warm, loving relationship, there really is no difference in sex before or after 60 (see pages 190–210). This is particularly true if you make love regularly, with a continued imaginative effort to please.

Even when you and your partner are no longer able or willing to complete intercourse, you should not draw apart physically. No one is too old for physical warmth and affection. Lovemaking in these more tranquil years is contact, communication, and physical reassurance in a love that has stood the test of time.

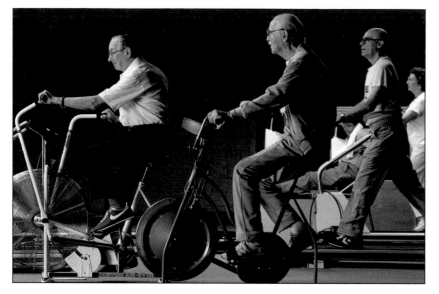

Energy breeds energy and physical activity keeps the body in tune and the mind alert. It preserves your sense of independence and your control over life.

Old age is usually considered as the time between 60 and 65, and death. Many people remain fit, alert, and vigorous well into their eighties, while others seem to be in their dotage in their sixties. It is hard to generalize about the medical and physiological implications of old age. The boundaries between different ages become blurred in the later years since there are no clear developmental stages. There is no specific age-range, for example, when people get their first gray hairs or wrinkles, and the rate at which people age varies greatly, although most people become frail from about 80 onward.

The cumulative effects of some aging processes that have been going on throughout your life or began in your middle years become noticeable only when you are at an advanced age, and for this reason they are considered symptoms of aging. They may take the form of disabilities or diseases.

Osteoporosis (see page 239) is the long-term effect of a process that usually begins before the age of 50, and osteoarthritis is a manifestation of the normal wear and tear sustained by major joints throughout life. In the cardiovascular system, the arteries slowly harden and arterial plaque clogs up the blood vessels, a process that can lead to strokes and heart disease. The old are more at risk, too, from respiratory infections because their lung tissue has lost so much of its elasticity and resilience.

Older people also contract some diseases apparently unconnected with the normal aging processes because they have been exposed to harmful factors for a long time and their general resistance to infection is low.

Resisting old age

Disease and disability are not, however, inescapable companions of old age. In fact, one of the greatest health hazards the elderly face is the widespread tendency to attribute their symptoms to old age. Often both doctors and patients hesitate to explore many symptoms that could be the signal of a treatable disease.

The body has a remarkable ability to adapt to the changes that come with age. Illness is no more normal in later years than it is at any other time of life. You should feel as fit and well as when you were younger, even if you are less resilient to sudden stress. You should always seek medical help for health problems.

It can sometimes be difficult for even the most enlightened doctor to know at what point normal aging shades into a decline caused by self-neglect or depression. Yet the distinction is critical, for most illness or injury can be successfully treated—or at least greatly relieved—at any age. It may take you longer to recover when you are elderly, but you do. Even the extremely old can be treated and comforted, and so regain the will to live and pass the time comfortably, to the end.

Common problems of aging

Medicines
Work in partnership with your doctor in pursuit of good health, and review the need for drugs regularly. Too many people buy over-the-counter drugs they do not need, but fail to fill prescriptions or take medicine as prescribed, and many find it difficult to keep track of dosages. To avoid any confusion, keep a simple schedule for regular medication. If certain medications are used infrequently, make a note on the containers of what each one is for. Do not hoard drugs indefinitely; many have a short shelf-life.

Illnesses
Heart disease is the main cause of hospitalization and death among people over 65. Next is cancer, and strokes account for the third largest share of disability and death.

Arthritis and rheumatism, while infrequently a cause of hospitalization, are second only to heart disease as the reason for visits to the doctor among the elderly. If you feel persistent joint pain and stiffness, seek medical advice to minimize the disabling effects of arthritis.

Memory lapses
Recent memory suffers more than long-term memory, and lapses from one minute to the next may become distressingly common. It often helps to make lists and to tackle tasks systematically, one at a time.

When apparent changes in memory, confusion, disorientation, or difficulties in reasoning appear, you should consult your physician to obtain a thorough evaluation of your symptoms. Such changes are not normal features of aging and might be related to medications, diet, sensory deprivation, or a treatable illness.

Impaired senses
All five senses are subject to some change with aging. The cumulative effects can prove most significant to safety, for example, when driving. It is, therefore, important regularly to assess whether you are fit to drive. The two most troublesome effects are difficulty with near focusing and a reduction in hearing acuity; both are correctable to some degree. Impaired sense of balance is often ignored and may lead to falls. Remember, too, always to bend from the knees when picking things up (see pages 138–139).

Incontinence
This is not an inescapable part of growing old and should not be accepted as such. However, urination becomes more frequent with age, and there may be a reduction in the efficiency and tone of the sphincter and the ligaments associated with the outlets of the digestive and urinary tracts. Incontinence should always be fully investigated, since it can usually be controlled and often cured.

Warning notes
The following symptoms are not normal consequences of aging. They need immediate investigation.

● Undue shortness of breath occurring at rest or during the night.

● Palpitations.

● Persistent or recurrent pain.

● Constant tiredness.

● Double vision.

● Persistent or loud ringing in the ears.

● Sudden weight loss.

● Persistent thirst.

● Persistent low-back pain.

● Loss of power in an arm or leg.

● Sudden change in bowel habits.

● Bleeding from any source.

Although there is no magic formula for eternal youth, medical science has done all it can to extend the human lifespan by banishing the epidemic diseases, such as smallpox, tuberculosis, and typhoid, that once killed most people by middle age. Over the last century, life expectancy has more than doubled. Even the conquest of other diseases is unlikely to extend the average lifespan of people in the developed world significantly. Instead, medical science is working toward making old age more active and enjoyable. The main thrust of the branch of medicine known as gerontology—the study of aging—is to establish the factors behind the normal process of aging, and to distinguish between the effects of age and those caused by lifestyle or disease. Its aim is to slow the decline in vigor that affects the body with increasing age.

Research of this kind has shown that the foundations of a robust old age are laid in youth; in making a positive investment toward good health through sensible use and care of the body. There is growing evidence that lifestyle may be a more significant factor in producing some of the degenerative diseases that are most common in old age than the aging process itself. Many illnesses of old age are attributable to years of smoking and heavy drinking (see pages 284–293), obesity (see pages 72–79), unhealthy eating habits (see pages 62–69), and a lack of exercise (see pages 96–97). One leading gerontologist estimates, for example, that almost a third of Americans die from chronic overeating.

You can begin to improve your health and well-being as soon as you break any of these bad habits. Obviously, the sooner you do it, the greater the benefits, but experiments have shown that a switch to a more health-conscious regimen can produce positive results even in people aged 70 and over.

It seems that society has seriously underestimated the human potential to lead a full and active life. The cultural expectation that older people should slow down means that many people eventually ask too little of themselves, and find that they can do less and less. Although you may not be as mobile or sprightly as in past years, the more you exercise, the more mobile you will remain. Even those confined to a wheelchair can, with their doctor's advice, do exercises for their arms and shoulders (see pages 254–255).

The science of gerontology cannot remove the fact of aging, but it can point the way to replacing dependency with extra years of vigor. It has already given a glimpse of a new era—when it might be abnormal for the old to be sick, frail, and vulnerable before they are 80. Now it is up to you, in modeling your lifestyle before and during retirement, to recognize that age need not necessarily "weary ... nor the years condemn."

A healthy old age

Food and drink
There is a great deal of evidence linking unhealthy diet with degenerative disease, including heart trouble, strokes, hypertension, late-onset diabetes, and certain cancers, so check your own diet.

● If your diet is high in fat and low in roughage, change it. To ward off constipation, add whole-wheat (or whole-grain) bread or bran, and fresh fruit and vegetables.

● It is a fallacy that elderly people should cut down their fluid intake. The recommended daily intake is 3 to 5 pints and even more in summer or if you are confined to a centrally heated home.

● If you are bored, don't resort to eating. Do some exercises or seek company.

● If you have lost interest in food, try to tempt yourself with your favorite meals, but keep your menus well-balanced with protein, carbohydrates, fat, fruit, and vegetables.

Keeping in motion
Society is at last beginning to recognize that a balance of work, play, and exercise is essential at any age.

● Everyone of retirement age should build some exercise into their daily round, but under a doctor's supervision. It will pay dividends.

● Make a point of walking or, possibly, bicycling to the store.

● Use the stairs instead of the elevator when possible.

● If you have no dog of your own, perhaps offer to take someone else's for a walk.

● Take up an activity that you enjoy, such as golf, dancing, walking, swimming, tennis, or gardening, at least 3 times a week and preferably every day. Follow the programs on pages 108–123 and do not exceed your safe maximum pulse (see pages 12–13).

● Start an exercise routine to mobilize your joints. Use the warm-up and flexibility exercise on pages 108–109 and 126–131.

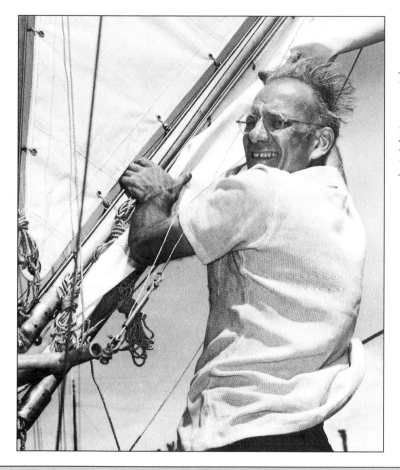

Lone yachtsman *Francis Chichester offered a perfect example of just what can be achieved in the later years of life. Having made a remarkable recovery from cancer, Chichester set out from Britain on his single-handed around-the-world voyage in August 1966, less than a month before his sixty-fifth birthday. Sailing is one of the many sports and activities open to you when you pass retirement age. With increased leisure hours, you have an ideal opportunity to take up new sports and fitness ventures.*

● A heart attack does not ban you from activity; exercise in moderation is advisable.

● It is never too late to start.

Routine maintenance
Go for regular health checks; it will either put your mind at rest or uncover any problems at an early stage. Your doctor can arrange this, or there may be a clinic in your area specializing in preventive care for the elderly.

● Flu injections may give a degree of protection and at least reduce the severity of the symptoms of an attack.

Vision: The vast majority retain more than adequate vision with the help of glasses all their lives.

● Keep your glasses clean and use good lighting for close work.

● Have your eyesight checked every year; your glasses might need changing and examination could detect a treatable condition such as cataract or glaucoma.

● Report any pain in the eyes or sudden deterioration in vision to your doctor without delay.

Hearing: Deafness is not inevitable in old age; wax accumulates faster, so syringing may help.

● If you cannot hear ordinary conversation, see your doctor.

Teeth: Neglected teeth or ill-fitting dentures can make you look older than your years, cause infections, and impair digestion.

● Have regular 6-monthly checks if you have your own teeth.

● Dentures should be checked at least every 5 years; they may need adjustment or replacing.

Feet: There is no point in becoming housebound because your feet hurt.

● Wear good, supportive shoes—avoid uncomfortable shoes and slippers for daily use.

● See the podiatrist if you have difficulty taking care of your feet.

FITNESS PROGRAM 65+

Regular physical exercise can help to maintain and improve the health of people over the age of 65, even most of those with illnesses or disabilities. Exercise helps you to move more easily and with less effort, improves your posture, and promotes relaxation. By maintaining bone strength, it might also help to slow down the process of osteoporosis. In addition to the general health benefits, physical activity promotes a sense of well-being and aids sleep.

A balanced exercise program should include:

● Flexibility, or stretching, exercises to increase and maintain the range of motion of the joints (see pages 126–131). Do them at least three times a week, but preferably every day.

● Aerobic exercises to increase endurance and stamina by conditioning the respiratory and cardiovascular systems. Do these for 30 minutes, three to five times a week. Walking briskly (see pages 108–109), using an exercise bicycle (see page 110), and swimming (see pages 116–117) are all recommended.

● Strengthening exercises twice a week to tone muscles (see pages 132–133).

If you have always been very active, age need not slow you down. At any age, stop and consult a doctor when pain or other symptoms appear and before starting a new physical activity. The exercises shown here will improve flexibility, posture, and breathing, and can be done standing or sitting in a chair.

FINGER STRETCH
1. Place the fingertips of each hand against each other. Press the palms and fingers together, creating tension along the fingers. Now relax the fingers. **2.** Squeeze the fingers together in tight fists. Relax the fingers and hands. Repeat 2 times, gradually increasing to 5.

BREATHING
1. Sit comfortably erect in a chair with your arms at your sides. **2.** As you inhale, gently raise your arms to a count of 4. Bring your palms together over your head and hold your breath for a count of 4. Exhale to a count of 4 as you lower your arms to the sides. Establish a rhythm of coordinated breathing and movement to this count of 4, and gradually increase to a count of 10. Repeat the exercise 3 times, and gradually increase to 10.

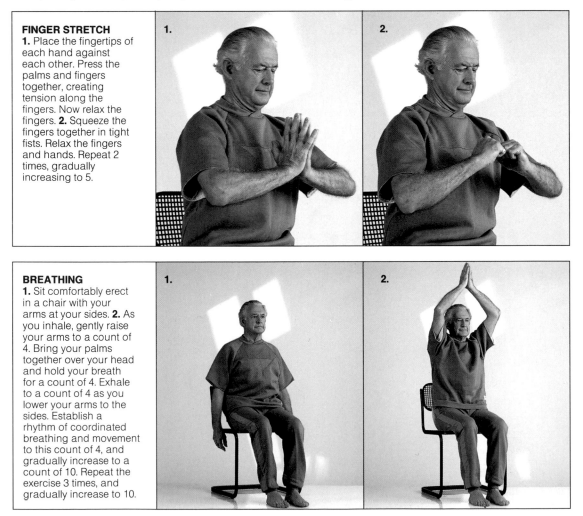

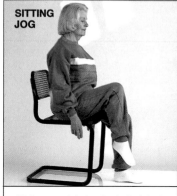

SITTING JOG

Sit in a straightback chair. Inhale as you begin to lift your right foot. Exhale as you begin to lower your right foot and raise your left. Jog 10 steps; increase to 50.

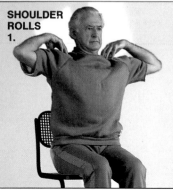

SHOULDER ROLLS
1.

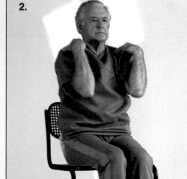

2.

1. Place your fingertips on both shoulders, elbows to the sides. Inhale as you circle your elbows up and back. **2.** Exhale as you

bring them forward and down. Repeat 4 times gradually working up to 10.

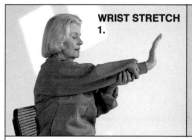

WRIST STRETCH
1.

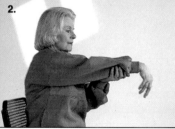

2.

1. Extend your right arm. Place your left hand under the right forearm. Spread the fingers of your right hand comfortably.

Flex the wrist back. **2.** Stretch the wrist forward and down. Repeat 2 times on each side, gradually working up to 5.

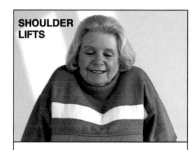

SHOULDER LIFTS

As you inhale, lift both shoulders. As you exhale, lower them and relax. Repeat 4 times, taking deep breaths between repetitions, and increase gradually to 10.

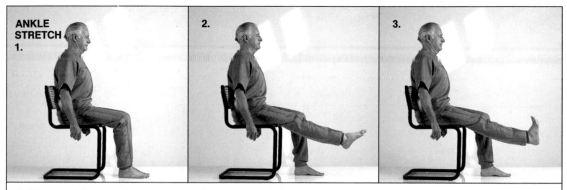

ANKLE STRETCH
1.

2.

3.

1. Sit comfortably erect in a straightback chair with both your feet flat on the floor. **2.** Extend the right leg forward and inhale as you raise it off the

floor, gently pointing your toe. **3.** As you exhale, flex your foot so that the toes are pointing toward the ceiling. Inhale again as you point your foot, and

exhale as you flex it. Now wriggle your toes, relax your foot, and return it to the floor. Repeat with the left leg. Gradually work up to repeating 5 times on each side.

Older people have as keen a sense of safety as anyone else. Moreover, they have more experience than younger people in anticipating, and avoiding danger. However, when you are older, you are clearly no longer as nimble and alert as you used to be, so situations you used to take for granted, such as crossing the road, can become hazardous.

Reduced mobility, and the combined effects of failing senses and longer nerve reaction times, can render you particularly vulnerable. Most people compensate for this by taking life at a more leisurely pace and becoming extra attentive in potentially risky situations. Unable to move quickly, for example, you are less likely to try to cross the street if the lights begin to change.

Accidents and injuries

Falls are the most common calamity for elderly people. Women's bones break more easily than men's, and about half the admissions to female orthopedic wards consist of elderly women with fractures caused by falls. Broken hips are especially common and notoriously slow to mend, but many respond well to surgery.

"Drop attacks" also pose a threat in old age. These are sudden episodes in which the legs become unaccountably weak, causing the victim to fall to the ground without losing consciousness. Their causes are not fully understood, but they are usually related to a fall in blood pressure or constriction of the brain's blood supply.

Injuries incurred by falls and drop attacks may be compounded by falling against something sharp or hot, such as the corners of cabinets, heating appliances, or stoves. There is the additional risk that if you live alone you might lie undiscovered for hours or even days. It is essential, therefore, to be alert to these dangers, to guard against falls, to consider an emergency alarm and response system in the home, and to see a doctor if you experience a drop attack.

Few people would want to live in an environment so safe and structured that it feels clinical, and when you are elderly you will probably manage as well in a place you know as you would in some custom-built home. However, it does pay to invest in safety, as it does in health, by eliminating some of the potential hazards before anyone gets hurt. The illustrations provide examples of some helpful gadgets and safety devices.

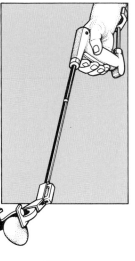

The hand reacher fitted with tongs on the end is ideal for picking up small and delicate objects that arthritic hands find it hard to cope with.

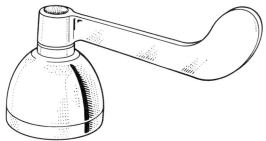

Long-bladed faucet handles that can be turned by the wrists or forearms are a great advantage if you have difficulty using conventional handles.

A jar opener that is screwed to the underside of a table or shelf enables you to open screw-top bottles and jars with one hand.

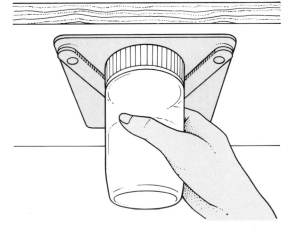

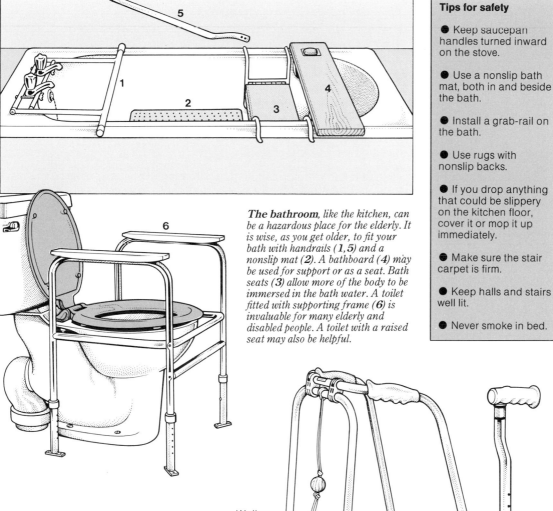

The bathroom, like the kitchen, can be a hazardous place for the elderly. It is wise, as you get older, to fit your bath with handrails (**1**,**5**) and a nonslip mat (**2**). A bathboard (**4**) may be used for support or as a seat. Bath seats (**3**) allow more of the body to be immersed in the bath water. A toilet fitted with supporting frame (**6**) is invaluable for many elderly and disabled people. A toilet with a raised seat may also be helpful.

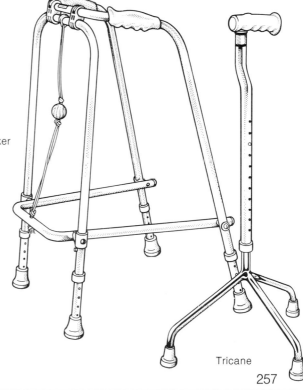

Walker

Tricane

If mobility becomes a problem as you grow older, it is sensible to use some kind of supportive device to help you get about. It is better to give in to your need for such aids than to be immobile or an accident victim as a result of your own pride. Walking sticks designed to give more support than the conventional cane come in many guises. The tricane (far right) gives extra support and stability at the base. Look for a model whose height can be adjusted and whose handle can be altered for use in either right or left hand. A walker is cumbersome but a better proposition than being confined to a bed or chair. It should be strong enough to support the entire body weight. Models such as the one illustrated (right) can be folded away for easy storage and transport.

A FIT MIND

The characteristics and foibles acquired in early life often become exaggerated with the passage of time, so that old age reveals a more fascinating mix of characters than any other age group. Some old people, however, develop into caricatures of their former selves, becoming mellow and nostalgic or miserably bitter and inward-looking. Yet, many remain wonderfully alert, vigorous, and unselfish, and are a valuable example to younger members of the community.

A positive philosophy

There is no magic formula for achieving a happy and constructive old age, but it is important to seek ways of priming the morale for the coming years. Most important of all is to realize that mental and physical stimulation are both essential and possible. Whatever your age, it is never too late to learn something new.

Another essential of the positive philosophy is to confront your fears about old age and to recognize that, if allowed to get out of hand, they can prove more diminishing to the personality than the aging process itself. The four principal fears common to most people are loneliness, physical incapacity, senility, and death. It may not be possible to banish those fears, but you must come to terms with them so they do not overshadow your life. Fear undermines and saps your vitality and resistance to disease.

Anxiety and depression can occur at any age, but remember, they are reversible. The incidence of total incapacity in the elderly population is surprisingly small and, since most old people continue to function efficiently to the end—albeit in a lower gear—everyone should look for fresh ways of gaining both experience and achievement in the later years.

Too many people fall into the trap of viewing old age as a waiting room for death. They gradually become what society expects them to be—sedentary and submissive. Instead of falling into unnecessary decline, you must take up the challenge of retirement.

Well-integrated older people capitalize on the advantage of a long life—knowledge, experience, wisdom, memories—and find that these help to compensate for the gradual physiological changes. Such people turn these later years into an Indian summer of joy and achievement. For them, after a full life, death intervenes as Leonardo da Vinci believed it should: as sleep comes after a hard day's work.

An expression of caring

Contrary to popular belief, death is, for most people, a calm rather than a painful experience. It is important to allow a dying person to choose his own style of death, and to encourage him to make the most of every living moment that remains to him. Even the dying have much to experience, and much to offer to those destined to outlive them.

For those with a deep sense of commitment to the people they love, discussion of death and its consequences is an expression of caring and not a morbid exercise. Bereavement is hard enough to

---

An aim for the elderly

The Nun's Prayer, written in the seventeenth century, is now well known across the world. Shot through with humor and compassion, it articulates the desire for the patience and restraint for which many people strive with advancing age.

"Lord, thou knowest better than I know myself that I am growing older, and will some day be old.

"Keep me from getting talkative and particularly from the fatal habit of thinking I must say something on every subject and on every occasion.

"Release me from craving to try to straighten out everybody's affairs.

"Keep my mind free from the recital of endless details—give me wings to get to the point. I ask for grace enough to listen to the tales of others' pains. Help me to endure them with patience.

"But seal my lips on my own aches and pains—they are increasing and my love of rehearsing them is becoming sweeter as the years go by.

"Teach me the glorious lesson that occasionally it is possible that I may be mistaken.

"Keep me reasonably sweet; I do not want to be a saint—some of them are so hard to live with—but a sour old woman is one of the crowning works of the devil.

"Make me thoughtful, but not moody; helpful, but not bossy. With my vast store of wisdom, it seems a pity not to use it all, but thou knowest, Lord, that I want a few friends at the end."

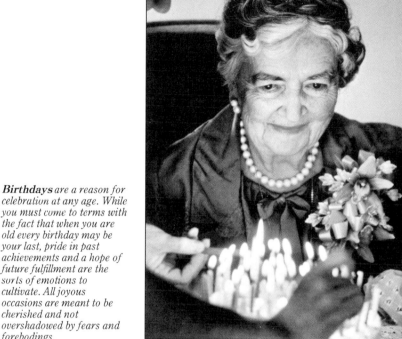

Birthdays are a reason for celebration at any age. While you must come to terms with the fact that when you are old every birthday may be your last, pride in past achievements and a hope of future fulfillment are the sorts of emotions to cultivate. All joyous occasions are meant to be cherished and not overshadowed by fears and forebodings.

Tips for mental fitness

● Learn to adapt to a lifestyle that is not governed by the need to earn a living.

● Recognize your own strengths and put them to work in new and fulfilling ways.

● Plan for the future so you have plenty to look forward to.

● Set yourself new goals.

● Stay tuned in to the outside world, including current events, the social scene, family life, and the arts.

● Hang on to your own identity, no matter what pressures there are to conform to the geriatric mold.

● Maintain standards of dress and behavior that add to feelings of self-respect.

● Keep self-pity and any other negative tendencies at bay so that you present a positive and purposeful image to the world.

● Be dignified, not submissive.

bear when it comes, and the survivors should not be burdened with the problems of trying to resolve practical affairs that could have been anticipated and dealt with well in advance. Partners should talk together openly about death, so that their wishes and the whereabouts of relevant papers—wills, insurance policies, and so on—are known to both parties, other family members, or close friends. This helps the surviving partner to cope in the first few disorienting months.

It is hard to be left alone late in life, and feelings of grief may be tinged with resentment, anger, and guilt. All these conflicting emotions need to be released, and family and friends must encourage the bereaved partner to talk about the loss until each successive stage of mourning is adequately worked through (see pages 298–299).

Grief distorts the human sense of perspective, so it is wise to resist any major changes, such as moving house, for some months after the loss of a partner or a live-in companion, housekeeper, or relative. Remember, the bereaved person is at risk, both psychologically and physically, for at least a year after the event.

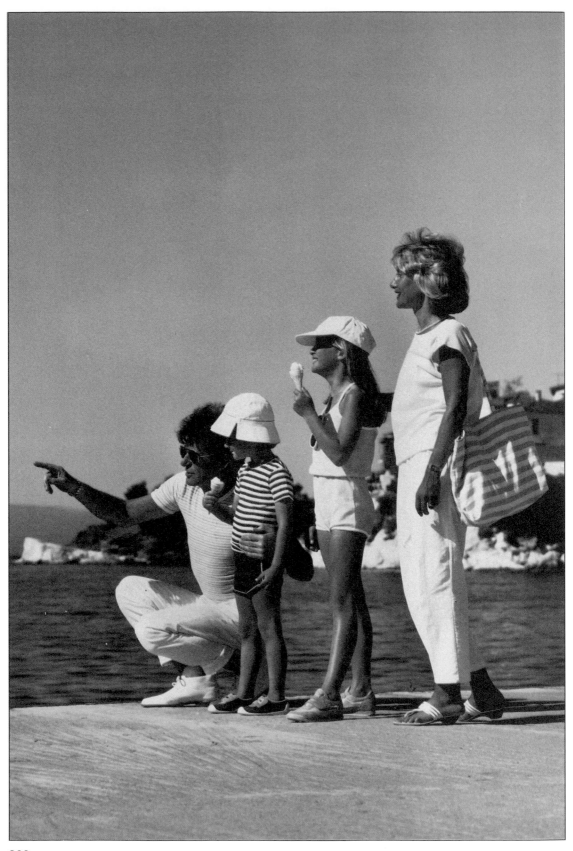

COPING WITH STRESS

People respond both physically and emotionally to stresses created by events and by the elements of their environment. This is because the mind and body work together in a complex way to create the whole person. While you need a certain amount of stress and challenge to fire you, to keep you alert and motivated, too much stress is linked with the development of a variety of illnesses. Therefore, understanding stress and learning how to deal with it need to be an integral part of both preventive health care and therapeutic medicine.

Sometimes the link between stress and physical symptoms is obvious. For example, it is quite common for children to get stomach pains or headaches before a dreaded examination or class. These symptoms are real enough, but will probably disappear quickly if the test or the feared class is canceled.

As you get older, the sources of stress in your life do not decrease. Instead, you get used to expecting certain stress-related symptoms and living with them. As you begin to master your environment, some of the events that once caused panic no longer do so. However, modern life is full of stresses—there is no limit to the circumstances that can create pressure, frustration, irritation, or anger. And compared with your forefathers, you live life at a faster pace and have much higher expectations of it.

Too often people attempt to escape their problems—or try to resolve them—by using props such as drugs, alcohol, or cigarettes. In the short run, these might provide some relief, but the costs are high. They can cause more problems, and stop people from effectively resolving the original cause of stress.

This chapter explores some of the physical and mental responses to stress, and the risks to your health and well-being that they involve. It will help you to identify the underlying causes, to analyze your reactions, and to seek new, safe, and sensible ways of problem-solving and relief from stress.

PERSONALITY

Personality is the individual hallmark of every member of the human race. No two people, not even identical twins, have the same personality. Your personality gives definition to your life and determines many aspects of it, including the things that please and displease you, the type of employment you choose, and the sorts of friendships and relationships you make.

Personality types

There are two problems in trying to classify a personality. First, there is no objective way to measure it. A physical characteristic, for example, can be measured according to absolute scientific standards. Personality, however, is a complex, inseparable mixture of mental, emotional, and behavioral traits, and the methods used to measure it—questionnaires, interviews, projective tests—are always subjective to some degree. Also, one person might be frank when completing a questionnaire, whereas another might say what he thinks is expected, even if it isn't accurate. To complicate matters further, two interviewers might differ in their observations of a person's personality or actions.

The second problem is that personality is not consistent. Different aspects of personality emerge depending on the circumstances, and can change with a person's mood. The danger in labeling personality types is to assume that a person will always react in the same way and in all situations.

With these limitations in mind, psychologists and psychiatrists try to categorize personalities by analyzing people's behavior and experiences. They group personality traits that have something in common and give them a name to describe their broad characteristics. If, for example, a person likes to be organized down to the last detail, from the placement of papers on the desk to the arrangement of clothes in the closet, or positioning the car in the garage, that personality type might be described as obsessive. This does not necessarily mean that the person is obsessive about everything, only that he has a tendency to be.

In many ways, personality determines people's reactions to certain situations, and has a bearing on their physical and mental fitness. The labels—obsessive, introspective, passive, compliant, aggressive, repressive, and so on—are a useful shorthand that helps in the definition and treatment of problems.

Some personalities, for instance, can be described as anxious. Whatever the situation, such people always find they have a higher than average level of anxiety. They might feel worried about going to social events or meetings, even if they are on good terms with all the other participants. And they often suffer from phobias, such as fear of crowded areas or open spaces, or of traveling in elevators.

Anxious personalities are not the only ones to be prone to a potential overload of stress. Obsessive personalities create stress by their meticulous attention to detail, and by their unhappiness at the imperfections that surround them. Introspective types can fret about every event and decision, and worry about their implications for themselves and others to the extent that they might end up convincing themselves to do nothing.

How personality is formed

It is not clear to what extent you are born with a certain type of personality and to what extent your personality is determined by your experiences. It seems fairly certain that you are born with a tendency toward particular traits, which are molded and changed by experience, and that other traits are learned.

Anxious personalities are often born with a genetic loading toward anxiety; their parents and close relatives usually suffer from similar problems. As children they are often bedwetters or nailbiters, are afraid of the dark, and are frightened of animals or people. Most children might have some of these problems, but anxious children suffer from many of them.

Other personality traits, such as low self-esteem or repressed behavior, are probably learned. Children who grow up in an environment in which they are not allowed to express feelings of anger and frustration find, as adults, that they cannot easily express these emotions. The conflict between their inner feelings and outward behavior creates stress. Children brought up in homes where there is little show of affection later find it difficult to express love or accept it. Children from homes in which both parents are highly successful often find themselves under severe pressure to become achievers because achievement is the one thing for which they have been rewarded in the past

Physical factors, such as height or weight, can also influence the development of personality. A boy who is significantly smaller than his peers often tries to compensate by becoming aggressive and determined to succeed. His motive might be to acquire the status and authority among his peers that his height denies him. An overweight child might act in an extroverted way in an attempt to cope with the jibes of peers and to be accepted by the crowd.

Self-esteem

One of the most important factors influencing stress-prone personalities is self-esteem, that is, the value you place upon yourself. Even if you are born with a genetic loading toward high anxiety, you will not necessarily suffer from stress, provided you feel that you are lovable and have worth, and do not need to prove yourself all the time. Problems begin if you have high anxiety and low self-esteem. You may put so much pressure on yourself that you become an extreme type A personality (see the chart at right).

It is important for parents to encourage children to develop a sense of self-esteem, so that they are able to grow up feeling loved and secure. The goals that you set for your children should be consistent and attainable, and should not be adjusted upward as soon as they have been reached. Let your children know when they have done well; don't make them feel that they are a constant disappointment to you.

Children who grow up with self-doubts often distrust others, resent injustice, and fear betrayal. They continually pressure themselves to achieve, to be more aggressive and more competent than others. They find it difficult to form stable relationships with others for fear of being betrayed by them.

Can personality be changed?

Although it is impossible and probably undesirable to completely remake your personality, it is possible for you to modify it.

The first step is to take a close look at yourself; what you are, the way you think. There is little point in trying to overcome an inborn tendency toward anxiety, for example, by sheer willpower. The harder you try, the greater your anxiety

about failure will be. And the greater the anxiety, the worse will be your performance. The best course for anxious personalities is to be aware of their limitations and to make a careful choice of job, living environment, and the like, so that they don't expose themselves to high levels of stress.

Try to spot how you may be adding to your own stresses and difficulties by the way you react. If you feel that there are aspects of your personality that you would like to change, then follow the techniques described throughout this chapter, and elsewhere in the book, to help you make a change. You'll never be perfect, but by thinking positively, and altering some aspects of your life, you can improve the quality of your life. Always remember that stress, if it is out of control, makes life significantly less pleasant for you, as well as for those around you.

Personality types

In the 1960's, two American scientists, Mayer Friedman and Ray Rosenman, devised a way of classifying personalities that has important implications for the way people deal with stress.

Type A	Type B
1. Unremitting urge to compete.	**1.** Do not feel the constant urge to compete.
2. Easily aroused to anger, irritation, aggravation, and impatience.	**2.** Relaxed, not easily roused to explosive reactions.
3. Aggressive with people who get in their way.	**3.** Tolerant toward others.
4. Cannot bear delays or waiting in lines.	**4.** Able to wait patiently.
5. Speak in a loud staccato. Tend to interrupt and to finish other people's sentences for them.	**5.** Speak slowly and calmly, do not interrupt. Good listeners.
6. More likely to smoke cigarettes.	**6.** Less likely to smoke cigarettes.
7. Twice the risk of coronary heart disease and death from heart attacks as type B personalities.	**7.** Half the risk of coronary heart disease and heart attacks as type A personalities.

The implication of these findings is that type A personalities need to learn relaxation to modify their behavior. Physical relaxation and self-talk (pages 272–273), meditation (pages 328–329), and biofeedback (pages 326–327) are among the many helpful techniques that can be used.

YOUR PLACE IN THE WORLD

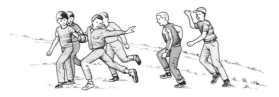

Balancing your needs with those of others, within the accepted norms of society, is crucial to any successful relationship. From the time you are born, you are taught to conform to the behavior accepted by your family, in particular, and society, in general. It is human nature to want approval and avoid doing things that will make you unpopular with others. But there may be times when you feel that you do not fit in, that what you believe is completely different from what the rest of your family, friends, colleagues, or society feels. This is natural, for few people are totally without conflicts. Usually you are able to express your individuality within the broad boundaries of conformity and cope with the occasions when you seem to be out of step with the rest of the group. Your problems begin when you are prepared to sacrifice your identity for the sake of others' approval.

Realistic goals

Many more people than you think are made uncomfortable by fears, self-doubts, and repressed thoughts similar to your own. One survey, for example, suggests that possibly 60 percent of individuals have significant sexual difficulties for a substantial period of their lives, and those who have never experienced any sexual problems are in the minority. Yet you are wrongly led to believe that other people are better adjusted or more confident in this area than you are. The "ideal" person portrayed by the mass media presents images and standards that have little chance of being lived up to.

Most people fit into society well enough most of the time, either because they are flexible, or because their attitudes or temperaments happen to agree with those of their neighbors and colleagues. If you don't fit in easily, you have to decide how to cope. If you try desperately to conform, you can put yourself under a great deal of stress, particularly if others seem aware that you still are not "one of them." You can decide not to try to conform at all, which will be seen as rebelling. Outward rebellion may seem an easy

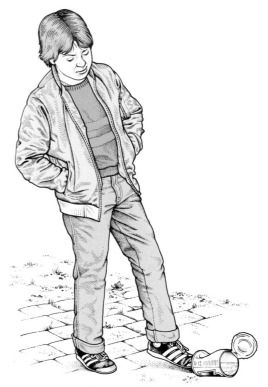

A child *who genuinely has a different outlook on life from that of his peers or his parents is likely to be a "loner." Any unhappiness experienced will be exaggerated if a child is pressured to participate in activities he considers worthless.*

option, but it can leave you isolated, which also produces stress. Inward rebellion masked by outward conformity is harder to sustain.

The halfway approach

Adopting the halfway approach means conforming to some rules and not to others, and requires a great deal of self-confidence. For example, a woman who does not like to cook might feel obliged to give a dinner party for her business associates. She might decide that the best compromise between her dislike of cooking and her guests' expectations is to hire caterers or to invite each guest to provide a dish. Some people would probably regard her as an outsider because of her unconventional behavior, but others might admire her courage and even follow her example.

The halfway approach must be thought out intelligently: if you turned up at the firm's annual dinner dance in a smart shirt and tie, but also wearing a pair of jeans, it is the latter you will be

A workable philosophy

If you are by nature a nonconformist and you try to conform, you might be exhausted by the effort. If you choose not to conform, you will have to subject yourself to pressure and rejection from others. Both choices are stressful.

The most effective course involves a change of philosophy, summed up in this prayer:
"Lord, help me to change the things I cannot bear. Lord, help me bear the things I cannot change. And, most important, Lord, grant me the wisdom to know the difference."

To get to this point, try the following steps:

● Decide what you have to do to get along with the outside world and make a list.

● Carry out these plans with good grace and, if possible, without compromise.

● Eliminate from your list those activities you are doing simply from duty. Do not be ashamed, embarrassed, or apologetic for not carrying them out.

● Remember: it is *how* you present yourself, and your degree of self-confidence and sensitivity to other people's feelings that determine how they will respond to you.

judged on. In this case, your compromise will be seen either as a halfhearted attempt to flout convention or as a lamentable lack of dress sense.

Children who do not fit in

Children who, from an early age, genuinely see things differently from the majority will suffer if their parents try to pressure them to conform. Such children are aware of their differences and usually realize that attempts to change them are doomed to failure. They will be under stress from the conflict between the way they know they are and the way their parents want them to be, and may come to believe that there is something wrong with them. But being different is not necessarily wrong, any more than conforming to the crowd is automatically right. Parents can help children who are misfits by encouraging them to explore the world as they see it, by making clear the choices open to them, and by pointing out the advantages and disadvantages of specific courses of action.

Children who are anxious or lack self-confidence also have trouble fitting into society. Again, pressure from parents and other adults is counterproductive. Setting up an active social calendar to get children used to situations they fear is rarely successful, and often increases their basic anxiety. The best course is to help these children to build up their social confidence gently and steadily by organizing occasional small gatherings or encouraging them to invite their friends to come around.

Children who are rebelling also suffer from alienation. Most children go through phases of rebelling against specific parental rules as they try to broaden and define areas of their independence. But there are some children who seem to rebel against all adult rules and standards. These children are usually conforming to peer group pressure.

Confrontation is unlikely to produce any positive results. It often leads to intensely emotional arguments, which force children to maintain their position. Instead, parents should be tolerant, bearing in mind that adolescent rebellion usually represents an attempt to assert individuality and independence, rather than just a crude rejection of parental values. Parents need to be supportive at a time when the demands of adulthood are putting pressure on their children.

How to deal with a rebellious teenager

● Try a contract. If your child wants something from you, you are entitled to ask for something in return. But remember, blackmailing a child into changing by withholding money is unlikely to work.

● Ignore the behavior if you can. Rebellion usually continues because it is reinforced by a disapproving reaction.

● Is the rebellious behavior *really* so deserving of criticism? It is often a response to peer group pressure.

● Remember that teenage revolt is usually temporary.

● If you can tolerate the behavior, you might try encouraging it; this will make rebellion lose its appeal.

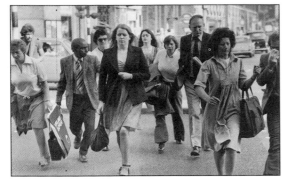

Stress is usually thought of as a particular response of the body to threatening external events. Surprisingly, perhaps, stress is the body's general response to any demand made on it, regardless of whether that demand is pleasant or unpleasant, and whether it is emotional or physical. The stressful effects of accidents or bereavements, or of simply trying to keep up with the many tasks you have to accomplish during the day, are obvious. But the physiological responses to happy events, such as getting married, having a baby, receiving an increase in salary, or falling in love, are strikingly similar to those brought about by unhappy events.

Is stress necessary?

All living creatures need challenges to keep them stimulated, and human beings are no exception. Without challenges, people become dull and apathetic, and lose the will to live life to the fullest.

The hectic pace of life, particularly in crowded towns and cities, induces stress by activating the nervous system and preventing muscles from relaxing.

The soft life is not as attractive as it might sound. In fact, it may hold as many potential dangers to fitness and well-being as one in which there is a high degree of stress.

For primitive humans, the challenges of life were largely physical. In modern society, however, physical challenges are few, and the ones that exist tend to be self-created, such as those of sports. But you are regularly faced with emotional challenges. These emanate from your work and your homelife, and from your relationships with other people.

Challenges can also be enjoyable and raise your performance to unexpected heights. Tackling a difficult job successfully, taking part in a high-risk sport, or watching a horror movie can all provide you with an inner thrill. And anxiety, so long as you can keep it under control, can help you to perform at your best in all kinds of tasks, from taking examinations to handling business meetings or competing in a tennis tournament.

Stress thresholds

Overt, damaging stress occurs when challenges become impossible to cope with. In this sense, stress is a protective reaction to too much challenge. The effect of excessive stress can manifest itself in a variety of ways; it can cause potentially harmful changes in behavior and undermine

Mass transit is one stressful aspect of modern city life. Fear of strangers is a constant source of inner anxiety, particularly for concerned and caring parents.

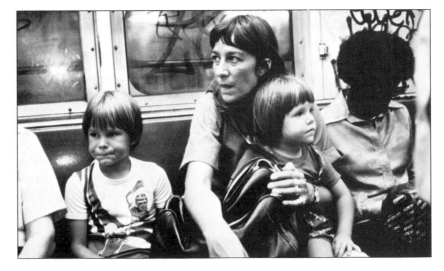

Stress is nothing new, but the 20th century has produced many changes that have increased the amount of stress people experience.

● Any change that upsets your accustomed pattern of life can cause stress.

● Advances in technology have increased the pressure on everyone. In an age of speed and instantaneous worldwide communication, there is greater need for quick responses than in the past.

● More decisions have to be made nowadays. The average person has a high degree of responsibility and accountability.

● You have a wider range of choices at all levels of your life, in work and in leisure.

● Overcrowding, noise, and pollution have resulted from an increase in population.

● People have come to demand a higher quality of communication and understanding in all their relationships.

● Technology has affected work, leisure, and social relationships. Human contact is decreasing as a result.

both physical and mental health (see pages 268–269).

Apart from being deprived of basic necessities such as food or sleep, there are no situations or circumstances that are universally stress-inducing. People vary widely in the amount of challenge they can tolerate before they begin to experience adverse effects. While some people cope easily with the demands of a job that involves regular international travel, others find it intolerable.

Similarly, the threshold at which potentially harmful stress occurs in any individual varies with the circumstances. Thus you might find it easy to cope with the stresses of office life but difficult to cope with the demands of parenthood, of managing your personal finances, or of maintaining a loving relationship with your partner. Or you might find your work a breeze when you are alone, but difficult or impossible in a noisy, crowded office.

There are many factors that determine stress thresholds. They include personality, self-discipline, and the discipline imposed by society and by circumstances. As a rule, people whose lives and relationships can be labeled "stressful" are also those with the highest tolerance for all kinds of stress.

These people have learned not only how to cope with stress and overcome it, but also how to adjust their aspirations to the realities of life. Their success is not necessarily measured in material terms. They might be tired at the end of the day, but their morale is high, and their health is not likely to be suffering.

Stress and fitness

The way in which damaging stress manifests itself in the body varies from one individual to another. And one of the important aspects of dealing with stress is knowing the way your body reacts to challenges that are too severe. These reactions are automatic and subconscious, and might range from being irritable to overeating, breaking out in hives, developing a migraine headache, or having heartburn. However, once you understand the stresses operating in your life, you can begin to cope with them. You should find that eventually, with practice, it is possible for you to control your stress-related symptoms (see pages 268–269).

As long as you feel that there is a good correspondence between the world as it is and the world as you expect it to be, your expectations are unlikely to be a cause of stress. Stress emerges if reality and the fantasy of what life should be are widely different.

When assessing your expectations in life, and the amount of stress they provoke, remember:

● Expectations are taught from earliest childhood. To lessen stress, it might be necessary to "unlearn" some of them.

● The nature of the society in which you live brings with it certain expectations. You are expected to be competent, to achieve, and to conform.

● Your expectations are subtly molded by what you see and read. The expectation of perfection induces stress if you try too hard to live up to it.

● Your feelings of self-worth are likely to depend on whether you live up to your standards. Within limits, it is important to learn to live with yourself as you are.

REACTIONS TO STRESS

Throughout life, the component parts of the body strive to work together in efficient harmony, reacting constantly to the demands made on them from within and without. Many of these demands pose a threat to the body. The body's response, which is both universal and primitive, is to prepare itself for fight or flight. First, in a reflex action, the muscles become tense. After this, a whole series of reactions comes into operation, as described below.

The hypothalamus at the base of the brain becomes activated and stimulates the pituitary gland to release hormones. These stimulate the adrenal glands above the kidneys to produce other hormones, which have wide-ranging effects on the body. Some body activities are increased, others decreased.

Muscles might ache. Pain might also result from the slow mobilization of lactic acid.

The liver discharges sugars into the blood to provide muscles with extra energy. It might also produce and release excess amounts of cholesterol.

The skin becomes pale as blood is drained away from it and sent to the muscles.

Sweat production is increased, ready to cool down a body overheated by the exertion of fight or flight.

The pupils of the eyes dilate.

The salivary glands stop secreting saliva, making the mouth feel dry.

Breathing rate speeds up to supply more oxygen to the muscles.

Heart rate increases to supply more blood to the muscles.

Blood pressure rises.

Adrenal glands release adrenaline.

Kidneys work less efficiently because their blood supply is reduced.

Digestion ceases or slows down.

Defecation and urination are prevented by the tightening of muscles. Alternatively, diarrhea or uncontrolled urination might occur.

The immune system is impaired, making a person susceptible to disease or to an allergic reaction.

Do you recognize two or more of the following in yourself or someone close to you? If so, the problem needs to be tackled immediately (see pages 272–275).

● Have your eating habits changed?

● Has your sleep pattern altered?

● Is your digestive system upset?

● Have you developed any nervous habits, such as fidgeting or touching your hair and face repeatedly?

● Is your blood pressure raised?

● Do you have frequent headaches, cramps, and muscle spasms?

● Have you become hyperactive?

● Have your sexual performance, drive, and enjoyment deteriorated?

● Are you drinking or smoking more?

● Has your child reverted to an earlier, outgrown habit, such as bedwetting, temper tantrums, or thumb-sucking?

The body's first reaction to any potentially harmful demand is to prepare for action. It gets ready to face danger (fight) or to run away (flight). The illustration opposite shows how the various parts of the body respond.

The two key areas are the heart, which needs to be able to pump more blood to the muscles, and the muscles themselves, which make the body ready for physical action. The lungs provide more oxygen to the muscles for energy and to the brain for alertness. Stored sugars and fats are released into the blood, but because of the overriding need of the muscles, the blood flow to some organs, such as those of the digestive system, is cut off.

When immediate danger passes, this gearing-up process is reversed. And it seems that the act of fighting or running away actually helps the reversal process. In your everyday life, however, you encounter many threatening situations in which you cannot fight or flee. Since there is no physical action you can take, the reversal does not occur, or occurs incompletely, and you stay "wound up." This is one reason why exercise is so effective in relieving stress.

Adaptation and exhaustion

When the body is subjected to stress over a long period, it remains in a prolonged state of preparedness for fight or flight. Blood pressure is permanently raised, continuing muscular tension leads to digestive problems and aches and pains, and the body's resistance to disease remains suppressed.

Unless action is taken to alter either the stress factors or the body's reaction to them, the consequence will eventually be exhaustion. How long it takes before this exhaustion occurs depends on a person's physical constitution, which is determined partly by heredity and partly by health habits such as diet and exercise; on personality and attitudes; and on social relationships. When the body is no longer able to cope, a major physical or mental breakdown results.

In order to combat stress, you have to be able to recognize when it is affecting you. Use the physical and mental symptoms listed on this page to help you discern whether stress is affecting you; but remember that many of them can have other causes and it is the *changes* in behavior that are significant. If an activity is ingrained, it is a habit, not a sign of stress.

Do you recognize two or more of the following in yourself or in someone close to you? If so, stress might be reaching a potentially dangerous level. Remember, however, that these can also be symptoms of other problems, such as physical illness.

● Have you begun to suffer from a phobia or obsession?

● Have you lost self-confidence and self-esteem?

● Do you constantly feel guilty?

● Do you dread the future?

● Have your memory and concentration deteriorated?

● Do you find yourself unable to finish one task properly before having to rush on to the next?

● Do you feel constantly irritable and angry?

● Do you feel isolated?

● Do you fill the day with trivial tasks?

● Do you find it hard to make decisions?

● Do you often cry or feel like crying?

● Does your mind race so that you cannot focus on one task or thought?

TRAVEL STRESS

Whether you are a driver or a passenger, travel can be a major source of stress in your life. Although many people find that going for a drive can help them unwind when they feel tense or angry, research suggests that driving can be enormously stressful.

Drivers and passengers

The stress associated with driving is caused by many factors, including noise and vibration, the behavior of the passengers, and frustration with the traffic. Studies of rush-hour drivers show that they experience marked rises in heart rate, blood pressure, and sweating on the palms (see page 326), all of which are reliable indicators of inner stress.

The very act of driving seems to create personality change. While it may be expected that aggressive people become even more so when driving, it is surprising that people who are normally restrained, calm, and unassertive often become aggressive as soon as they are behind the wheel of an automobile. It has been suggested that inside their cars drivers feel secure enough to reveal an otherwise controlled aggression because they are not involved in any face-to-face confrontation.

Some drivers respond to traffic with mounting irritability and hostility, and act as if someone has to be blamed for the problem. You may take it as a personal affront if someone passes you or prevents you from getting ahead. And these feelings are intensified if you feel envious or dismissive of either the driver or the other car. Furthermore, your "fight or flight" response (see pages 268–269) will make you try to release your tensions through more aggressiveness and risk-taking. Add to all this the frustrations and exhaustion of a hard day's work at the office, and your "stress total" can be excessive.

No matter what the form of transportation, as a passenger you might not fare much better. Frustrations arise as you wait for bus, train, or taxi, and mount the longer you wait. Your frustrations might be exacerbated by people who are also stressed and who, not waiting their turn, rush ahead of you, perhaps taking "your" taxi or preventing you from getting on the bus or train. If you are worried about arriving at your destination in time for an appointment, your anxiety will intensify with each delay.

Other passengers are also a source of stress. You might resent the fact that they have a seat on public transportation and you do not, and be irritated by being jostled in a crowd of other standing passengers. By the end of such a journey, even a simple act, such as someone coughing, can be enough to infuriate you.

Add to these stresses those brought about by bureaucratic procedures, such as checking in at an airport or being woken up in a train to check for a ticket, and it is no wonder that you arrive at your destination harassed and irritable. And the cup of coffee offered on arrival to calm you down has the effect of exacerbating, rather than reducing, stress symptoms (see page 269).

Reducing travel stress

There are many practical ways to reduce the amount of stress you experience when traveling, especially when driving.

● Learn to calculate travel times sensibly. Add on extra time for delays.
● Resign yourself to the fact that there is no way of speeding up arrival times.
● Sit as comfortably as you possibly can, especially behind the wheel of a car. Check that your shoulders are not hunched, your teeth are not clenched, and your hands are not gripping the wheel too tightly.
● Reduce neck tension with relaxing movements of the head.
● Do not drive for more than two or three hours without a break. At breaks, take a short walk or a nap, and eat a light snack.
● Change your position regularly.
● If children or other passengers create a disturbance, stop the car and explain that it is unsafe to continue.
● Learn to suspend, rather than give in to, frustration. Use your imagination. Try labeling a reckless driver as "probably someone whose loved one is on the danger list in the hospital," the poor driver as "someone who is on a once-a-year outing."
● Find a less frustrating means of travel.

Coping with jet lag

Many business trips and family vacations have been marred by jet lag, the result of traveling by airplane across several time zones. Your 24-hour

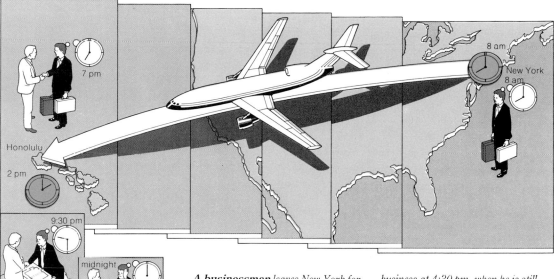

A businessman leaves New York for Honolulu at 8 am. He travels 5,000 miles across 5 time zones in 11 hours. He arrives at his destination at 2 pm Honolulu time. His body clock registers 7 pm New York time. Arriving at his Honolulu office at 2:30 pm, having eaten on the plane, he concludes his business at 4:30 pm, when he is still performing at peak level. At 7 pm Honolulu time, he goes out to celebrate. By this time he is too tired to enjoy himself and the drink quickly goes to his head. It would have been more sensible for him to have eaten a light meal and to have gone to bed early.

Training for local time

Cope with jet lag by preparing your body beforehand.

● Calculate the time difference between home and your destination.

● For a few days before your journey, start going to bed an hour earlier or later each night (depending on whether you are traveling west or east).

● Rise an hour earlier or an hour later each morning.

● Adjust your meal times to the new schedule.

cycle of sleeping and waking is largely controlled by a gland in the brainstem and synchronized with the day-night cycle of your environment. When you move to a very different time zone your body rhythms will usually take several days to a week to adjust to it.

Don't try to ignore jet lag in the hope that you can overcome it by sheer effort or with sleeping pills. Instead, either keep to home time or train yourself for the new local time before you travel. If neither of these is possible or practicable, try to find a compromise.

If possible, choose your flight so that events at your destination will fit in with your own home rhythm. An early or mid-afternoon flight from New York, for example, will bring you to Hawaii in the evening. If you have slept on the plane, as your body clock would tell you to, you will arrive reasonably refreshed and ready for an evening meal. Go to bed at a reasonable hour local time, and you should be able to sleep and be refreshed the next day.

Decision-making

After a long flight:

● Schedule important decisions to fit in best with your body clock.

● Do not make decisions when your body clock says you should be asleep.

● Do not make decisions until you have had at least one good night's sleep following your arrival.

● Do not make a decision until you have adjusted sufficiently to the new time zone.

MANAGING STRESS/1

Two important strategies in dealing with stress are learning to relax and learning to modify your behavior in order to avoid stress or alleviate it. Relaxation helps reduce stress by distracting your mind· from stress-provoking thoughts. It also helps to counter the effects of the "fight or flight" reaction (see pages 268–269). Learning to relax takes considerable practice, and mastery comes slowly; follow the tips given in the illustration opposite.

As an alternative to physical relaxation, use your imagination. For example, imagine a pleasant, peaceful scene, such as a sunny, deserted beach. Close your eyes and concentrate on all the colors, smells, and sounds. Put yourself in the picture in a relaxed position. Continue imagining yourself on the beach for 10 to 15 minutes. You might find a sound-effects tape helps to increase the reality of the scene. You could also try techniques such as meditation (pages 328–329), yoga (pages 148–153), massage (pages 308–311), or biofeedback (pages 326–327).

Exercise, diet, and sleep play an enormous part in reducing stress, as well as in maintaining more general bodily fitness. It is very easy to become so involved in the serious business of living that you never find the time or energy to play. Make sure that you regularly do things just for fun. It may be as simple as taking a walk in a park, going to the movies, or even doing something you would normally think of as childish, such as jumping into a pile of fallen leaves or splashing in puddles. If life seems to be full of worries, try to see the lighter side. Laughter is a great antidote for stress, and if you can laugh, those around you will also feel less stress when they are in your company.

A change of routine
Breaking routines helps to remove the stress that is bound into your personal rituals. For example, try coming home by a different route. Pick up a small gift for yourself or a loved one on the way. And when you arrive, don't always do the same thing. If you usually sit down in front of the TV with a drink, try doing 10 minutes' exercise and taking a shower first. Similarly, on weekends it is just as important to vary your activities as much as you can.

As a rule, increasing your level of activity is beneficial in reducing stress. The list of possibili-

ties is endless; why not start with simple activities like walking, singing, window shopping, cooking, painting, or gardening. Choose something you think will be fun, and if it isn't, try something else. Although no single activity is guaranteed to remove all stress, if you do nothing and change nothing, your stress will certainly persist and probably increase.

You might find that volunteer work helps to relieve your stress. This is not because seeing people with greater problems than your own puts your life in perspective (although that might be a bonus), but because helping others involves new social interactions, and the use of talents that otherwise remain untapped. If, however, you find volunteer work competitive, too time-consuming, or emotionally demanding, have no qualms about stopping at once.

Letting off steam is a good way of relieving tension. It is best to express your frustration or anger when it occurs; if you always bottle things up, you are more likely to suffer from the physical illnesses associated with stress or to explode with pent-up rage. If you want to yell to let off steam, go somewhere, such as a basement or a garden, where you cannot easily disturb others.

One of the best, but most difficult, stress-relieving strategies is to change your responses to the events around you. In a traffic jam, for example, instead of honking your horn and fuming, try leaning back and relaxing. Wind down the window and see if you can catch someone's eye and make him or her smile. If your first attempt isn't successful, don't give up—try something different.

Self-talk
When you watch children carrying out tasks such as tying their shoelaces, you will see that they talk themselves through the action. Without this chatter, the task is difficult to learn and perform. Recent research has suggested that this approach is also useful to adults, especially when they switch from negative to positive talk.

As you talk to yourself, use the examples given opposite to help you. Be sure to concentrate on the positive aspects of the problem or situation. Don't become self-conscious if you discover you are talking aloud to yourself. Finding a way to deal with stress is more important than temporary embarrassment.

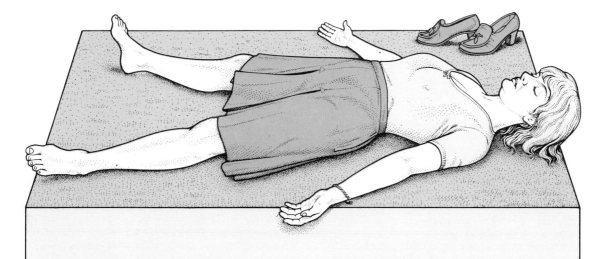

LEARNING RELAXATION

1. Do not try to learn relaxation when you are feeling tired. You will learn better and more effectively when you are alert.

2. Try to minimize background sources of stress such as noise and the presence of other people.

3. Do not rush or watch the clock. If you are worried about going on too long, set an alarm to ring after a period of, say, 20 minutes.

4. If you are not succeeding, *do not* try harder. This will only make you more tense. Instead, give yourself a rest for a couple of days and start again, giving most emphasis to the parts of the exercise you found most effective.

Before you begin

1. Choose a quiet, comfortable place.

2. Loosen any tight clothing and take off your shoes.

3. Sit or lie as comfortably as possible.

4. Close your eyes, uncross your legs, and rest your hands flat, palms upturned.

Relaxing each body part

Tense each part of the body as described below for a count of 10. Take a deep breath in, feel the tension, then let the tension go as you breathe out, quietly saying the word "relax" to yourself as you do so to reinforce the message of relaxation.

Toes: Curl your toes toward you or down to the floor.

Calves: Point your toes toward your face.

Buttocks: Push your buttocks hard against your chair or bed, at the same time trying to make your body feel as heavy as possible.

Abdomen: Tense your abdomen, as if preparing to receive a punch in the stomach.

Shoulders: Shrug your shoulders as high as they can possibly go.

Throat: Use your chin to press your throat hard.

Neck and head: Press your neck and head against the backs of your shoulders, stretching your neck as you do so.

Face: Tighten as many facial muscles as possible, including forehead, jaw, chin, and nose.

Quick relaxation

If there is no time to complete the full procedure, or it is not convenient, use the following actions, tensing and relaxing as above. You can perform such actions unobtrusively in all kinds of situations.

1. Tighten and tense the whole of the upper part of your body.

2. Pull in your abdomen or tense your buttocks.

3. Try to force your body off the chair by pressing the soles of your feet hard against the floor and trying to lift your body using your calf and other leg muscles.

Self-talk

Use the following examples to work out some possibilities for yourself:

1. "It might be difficult, but I am going to go through the argument with them again."

2. "I must turn down that extra work. I can cope now, but with extra I will be overloaded."

3. "I know I am being yelled at, but she is under stress too and has probably had a bad day."

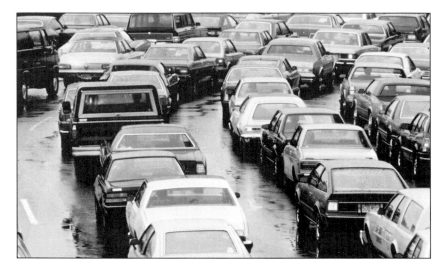

If car travel is an essential part of your daily routine, try to minimize the stress it involves. Use delays and traffic jams to advantage by taking the time to relax. Don't let yourself become agitated by a situation you have no power to change.

Stress is often the result of a conflict between unrealistic expectations and reality. Some expectations may be imposed on you by your parents and teachers; others you learn from your peers and from the society in which you live. If you accept these attitudes uncritically, and don't allow for your own and others' abilities and shortcomings, your expectations are likely to be unrealistic. Psychologists refer to such expectations as myths. How many of the following statements do you believe are true and influence you?

● I must be competent and win the approval of people I think are important to me.
● I must please everyone.
● Happiness comes from the outside.
● Life must deal justly with me.
● Others must reward me and support me whatever I do.
● There is always a clear-cut and identifiable solution to any problem.
● I must never make mistakes.
● I must never fail.

All of these statements represent unrealistic expectations—they are myths.

The consequences of myths

Stress is invariably the consequence of myths such as these. If you feel that you must win the approval of everyone around you, you will spend a great deal of time doing what other people want—or what you *think* they want. Since it is impossible to please everybody, your actions will be inconsistent and arbitrary. Even more important, you will always be frustrated.

If you regard happiness as coming from the outside, you will waste a lot of time chasing it, because all the evidence suggests that happiness comes from within yourself. You will be similarly disappointed if you always expect life to be just to you. And believing that there is always a clear solution to a problem means that you will often spend a great deal of time seeking nonexistent answers.

To believe that you must never make a mistake means you will spend a lot of time checking everything you do. You will probably be intolerant of other people's errors, and find it impossible to admit your own. If you believe that you must never fail, then the stressful conditions you create for yourself will make you much more likely to do so.

To reduce stress resulting from myths, you must learn to identify the myths and accept the realities of life. Use a step-by-step approach. First, ask yourself what your own "shoulds" or "musts" *really* are, and write them down. Then challenge your own expectations, asking yourself, "Why do I believe that? Is it possible to live up to this rule? What will happen if I don't? Will I really lose the approval of others?"

Next, revise your rules to make them more reasonable. Use self-talk methods, making statements such as, "It would be nice if others thought well of me. I certainly would feel uncomfortable if everyone did not like me. But I can accept that some people may not like me. Besides which, I like myself, and my friends like me, even if other people do not."

Solving problems

The first stage in solving stress-inducing problems is to *define* them clearly. Ask yourself whether a problem is related to a particular situation or is a general reaction. For example, is it all criticism that upsets you, or only criticism from particular people? Look, too, for the reasons underlying other people's reactions rather than assuming that it is you who are at fault. Then think out a wide range of possible solutions, rejecting those that you know from experience do not work. Do not delude yourself into thinking that if you try hard enough, a chosen solution must work. This is not true. It is the *quality* of effort involved in seeking out feasible solutions, not the *amount*, that is important.

Now ask yourself how other people might respond if asked to solve a problem similar to your own. This will generate more ideas, and will also help put the problem in perspective. Next, rank each suggested approach in order of desirability and try the most feasible. Evaluate the results, and use any failures as feedback for attempting a different approach.

Coping with failure

No one can cheat the laws of chance and win all the time. That is a fact of life. But when some people fail, they sink into a state of "learned helplessness," an attitude that implies they are incapable of succeeding at anything. People with a keen sense of failure also tend to consider every situation to be more important to their own self-esteem than it really is. And because they are often afraid to ask others for help or favors, or refuse to delegate, they do not make the most of the resources available. It is not whether people fail that determines their success, but how they cope with failure.

Change your responses if they are not resolving your difficulties. You are the only person who can improve your performance. There is no sense in blaming past events or other people for everything that goes wrong. You might get sympathy, but you will not achieve the results you want.

SLEEP AND DREAMS

Sleep is an activity essential to fitness and well-being. Yet many people have trouble in sleeping well, or worry that the amount of sleep they do get is inadequate for their needs. The massive consumption of sleeping tablets is alone a testament to this fact.

The amount of sleep that people need varies widely. It is the quality rather than the quantity of sleep that seems to be significant. And too much sleep can make people as irritable and impair their concentration as much as too little. Some can manage with as little as five hours a night, others need eight or even nine hours. It does seem, however, that the symptoms resulting from lack of sleep are due as much to feelings of being deprived of sleep, as to actually having lost necessary sleeping time.

Sleep and stress

Stress is probably the largest single cause of sleeplessness. What is worse, stress not only leads to insomnia, but insomnia increases stress by producing worries about whether you are getting enough sleep to cope with the next day's problems—and so a vicious circle begins.

People vary in their basic levels of anxiety, and this has a bearing on their sleep patterns. Low-arousal people remain calm in most situations and have few, if any, sleep problems. High-arousal people—the worriers—are the ones who lie awake with alert, anxious minds at night. If they fall asleep and then wake during the night, the anxious thoughts and worries reappear almost immediately, and they find it difficult to drop off to sleep again.

Most people fall between these two extremes, and it is only the occasional worry that disturbs their sleep. Unfortunately, the greater the worry, the more they try to forget it and the more it affects their sleep. When people are under stress, they might, therefore, have difficulty in getting to sleep and have long periods of wakefulness during the night. People suffering from depression, however, usually find, by contrast, that they wake up too early in the morning rather than have trouble getting to sleep.

Whenever the mind is unoccupied—as it is immediately before sleep—the "gap" is filled by worry. Short-term worries, such as moving house or an important business meeting, can cause temporary insomnia; the normal sleep pattern returns as soon as the problem is solved. Long-term worries, however, such as losing a job, emotional upheavals, or serious illness in the

STAGES OF SLEEP

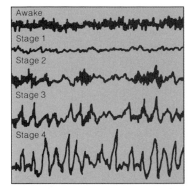

Sleep consists of several stages, which can be recorded from the brain as electroencephalograms, or EEGs. On the average, a person lies in bed for 15 minutes before falling asleep. Blood pressure, heart rate, and body temperature fall. Consciousness shifts from one subject to another. This is Stage 1 sleep. Soon Stage 2 sleep appears. The sleeper is unconscious and heart rate has slowed further. Stage 3 is deeper still, and Stage 4 the deepest.

Some 60 to 90 minutes after the onset of sleep, the heart rate increases, and the eyes dart about beneath closed lids. This is rapid eye movement, or REM, sleep (see below), which is associated with dreaming. The sleeper then descends to Stage 2. The next move is to Stages 3 and 4, back through 3 and 2, and into another REM period. The cycle from deep sleep to REM and back again usually repeats itself four to six times during the night.

It is known that Stages 3 and 4 are essential to avoid feelings of lethargy the next day. Loss of REM sleep leads to aggressiveness and irritability. Sleeping pills and other drugs interfere with Stages 3 and 4, and with REM sleep.

RAPID EYE MOVEMENT (REM) SLEEP

Getting a better night's sleep

Although the same strategies are not equally successful for everyone, there are some do's and don't's that should be helpful to most people.

Do:
● Set up and follow pre-sleep routines. A ritual and gradual "winding down" seems important for many people. This might consist of light exercises followed by a hot bath, a warm drink, and a short period of reading.

● Exercise regularly.

● Get up earlier.

● Make your sleep schedule as regular as possible. Go to bed at about the same time each night and, more important, get up at the same time each morning, even if you feel you would prefer to stay in bed a while longer.

● Keep warm.

● Drink a glass of milk or a milk drink. Milk contains tryptophan, a substance that promotes sleep.

Don't
● Eat food that leads to the production of gas in the stomach a few hours before going to bed. Such foods include fruit, beans, nuts, and raw vegetables. Don't eat high-fat foods, which keep your digestive system active.

● Drink alcohol. A small amount can help sleep, but too much can rob you of important REM sleep.

family, can cause the insomnia to persist even when the original cause is removed. In chronic insomnia anxiety shifts away from the basic problem to whether or not sleep will arrive. It leaves the sufferer exhausted and is a problem that usually requires medical help.

Surprisingly, for some people anxiety or misery can lead to more sleep than usual. In this situation, sleep seems to provide a means of escape from problems.

Sleeping pills

Pills are useful for curing short-term, acute insomnia, but they can impair the quality of sleep and produce feelings of a "hangover" the next day. They are not advisable for chronic insomnia because they create dependence.

If you want to stop using sleeping pills, which is recommendable, try to cut down your dosage gradually, and be prepared to experience more restless sleep than you have been used to. Getting back to your normal sleeping pattern could take several weeks, and it will also take you time to overcome your physical and psychological dependence on the drugs. Remember, too, that exercise will help, since physical tiredness helps override anxiety.

Dreams and sleep

Everyone dreams, but people often quickly forget their dreams on waking. It might be that you are most likely to recall the dreams that have the most meaning to you. Also, dreams are easiest to remember if you are awakened immediately after a period of REM sleep (see diagram opposite).

Dreams are now thought not to be essential ingredients of sleep. Rather, it is REM sleep that is critical. But, from the Old Testament prophets to modern psychoanalysts, dreams have been thought to convey truths, albeit hidden in strange symbolism. However, there is no one method for deciphering dreams, and their value cannot be proved by strict scientific method.

Nightmares may be caused by anxiety. While there is no evidence that they are caused by eating particular foods, such as cheese, before sleeping, they might be induced by too much alcohol. If you are anxious or depressed, and having frequent nightmares, there is probably an underlying problem which you should tackle, perhaps with the initial help of your doctor.

If you are having difficulties in getting to sleep:

● Avoid taking naps; they aggravate the problem.

● Try relaxation. For most people, muscle relaxation or psychological relaxation (shifting your mind to pleasant events) will help.

● Change your nightly routine. For example, change your bedtime, go out in the evening, or don't read in bed.

Other strategies
If the above measures do not work, try the following.

● If your mind wanders while you try to accomplish a mental task, change to one that occupies you but does not increase your anxiety. For example, try to take yourself on a guided tour of a house you lived in as a child. Try to imagine a favorite piece of music or plan a vacation. Imagine a favorite walk, step by step.

● Deliberately try to stay awake. If you are sleepless for more than about 15 minutes, get out of bed. You might try attacking a task you have put off, such as writing a letter.

● Don't worry or panic about lack of sleep. You are unlikely to miss so much sleep that your performance will be impaired.

● Don't smoke or drink coffee at bedtime or if you wake during the night. Both are stimulants.

STRESS AND ILLNESS

Stress plays a significant part in producing, maintaining, and worsening illness. When your body is constantly on "red alert," prepared for fight or flight, it continues to produce higher levels of certain hormones. When you are under stress, you not only tend to eat more hurriedly and pay less attention to your diet, but you also digest food less efficiently and your body doesn't derive the maximum nutritional benefit from it.

What happens is that the liver discharges more sugar and fats into the blood, but your body cannot utilize these substances, unless you release your stress by physical activity. As a result they are redeposited in the body, usually in the coronary arteries. In addition, your intestines and kidneys work less efficiently and so do not remove all the waste and toxins from your body. And because your immune system is impaired, you are more vulnerable to illness and less capable of combating it once you have it. Constant muscle tension produces aches and pains, which can develop into chronic conditions.

If you are under constant stress, you may suffer from frequent indigestion and heartburn, constipation or diarrhea, insomnia, a tendency to sweat for no apparent reason, headaches, backache, nausea, and breathlessness. It is known that stress is a contributing factor in stomach and duodenal ulcers, high blood pressure, and heart and circulatory disorders. It is also implicated in asthma, rheumatoid arthritis, and eczema.

Hypochondria

A hypochondriac is someone who has an abnormal interest in, and anxiety about, his state of health. He or she is usually a person who constantly goes to the doctor with symptoms for which there are no physical causes, and bothers family and friends by describing imagined illnesses. True hypochondriacs are very insecure people who revel in being ill because they need to feel that someone is concerned about, and will take care of, them. Someone with "illness phobia," however, is terrified of contracting a fatal disease, and takes extravagant steps to avoid exposure to health hazards.

Many people go to their doctors to discuss a long series of minor ailments because they are too frightened to reveal a major source of worry. This is particularly so in the case of stress-related disorders, and marital and sexual problems. Once the major problem has been identified and solved, the minor ones often disappear. Many people suffer from psychosomatic illnesses, which are often stress induced. Although there may be no organic cause for this type of illness, the symptoms are just as real and uncomfortable.

Depression

Everyone can be depressed from time to time, for a few minutes or for days or weeks. Often people can identify the cause of their depression: divorce or the breakup of a relationship, children leaving home, failing an exam, or being passed over for promotion. They might become depressed because of their inability to manage their finances, to cope with life's demands, or in anticipation of a crisis, which often results in anxiety as well. The loss of employment, serious injury, severe or chronic illness, childbirth, and the use of certain drugs are other typical causes of depression. Such depression is a normal part of life.

Depression becomes a problem only when it gets out of proportion. For example, it is considered normal to become deeply grieved over the death of a loved one. Usually after an initial period of intense sadness, people gradually come to terms with the loss. If they do not, their depression is not alleviated, but may become a problem itself rather than a reaction to an event.

Exogenous depression

Depression caused by external forces is termed exogenous and produces changes in behavior. Depressed people find it difficult to concentrate or receive pleasure from anything they do. Their perception of the world becomes distorted, and events that they would normally take in their stride seem to be overwhelming problems. As stress is magnified, they become more frantic and less effective in their attempts to cope. Each failure seems evidence of their incompetence and worthlessness, a sign that emerging from the "black pit" is impossible, and so their depression deepens.

The belief that there is no escape is characteristic of chronic depression. As the ability to concentrate seems to disappear, memory becomes impaired, and the downward spiral of depression continues. Having lost their faith in their ability to surmount their problems, people lose the will to even try; they stop fighting. In this state people

Try the following:

● Seek out the source of the depression and ways to change it. If you can't make a large change, a small one might suffice.

● Seek support. The support of friends and family is important to help overcome depression in its early stages. Make the effort to talk to people. Even if their advice is misguided, social contact will distract you from the problems of the moment. Every minute's respite from the depression helps you in your quest for control over your life.

● Change your pattern of living. Take up a hobby or take regular exercise which is an antidote to depression.

● Do not try to solve all your problems at once. This approach is doomed to failure, and will maintain the depression. Instead, consider your problems one at a time.

● Eat regularly. Depression tends to reduce the appetite. If you are to increase your level of activity, you need adequate energy supplies.

● Realize that many of the thoughts you have and the actions you are taking stem from your depression. When you are depressed, it is easy to become trapped into seeing all events as evidence of personal inadequacy.

might cut themselves off from all activities and relationships, become housebound, and eventually even find it difficult to get out of bed. Their feelings of inadequacy and worthlessness can become so overpowering that they might contemplate suicide. Contrary to popular belief people who discuss suicide often attempt to commit it.

Endogenous depression

Not all depression is precipitated by easily identifiable events. Endogenous depression seems to come from within the body. Medical and psychiatric experts believe that it is caused by biochemical abnormalities in the brain. It tends to occur suddenly and for no obvious reason. It is often associated with disturbed sleep patterns, particularly early morning wakening, and with weight changes. Endogenous depression can be treated with antidepressant drugs (see pages 280–281).

Consult your doctor if you are suffering from depression. An accurate diagnosis is important. The tips on this page can help you to cope with mild depression, but professional medical treatment is necessary for endogenous or chronic exogenous depression.

Phobias, obsessions, and ruminations

A phobia is an irrational fear—accepted as such by the sufferer—of an object or a situation that severely disrupts a person's life. Agoraphobia, the fear of going out or of open spaces, can make someone a prisoner at home; claustrophobia, the fear of enclosed spaces, can make it impossible for a person to use public transportation.

Obsessions are also the result of fear. Someone with an obsession will perform complex or elaborate rituals to avoid the object of his fear. For example, a person with an abnormal fear of dirt may repeat complicated cleansing procedures over and over.

Ruminations will involve anxiety-provoking thoughts such as "I'm going to jump out of the window," although the action is not carried out. The thought is the touchstone that prevents the deed being committed; it is so frightening that the sufferer takes action to avoid it.

Phobias, obsessions, and ruminations are at their worst when the sufferer is anxious, tired, or depressed. Trying hard to cope can make the problem worse, and professional help is essential (see pages 332–337).

At home or at work, look out for someone who shows a change in behavior. When dealing with them, remember:

● Emotional pain is as bad as physical pain.

● Do not tell someone to "pull themselves together" or to "snap out of it."

● Do not report to a person all the features of his of her life that need improvement.

● The earlier help is sought, the better. Encourage anyone who is depressed to seek help from a psychiatrist or psychotherapist.

Phobias and obsessions: getting help

It could be time to seek help when one or more of these apply to you:

● The fear is becoming too great to manage.

● Your life is being disrupted by your symptoms.

● Life is becoming unbearable, either because you are fed up or because you know that the cause of your anxiety is unavoidable.

● You have many symptoms of anxiety or depression, such as trembling hands, palpitations, and strange aches and pains.

● Others are urging you to seek help.

PRESCRIBED DRUGS

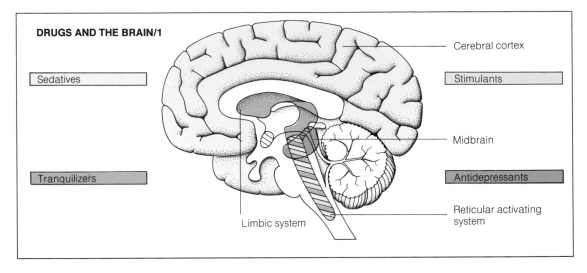

DRUGS AND THE BRAIN/1

Sedatives

Tranquilizers

Cerebral cortex

Stimulants

Midbrain

Antidepressants

Reticular activating system

Limbic system

Groups of prescribed drugs alter the activity of many parts of the brain. They are designed to have a therapeutic effect by acting principally on the areas indicated. Sedatives lower the level of the conscious experience by acting on the cerebral cortex. Tranquilizers work on the limbic system, which is involved in determining mood and in memory. They also work on the reticular activating system (RAS), whose activities are crucial to the maintenance of consciousness. The RAS is also affected by stimulants and antidepressants. The latter also act on the midbrain to alter mood.

Doctors have a vast array of drugs that they can prescribe for the treatment of physical disorders, ranging from analgesics to eliminate pain and antibiotics, which fight bacterial infection, to antiserums that prevent specific diseases and antiviral drugs, which fight virus infections. It is essential to take medication exactly as your doctor prescribes; be sure you understand exactly how much to take, as well as when, and for how long, to take it. Some drugs are ineffective if you do not maintain a certain concentration in your body by taking the correct dosage at the scheduled time. In other cases, a medication must be taken for a certain period to ensure that it has cured the illness, although you might feel better before then.

It is also important to know what reactions and side effects you might experience, and if you need to take any precautions. Many antihistamines, for example, which are used to treat hay fever and other allergic reactions, can make you drowsy; you should avoid driving or operating machinery if you take them. Furthermore, the effica-

cy of some drugs is impaired by the presence of food in the stomach, while others can interact with food, alcohol, and other drugs to produce harmful reactions.

Store medications in a cool, dark place, and if you have young children, keep them out of reach in childproof containers. Always throw out drugs left over after an illness, and never take any medication that was prescribed for someone else.

Psychopharmacology

The branch of medicine concerned with drugs that affect thinking, feeling, mood, and anxiety is known as psychopharmacology. These drugs are used to treat stress, anxiety, depression, and mental illness.

Antidepressants are used to treat endogenous depression (see pages 278–279). They do not make a person "high" or unnaturally cheerful, but correct a relative shortage of neurotransmitters in the brain. The person's mood is changed from a depressed to a normal state. Antidepressants have no real effect on anyone not suffering from chemically-induced depression.

Eighty percent of the people who use drugs to reduce stress and anxiety take sedatives to help them sleep and tranquilizers, such as Ativan, Librium, Tranxene, Valium, and Xanax, to reduce tension and make them feel calm while they are awake. These drugs are valuable up to a point. They provide temporary relief by masking the symptoms, but they do not treat the source of the problem and the symptoms will persist. Used irresponsibly, they create other serious problems, such as hangover and dependence.

Beta blockers are anti-anxiety drugs that block the action of the nerves that make the heart beat faster and the blood vessels contract. They are not habit-forming, but they are not successful in treating all forms of anxiety.

Side effects

All drugs have a multitude of effects on the body. Sedatives and tranquilizers act on the areas of the brain responsible for arousal and, as well as making you relaxed, they can make you feel drowsy, lethargic, and weak. They can affect concentration and memory, making you slightly absentminded. Large doses taken over a long period can lead to slurring of the speech and double vision, especially in the elderly. In addition, people all respond differently to any medication and may experience other side effects because of individual sensitivities. In deciding which drug to prescribe, the doctor has to consider the symptoms, their severity, and the patient's medical history; but there is no way of predicting an individual's response to a drug.

Becoming dependent

All drugs that affect the mind produce dependence; that is, they are habit-forming. There are two types of dependence—physiological and psychological—but the dividing line is hard to define. Physical dependence occurs when the body's functions adapt so that they are efficient only in the presence of the drug. The body gradually becomes tolerant to the drug so that larger and larger doses are needed to produce the same effect. Eventually, changes occur in the body to compensate for the effects of the drug. If the drug is then withdrawn, body functions are disrupted, and the person experiences an intense craving for the drug and other withdrawal symptoms.

Tranquilizers produce physical dependence. The symptoms of withdrawal are often the same as, or worse than, those the drug was being used to treat in the first place. They include palpitations, cramps, loss of appetite, insomnia, and extreme tension. Unfortunately, there is no way of knowing how long a person has to take tranquilizers for dependence to occur, but taking them on a regular basis for more than a couple of months would probably put you at risk.

NONPRESCRIBED DRUGS

The most widely abused of the drugs acquired without prescription are those that produce euphoria. The price paid for this short-lived pleasure is almost invariably a feeling of depression after the effect has worn off and, in most cases, drug dependence.

Most people probably consider caffeine and aspirin innocuous substances; believe that marijuana, alcohol, and the nicotine in cigarettes are sometimes addictive; and accept that opium, heroin, LSD, the amphetamines, cocaine, and solvents are addictive drugs whose consumption has dangerous physical, psychological, and legal consequences.

In fact, all these substances are drugs and can be addictive and harmful. Drug-taking can destroy physical and mental health, and lead to criminal behavior as a means of meeting the increasing cost of regular supplies. Injecting drugs can result in fatal infection.

The range of drugs
Caffeine is the stimulant found in coffee, tea, and cola drinks. It increases blood pressure, pulse rate, and, when taken in excess, leads to hand tremors, dizzy spells, breathlessness, and feelings of anxiety; yet many people drink coffee to calm their nerves. If you drink more than five cups a day, you are likely to be damaging your health; try to cut down or drink decaffeinated coffee. Reduce the quantities gradually to minimize any withdrawal symptoms.

It is not unusual for people to become dependent on aspirin, often taking up to 20 tablets a day as a precautionary measure against headaches. This leads to a high risk of bleeding in the stomach and induces withdrawal symptoms.

Individual reactions to cannabis (marijuana, "grass," or "pot") can vary according to the quality of the drug, the taker's mood and metabolism, and the influence of companions. Experiences range from euphoria to depression; hunger, drowsiness, and distortions of time are common. Cannabis affects short-term memory, concentration, and motor performance.

Amphetamines stimulate the nervous system to induce wakefulness, a sense of well-being, boundless energy, and self-confidence. They also inhibit appetite and have been used to treat obesity. Dependence on them comes rapidly, with strong side effects, including irritability, anxiety, aggression, and tremors.

The stimulating effects of cocaine ("coke") and crack (a smokable form of cocaine) are similar to those of the amphetamines, producing a feeling of intense elation, a sense of great physical strength and energy, and loss of appetite. Cocaine creates a rapid tolerance so that larger doses need to be taken; long-term use can damage the mucous membrane lining the nose and cause restlessness, overexcitability, fear, and delusions of threat.

Opiates, solvent-sniffing, and LSD
Opium, a drug produced from the poppy *Papaver somniferum*, and its derivatives, heroin and morphine (which is used medically to control severe pain), are known collectively as opiates. They give an almost instant feeling of elation, and produce addiction rapidly. A new dose relieves withdrawal symptoms almost immediately.

Solvent- or glue-sniffing is used mainly by teenagers to get "high." The effects are similar to drunkenness, and include euphoria, confusion, loss of inhibition, and altered perceptions, leading to hallucinations, aggression, drowsiness, fits, and nausea. Death is common, generally due to heart failure, liver and kidney damage, or accident while under the influence of the drug.

Even a single dose of lysergic acid diethylamide (LSD) can be dangerous. It produces ecstatic and mystical experiences, hallucinations, panic, and complete loss of control. Although a large proportion of the experiences are unpleasant, users of psychedelic drugs continue to take them. Long-term use disturbs the concentration, memory, and perception.

How drug-taking begins
Simple curiosity, often coupled with peer-group pressure, leads most people to their first experience with drugs. Some people come to drugs in their search for an inner self, but find that any drug-induced truths they experience become meaningless after the "trip" is over. Others use drugs to escape from everyday problems. Many people experiment with marijuana, which is believed to be psychologically, but not physiologically, addictive. The greater danger begins when they move up to more powerful drugs. Although using marijuana does not necessarily result in taking harder drugs, most people on hard drugs started with marijuana.

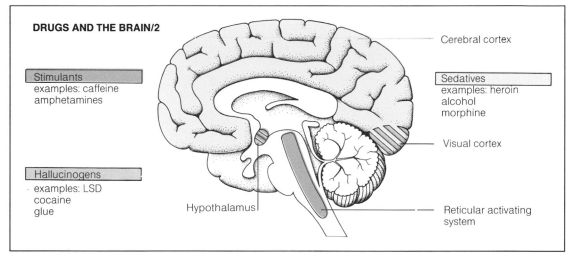

DRUGS AND THE BRAIN/2

Stimulants
examples: caffeine
amphetamines

Hallucinogens
examples: LSD
cocaine
glue

Hypothalamus

Cerebral cortex

Sedatives
examples: heroin
alcohol
morphine

Visual cortex

Reticular activating
system

Groups of nonprescribed drugs alter the activity of many parts of the brain. They are designed to have a therapeutic effect by acting principally on the areas indicated. Stimulants press the reticular activating system (RAS), responsible for consciousness, into greater activity. They also act on the hypothalamus to produce typical "fight or flight" reactions, which occur in stress. Sedatives act on the cerebral cortex to lower conscious awareness. Hallucinogenic drugs produce their bizarre visual effects by interfering with the working of the visual cortex, which is responsible for interpreting signals from the eyes.

Addiction

Personality is a significant factor in drug addiction. The people thought to be most at risk of addiction are those who lack self-esteem, those whose expectations are in conflict with reality (see pages 274–275), and those who feel alienated from society.

The longer a person continues to take a drug, the greater his dependence on it becomes. It is difficult to break a physiological dependence because the body's functions are disrupted, and the withdrawal symptoms can be very unpleasant (see pages 280–281).

A psychological dependence is often as strong as a physical one. People who usually feel inadequate derive a sense of belonging from the secretive behavior and special jargon of the group. This feeling, combined with the ritual pleasure of preparing for a "fix," *and* the euphoric effect are strong incentives to continue. The group will exert powerful pressure to prevent someone from breaking the dependence, since his success is a rejection of the group, and belies the excuse that it's impossible to kick the habit.

What to do if you think you are becoming dependent

● Be sure you want to stop; otherwise you will find it impossible to deal with withdrawal.

● Ask your doctor for referral to a specialized treatment center. There you will be told what to expect and given relief from some of the pain of withdrawal.

● If you decide on self-help, take time off and gather: an around-the-clock supply of friends to help you, a small supply of tranquilizers in case the pain is unbearable, and a plan for when you have kicked the habit.

● Give yourself substitute rewards through friends not connected with the drug-taking culture.

● The first two weeks are the most painful, but the real difficulties of coping begin *after* two weeks.

What to do as a parent

Remember:
● Few children modify their behavior because parents are critical of them; criticism not only gives them an excuse to continue, but also traps them into maintaining such behavior for fear of admitting they are wrong.

● Nagging, threatening, cajoling, bribery, and ignoring never work.

● The best chance of success is to arrange a meeting between the child and an outside expert, to be carried out as part of a contract in exchange for something the child wants from you. Choose the expert for his personality and track record, not only his qualifications.

● Regard your child as an adult in his relationship with his counselor.

THE DANGERS OF SMOKING

Cigarette smoking is always unsafe. The figures speak for themselves. On average, people who smoke more than 20 cigarettes a day take twice as many days off work each year than nonsmokers. Of men now aged 35, the proportion that will die before reaching retiring age is 40 percent for heavy smokers, but only 18 percent for nonsmokers. Smoking causes about 400,000 deaths a year in America alone. The illustration shows the parts of the body affected by smoking in both sexes. Women run an additional risk, however. Their unborn babies can be damaged by smoking, and smoking increases the risk of cervical cancer.

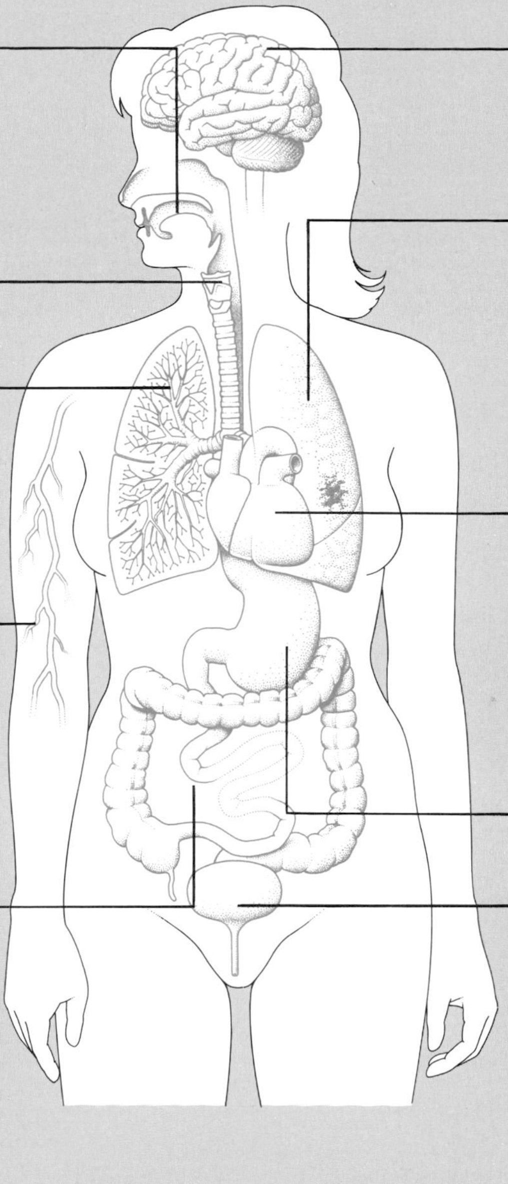

Mouth and throat: Cancer is the major risk. Tobacco smoke can also cause gum disease and tooth decay. The teeth become yellow and unsightly.

Esophagus (gullet): The tars in smoke can trigger cancer.

Bronchi: Smoke contains hydrogen cyanide and other chemicals, which attack the lining of the bronchi, inflaming them and increasing susceptibility to bronchitis.

Circulation: Nicotine raises blood pressure. Carbon monoxide leads to the development of cholesterol deposits in artery walls, causing heart attacks and strokes. Loss of circulation in limbs can necessitate amputation.

Intestines: Ulcers are a risk. Smoking can also cause diarrhea.

Brain: Headaches are common. Lack of oxygen and narrowing of blood vessels can lead to strokes.

Lungs: People who inhale cigarette smoke are 10 times more likely to get lung cancer than nonsmokers. Mucus secretion is increased, causing chronic catarrh and smoker's cough. Increased susceptibility to infection can lead to emphysema.

Heart: Nicotine in cigarette smoke makes the heart beat faster and so work harder. It makes the blood clot more easily, increasing the risk of heart attacks. Carbon monoxide robs the blood of oxygen, again increasing the risk of heart attack.

Stomach: Increased acid secretion can lead to ulcers.

Bladder: Excreted carcinogens can cause cancer.

Cigarette smoking is the major cause of serious illness and premature death in Western society. Every cigarette you smoke can shorten your life by an average of five and a half minutes. Yet people who smoke either cannot believe that such illnesses will afflict them or are unable or unwilling to give up the habit.

Tobacco smoke is dangerous because of the nicotine, carbon monoxide, tars, and poisonous substances it contains, as the diagram opposite shows. Even "passive" smokers, who inhale the smoke of others, are at some risk. It has been suggested that exposure to other people's smoke involves about a third of the risk associated with smoking a cigarette yourself.

Lung cancer among nonsmokers who live with heavy smokers is twice as high as in nonsmokers who live in nonsmoking households. Nonsmoking spouses of cigarette smokers die, on the average, four years younger than the nonsmoking spouses of nonsmokers. Small children are especially at risk from cigarette smoke, which can cause respiratory infections that leave the lungs permanently damaged.

Low tar cigarettes have been marketed as "safer" than high tar ones, but there is no evidence that reducing tar or nicotine intake per cigarette makes any difference to the development of smoking-related illnesses. This is largely because tar and nicotine have no effect on the carbon monoxide that deprives the blood—and thus all body organs, but significantly the heart—of oxygen. And people who smoke "low dose" cigarettes might smoke more to raise their blood nicotine levels or because they think such cigarettes are safer.

Changing to a cigar or a pipe can, as long as the smoke is not inhaled, reduce the risk of lung cancer. However, the risk of developing cancer of the esophagus, mouth, or throat is just as great.

The reasons why people start smoking are often markedly different from those that sustain the habit. Curiosity, the desire to impress or appear adult, and pressure from peers are all common reasons.

Research suggests that people with anxious, or type A, personalities are more likely to smoke heavily than "passive" B types (see pages 262–263). Smokers also associate certain benefits with their actions: if a smoker truly believes that a cigarette will increase alertness, relaxation, or confidence, then it probably will.

Nicotine is addictive and smoking is a drug addiction. Smokers regulate the dose of nicotine in their blood automatically, and smoke more or less accordingly. Smoking also causes psychological dependence, which makes giving up even harder to achieve.

Why do you smoke?
Finding out why you smoke is a good first step toward giving up. Read the statements below, based on research conducted by the US Public Health Service. Score as follows:
Always true: **5** points; Frequently true: **4** points; Occasionally true: **3** points; Seldom true: **2** points; Never true: **1** point.

Stimulation
"Smoking stops me slowing down."
"Smoking perks me up."
"Cigarettes give me a lift."
Stimulation results from the physiological effects of nicotine.

Handling
"Handling a cigarette is enjoyable."
"I enjoy the lighting-up routine."
"I like watching the smoke."
The ritual of smoking is an important, pleasurable element of the habit for some people.

Relaxation
"I find smoking pleasant and relaxing."
"Smoking is pleasurable."
"I want a cigarette when I am most comfortable and relaxed."
One of the paradoxes of smoking is that it can be both calming and stimulating. This might have something to do with the rate and depth of inhalation, but is unproven.

Tension reduction
"I smoke when I am angry."
"I smoke when I am uncomfortable or upset about something."
"Cigarettes take my mind off my worries."
Many people use smoking as a "crutch" to help them deal with stressful situations. This leads to psychological addiction.

Craving
"I cannot bear to be without cigarettes."

"I am consciously aware of the times when I am not smoking."
"I get a gnawing hunger for a cigarette when I haven't smoked for a while."
Nicotine can cause true physical addiction.

Habit
"I smoke cigarettes automatically without being aware of it."
"I light up when I already have a cigarette going."
"I have smoked without remembering lighting up."
Smoking can become an almost automatic response.

Scoring: A score of 11 or more in any category is high; 7 is low; any score in between is average. A string of high scores means that your reasons for smoking are complex and that it might be hard to give up. For help with giving up smoking see pages 286–288.

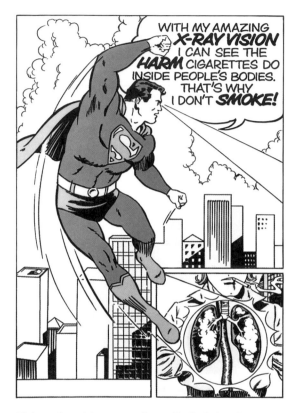

This antismoking poster is specifically designed to counteract the cigarette advertising aimed at children and young teenagers.

The best way to save yourself from the many illnesses associated with cigarette smoking, and from the difficulty of giving it up, is not to start in the first place. It is, however, extremely difficult to teach children and young adults to say "no," when there are so many pressures on them from their peers and the media to start the habit.

The figures show that children are more likely to smoke if their parents smoke. A teenager whose parents or older brother or sister smoke is four times as likely to take up smoking as a teenager from a nonsmoking family. In smoking families, children are used to absorbing the noxious substances in cigarette smoke passively. As a result, they may be less powerfully affected by unpleasant side effects when they smoke their first cigarette.

Children and teenagers, especially girls, are also the target audience of advertising. Tobacco manufacturers promote smoking as a symbol of maturity, and social and material success—very appealing qualities to adolescents striving for independence and self-confidence. In addition to spreading this message through the mass media, they also sponsor sporting events and use famous personalities admired by young people to promote their products.

The usual health warnings probably have little impact on children because heart disease and lung cancer, to which they refer, take many years to develop and are too remote to be perceived as threatening by young people.

One effective way of stopping children from smoking is to make a deal with them that provides attractive rewards for not smoking. A teenager might, for example, be offered a car and driving lessons as a seventeenth birthday present if he or she does not smoke. A child should be honorbound to keep to the contract—pressure, suspicion, inquisitions, and nagging will quickly negate it. If he has admitted smoking occasionally during the period of the contract, the lapse can be ignored; it is still worth giving the child the car so that he can boast about it at the end of the day and convince himself and his peers that smoking is not worthwhile.

Barriers to giving up

The dramatic decrease in deaths from heart disease in North America since the mid-sixties is almost certainly due to the fall in the number of smokers. But despite overwhelming evidence that cigarette smoking is harmful, people are, it seems, only likely to give up if they feel that the evidence applies to them.

A reason people often give for continuing to smoke is that giving up will make them gain weight. Most people who give up smoking do put on some weight. Their appetite for food increases because food supplies the oral stimulation once given by cigarettes, and because the "set point" for body weight is reset at a higher level in which there is more body fat. Remember that the mortality risks of smoking are more than double those of being overweight and that the problem of overweight can be dealt with later.

It is never too late to give up smoking. Even if you have been smoking for 20 or 30 years it is worthwhile. From the day you stop smoking, you start improving both your life expectancy and the quality of your life. You will immediately smell better, look better, and have more resistance to disease. Your heart and lungs will be more efficient, and your risk of heart disease, bronchitis, emphysema, and cancers of various kinds, but most significantly lung cancer, will decrease.

How to stop smoking

Motivation is the real key to giving up smoking. You must convince yourself that it is an unhealthy, dirty, expensive habit and unworthy of you. Like giving up any other addictive drug, there is little chance of success unless you are convinced that you want to give up. Indeed, the only course of action might be to say to yourself, "I will never put a lighted cigarette between my lips again." It might help to decide well in advance on a date on which this will take effect so that you can prepare yourself mentally. Finding they are

pregnant motivates many women to give up, in many cases for good.

Not everybody is strong-minded enough to be able to take, and keep to, such an all-or-nothing decision. If you prefer to try to give up gradually, use the smoker's diary below to see which cigarettes you need least, and cut these out first. Set yourself a target date for stopping completely and aim to cut down consumption by about a quarter each day or each week.

Whatever method you plan to use, begin by making a smoker's diary. This will warn you of where the greatest difficulties lie. Then consult the questionnaire on page 285 to discover why you smoke. Your answers will determine which of the strategies outlined on page 288 might be the most helpful to you.

SMOKER'S DIARY

Draw up a diary based on the example given here. In the column headed "Importance" score as follows:
0: "I lit up without realizing it."
1: "I just felt like it."
2: "I wanted a cigarette fairly badly."
3: "I was desperate for a cigarette."
Your answers will give you an idea of how much you smoke and when, and of the relative importance each cigarette has for you. It will provide clues as to which cigarettes will be easy, and which difficult, to give up.

MONDAY, AUGUST 10

TIME	TRIGGER	IMPORTANCE	THOUGHT AND FEELINGS
7:50	Having breakfast	3	I can't start the day without a cigarette.
8:20	Driving to work	2	Annoyed at being stuck in traffic.
9:00	Cup of coffee	1	Made me feel more relaxed.
9:35	Making a phone call	2	Needed a cigarette to calm my nerves.
10:10	Offered a cigarette by a colleague	0	Acceptance made me feel more sociable.
11:00	Heavy load of work	2	Helped me to concentrate.

Motivation

Any technique that can keep you motivated to persist without cigarettes is worth trying. Some of the following might help:

● Tell everyone you are about to give up. This places social pressure on you to keep to your plan. But remember that other smokers are not likely to be your allies. They have a vested interest in your failure; if you can give it up, they might be under pressure to do so too.

● Give yourself forfeits for failure, such as carrying out unpleasant but necessary chores. Either way you win— you give up cigarettes or get the chores done.

● Keep reminding yourself of the benefits of giving up and the penalties of continuing. Keep in your mind a picture of someone with lung cancer or chronic bronchitis.

● Think how much money you are saving and promise yourself a gift with what you have saved. Put the money you saved aside in a special jar, marked "vacation" or "gift."

● Remember that there will be times when you are tense, feel uneasy, and are unable to concentrate.

● You might feel dreadful now, but always keep in mind that *you will feel better soon.*

If you smoke for pleasure or relaxation, try to find a more healthy substitute. Distract yourself by listening to music or reading a book, or with a relaxation technique (see pages 272–273). If smoking provides the stimulation you need, try taking up a vigorous exercise or sport to give you a "high" instead, or find something more interesting to do, if only temporarily.

Doing something with your hands, such as doodling, knitting, fiddling with coins, paper clips, or pencils, can help you to overcome the problem if handling is important to you.

If you smoke to reduce tension, try other means of coping with your problem, including exercise, chewing sugar-free gum, or using relaxation techniques. Whenever possible, try to avoid stressful situations. If you cannot, then be aware that these are danger times.

If you crave the "buzz" that nicotine provides, you will simply have to bear the trauma of giving up. Nicotine chewing gum (available through your doctor) might help. If, however, you have a real craving for nicotine, you are advised to give up smoking at a single attempt rather than to cut down gradually.

You will find it most helpful to change your everyday routine if you smoke out of habit. Watch out for situations, such as drinking coffee, writing letters, or telephoning, which from habit you find conducive to smoking. Try substituting glasses of orange or grapefruit juice for some of those cups of coffee, since citrus juice seems to remove the desire to smoke.

Patronize restaurants that prohibit smoking or have a smoke-free area. Avoid going to bars for a drink; smoking is probably still the norm in most of them. At home and in your car, clean and remove all the ashtrays, and vacuum carpets and upholstery to get rid of the stale odor of cigarettes. Always sit in the nonsmoking section on planes, buses, and trains.

Many smokers give up cigarettes without suffering any side effects, but some heavy smokers experience a variety of withdrawal symptoms. These can include a dry mouth and thirst, irritability, headache, poor concentration, upset stomach, constipation, sudden changes of mood, sore throat, and coughing. Although they are unpleasant, they are all positive signs that the body is cleaning itself out, and most of them will disappear within a few weeks.

Preventing relapses

People relapse into the smoking habit for three main reasons:

1. A negative emotional state such as anxiety, depression, loneliness, boredom, impatience, restlessness, tiredness.
2. Social pressures, particularly those of feeling "left out."
3. Personal conflicts.

To help you avoid slipping back into the smoking habit, use the following tips:

● Make sure you are aware of the situations that put you most at risk.

● Do not become complacent.

● Practice saying to yourself and others, "I have just given up smoking."

● Get everyone around you to keep congratulating you on having given up.

● Do not fool yourself that since you have returned to smoking after a period of nonsmoking, your body still needs nicotine and you are a hopeless case. If you have given up once, you can do so again.

● If you make a mistake and smoke a cigarette, try to find out what prompted you and practice avoiding the problem in future.

● Go back to being abstinent *now*. Do not say to yourself, "I will start giving up again this evening or tomorrow."

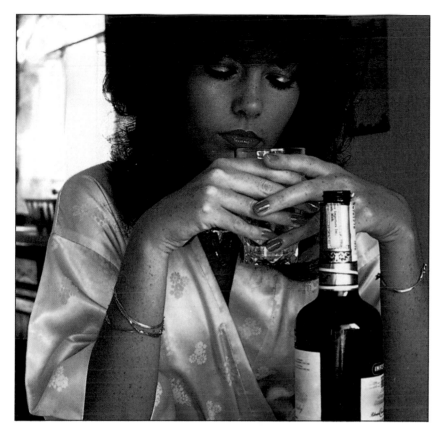

Alcoholism is a growing problem among women, particularly those who are in highly stressful jobs and those who are stuck at home all day and are bored.

Alcohol is generally thought of as a stimulant, making people talkative, aggressive, and uninhibited. In truth, however, it depresses the activity of the nervous system, and acts as an anesthetic. In extreme cases, depression of the respiratory center of the brain can be lethal.

People drink for many different reasons. In small amounts and for short periods of time, alcohol relieves tension, encourages a sense of well-being, and is unlikely to be harmful. However, some people mistakenly use alcohol to relieve major problems. This not only leads to alcohol tolerance so that larger and larger doses of it are needed but, unfortunately, also tends to exacerbate the problems. In large doses, alcohol can cause chronic depression, misery, and self-doubt, as well as many physical ailments, ranging from malnutrition to cirrhosis of the liver.

Social pressures are a subtle spur to drinking because a small amount of alcohol loosens the tongue and convinces people that their social interactions are improved. Advertisements for alcoholic beverages can reinforce this pressure by implying that the product will make you not only socially acceptable, but also attractive, interesting, and desirable, and might even suggest that it will enable you to do things you could not do otherwise. People also drink to give themselves rewards, to fill in empty hours, or to relieve tiredness, lethargy, anxiety, or stress. Consider your own reasons by keeping a diary such as the one for smokers on page 287.

Two different types of people may be most likely to develop a drinking problem. The first are those who lack self-confidence, have low self-esteem, and are often self-punishing. The loss of inhibitions from alcohol can lift them.

The second type also finds it hard to deal with the realities of life, but, unlike the first group, have often been overindulged in childhood. They resort to alcohol because they can't accept adult responsibilities. In both cases, the vicious circle which is created by alcohol abuse becomes the major problem.

THE EFFECTS OF DRINKING

BAL (Blood alcohol level) per 3½ fl oz	Effects	Drinks consumed
30 mg	Light and moderate drinkers feel relaxed. Heavy drinkers are unaffected.	20 fluid ounces of beer or 2 shots of whiskey or 2 glasses of wine
40 mg	Talkative and mild loss of inhibition. Increase in accidents.	1 quart of beer or 3 shots of whiskey
60 mg	Mood change. Judgment impaired.	1½ quarts of beer or 5 shots of whiskey
80 mg	Coordination impaired.	
100 mg	Deterioration in physical and social control.	3 quarts of beer or 10 shots of whiskey
150 mg	Staggering, slurred speech.	3¾ quarts of beer or 12 shots of whiskey
200 mg	Double vision, aggression, vomiting.	
300 mg	Loss of consciousness. Drinker is rousable.	¾ bottle of whiskey
400 mg	Coma, possibility of death.	1 bottle of whiskey
600 mg	Breathing stops. Death.	

mg/3½ fl oz alcohol in blood (0, 100, 200, 300, 400, 500, 600)

The amount of alcohol in the bloodstream, the blood alcohol level (BAL), determines how people behave after drinking. It is also the measure that the police use when deciding whether people should be charged with drunken driving. BAL is influenced by four factors. The first is simply the amount a person drinks. The second is the speed at which the alcohol is absorbed into the bloodstream. The type of drink determines the alcohol content and the speed of absorption. Whiskey is assimilated more quickly than beer, and carbonated mixers increase the rate of absorption. Eating a meal before drinking delays absorption. The longer a person takes to consume alcohol, the lower his BAL will be.

The third factor is body weight. Women, who generally have lower body weight than men, have higher BAL levels if they drink the same amount as men, and often have lower tolerance of alcohol. Any drinking that raises the BAL level to about 20 mg increases the chance of driving accidents. For someone with a light build and small frame, this level can be reached within one hour by having one drink.

The fourth is the speed at which the liver can remove the alcohol from the bloodstream by oxidizing it. A small percentage of the alcohol a person drinks is exhaled and/or excreted in the urine. The rest has to be broken down by the liver, which can oxidize, on the average, the alcohol

Are you developing a drinking problem?

Ask yourself the following questions, which are based on a questionnaire compiled by the National Council of Alcoholism.

1. Do you drink heavily after a bad day?
2. Do you drink more heavily when under pressure?
3. Can you drink more than you used to?
4. Do you have twinges of guilt about drinking?
5. Are you impatient for your first drink of the day?
6. Do you often feel uncomfortable without a drink?
7. Do you try to sneak a few extra drinks secretly?
8. Do you ever have memory blackouts after drinking?
9. Do others often discuss your drinking?
10. Have your memory blackouts become more frequent?
11. Have you tried to control your drinking?
12. Do you usually drink for an identifiable reason?
13. Do you often regret things you say or do when drunk?
14. Do you want to continue after others stop drinking?
15. Have your good intentions about cutting down failed?
16. Have you ever moved house or left a job to try to give up drinking?
17. Are you beginning to feel a little persecuted?
18. Have your financial and work problems increased?
19. Do you prefer to drink with strangers?
20. Do you eat irregularly when drinking?
21. Do you drink in the mornings to steady yourself?
22. Do you sometimes feel depressed and hopeless?
23. Are you sometimes drunk for days at a time?
24. Do you find you cannot drink as much as you once used to?
25. Do you see or hear imaginary things after drinking?
26. Do you sometimes feel terribly frightened after you have been drinking?

If you answered "yes" to any question, you could have a drinking problem. "Yes" replies in each of the following groups indicate the following stages: Questions 1–8 you are entering the risk area; Questions 9–21 you are in the middle stages; Questions 22–26 the final stage is beginning.

from a single shot of whiskey, or a glass of beer, in an hour. No substance has been proved to speed up the rate at which the liver works, but disease and malnutrition can slow it down.

Hangover

The most common symptoms of a hangover are headache, nausea, thirst, tiredness, dizziness, and upset stomach—either singly or in combination. Contrary to popular belief, there is no quick cure for a hangover. Drinking coffee or taking aspirin might exacerbate an upset stomach, although acetaminophen helps, while the "hair of the dog" merely delays the reaction. The best treatment is to relax, take acetaminophen for a headache, and drink plenty of nonalcoholic liquid.

A drinking problem

Alcohol tolerance, in which a person has to drink more and more to produce the same effect, develops rapidly. But there is no identifiable point at which someone becomes alcohol dependent. Rather, there is a gradual progression from occasional drinking to total dependence, and drinking problems begin well before chronic alcohol dependence sets in.

Like any other drug, alcohol, if taken in excess, has drastic effects on mental and physical health, and can reduce life expectancy dramatically. Cirrhosis of the liver, disorders of the digestive system, cancer, and brain damage are often the result of heavy drinking.

Before or after it harms the body, alcohol abuse can seriously affect a person's behavior. Some heavy drinkers have few behavioral problems, such as decline in memory and intellect, depression, breakdown, and notions of suicide, before the physical damage takes its toll. In others, the behavioral problems come first.

The effects of alcohol abuse—violence, child neglect, and, frequently, the break-up of relationships—can seriously disrupt people's lives. Even moderate drinkers can find themselves increasingly isolated and may soon prefer the company of a bottle to that of a friend. At work, their performance and attendance will gradually deteriorate.

Alcohol abuse can also destroy the lives of innocent people. For reckless behavior and impaired judgment can cause accidents at work, at home, and particularly with motor vehicles. In the U.S., for example, it has been estimated that at least 50 percent of deaths on the roads are associated with alcohol consumption.

Overconsumption of alcohol is a growing problem in many countries, and has become almost as prevalent among women as among men. There has, however, been much debate in scientific circles about whether heavy drinkers should control the amount they consume or stop drinking altogether. To date, no firm answer has emerged as to which is better. Early successes with alcohol-dependent drinkers who restricted their intake have been reversed, since many such drinkers have gradually returned to their old levels of drinking.

Evidence suggests that for most people who are heavily dependent on alcohol, total abstinence is probably the only way to achieve success. This is because it is far more useful to learn to do without alcohol altogether, and to discover different approaches to underlying problems, than to treat the symptoms by merely cutting down.

Whether you decide to reduce your intake or opt for total abstinence, you must be sure which course of action you are adopting and stick to it. Otherwise your attempt will be doomed to failure. Remember that cutting down is the harder of the two options, but if you are short on motivation, you will probably be unsuccessful whichever one you choose.

Total abstinence

Giving up alcohol is similar to giving up any other addictive drug. But a heavily dependent drinker should not equate it with giving up, say, cigarette smoking. Even if alcohol withdrawal symptoms do not amount to delirium tremens, with its shaking limbs and hallucinations, they can include aching muscles, sweating, rapid pulse, and fever. This means that medical help and supervision will almost certainly be needed. Some people find that they are able to "dry out" at home under a doctor's supervision. However, it is important to ask for medical advice before trying to give up drinking.

Many hospitals now provide detoxification centers for alcoholics. A patient is given tranquilizers and vitamins to prevent brain damage, and is monitored so that his condition and progress can be charted. Once the withdrawal symptoms have been overcome, a patient might be given drugs that induce physical illness if alcohol is drunk. The drugs are prescribed in pill form and are effective for only 24 hours after they are swallowed.

Unfortunately, a patient might forget—either deliberately or unintentionally—to take the drugs. The doctor might then ask another member of the family to supervise drug-taking; or he might implant a slow-release capsule beneath the patient's skin. This allows a constant dose of the drug to be absorbed directly into the bloodstream of the person in need of help, and removes the need for taking pills.

Drying out and drug administration are only short-term remedies. They do nothing to help combat the basic problems that lead to alcohol abuse in the first place, or to help maintain the state of abstinence. For people to stop or even control their drinking, sobriety must be made rewarding. They need long-term help in developing better work, social, marital, and family relationships. Research suggests that counseling is one of the most important factors in achieving and maintaining abstinence.

Alcoholics Anonymous (AA) is an organization that helps to provide support for ex-drinkers and those who want to stop. In itself, it is not a magic solution, but it benefits from the collective experience of thousands of drinkers. AA emphasizes self-help, individual motivation, and the fact that everyone is responsible for his own actions. Al Anon, for spouses, and Alateen, for children of drinkers, are part of the AA organization and provide valuable support and information for members of an alcoholic's family. Their numbers are listed in the telephone directory.

Young people at risk

To help a young person with a drinking problem, it is far better to get help from outside the family. Within the family, there is always a temptation to keep troubles private, but this can do more harm than good. If your child has a problem, try to arrange a visit to an expert who not only has good credentials but also a suitable personality and ability. Select someone who will talk to the child unpatronizingly, and who will not merely take the unwelcome role of a third parent.

People who drink to excess, whether young or old, usually do so for a reason. Unfortunately, parents are often the last people children or young adults feel they can talk to. Indeed, poor communication with parents might be the problem that is causing the drinking. Whether they are young or

Good excuses

The simplest way of refusing a drink is to say, "No thank you." There are, however, many social pressures on people to drink. Try some of the following excuses when you have to say "no." Present your case firmly and *do not* enter into a debate about the morals of drinking or try to change the drinking habits of another person.

● "I have given up drinking because I have been overdoing it." *If you repeat this message often enough, people will believe you.*

● "I am driving."

● "My doctor says I might be getting an ulcer."

● "My liver is not in very good condition."

● "I am taking antibiotics (or sleeping pills or any other drugs) and should not drink too."

● "The drink is making me feel sick."

● "I have to watch my weight."

● "I've had just about the right amount. If I have any more, I'll feel sick."

● "Drinking gives me a migraine headache."

● "I've stopped drinking at lunchtime; it ruins my concentration in the afternoon."

Remember, once people realize you are not going to drink, they will stop pressuring you.

old, people will not give up drinking unless they can see that it is worthwhile. Parents are often unable to supply the necessary rewards.

Rather than struggling with a situation they are incapable of controlling, parents should aim to talk to a child sympathetically, say that they are enormously worried and upset, and ask the child to make a deal with them to see an outsider. Enlisting the help of a close family friend, who can talk to the child adult-to-adult, might also be helpful.

Cutting down

The points system
Use the points system as an aid if you want to cut down your alcohol intake:

Aim for: a maximum of 24 points a week;
a maximum of 6 points a day *and*
no more than 4 drinking days a week.

Score as follows:
1 bottle of beer	= 2 points
1 small glass of sherry or fortified wine	= 1 point
1 fluid ounce of whiskey, gin, vodka, or brandy	= 1 point
1 small glass of wine	= 1 point

If your weekly score is currently more than 50 points, cut down by 10 points a week until you reach 40 points. For scores of 40 points a week and below, cut down by 5 points each week.

Helpful strategies

● Make a diary similar to the smoker's diary on page 288. Note when you are most at risk and which drinks you can cut out with ease.

● Remember that the distribution of your drinking is as important as the quantity. Do not drink to excess on any one occasion.

● List the reasons for not drinking more than your limit. Remember that you will be pressured into slipping back into old habits.

● Rehearse your excuses and coping skills (see panels left and right).

● Tell everyone you are cutting down because you are drinking too much; try to enlist their support.

● Try exercise or a new hobby to divert your attention from drinking.

● Get professional help to sort out your underlying problems.

Rehearse your coping skills

The first step in adopting skills to cope with cutting out or cutting down on drinking is to identify high-risk situations or cues. Then think of as many ways of coping with them as possible. Rehearse your actions mentally so that you will be confident when the time comes, and not be persuaded into changing your mind.

● At a party, stay for only 20 minutes.

● Drink tonic water or another mixer and pretend that you are drinking alcohol.

● Keep moving. If the pressure becomes too great, go somewhere else (e.g. another room) for a break.

● Rehearse saying "no" or offering the excuse of your choice.

● Rehearse going into a bar and having just one drink; this is one of the most difficult things to do.

● Rehearse ordering mineral water or fruit juice instead of wine with a meal in a restaurant.

When a crisis occurs, you could find yourself in one of two roles. You could either be the victim of a disaster, or you could be sorting out the troubles of others. Matters become blurred when crises and conflicts involve partnerships (see pages 298–299) or parents and children, but it is still possible to work out what your role will be.

The information on these pages is aimed particularly at helping you to cope with family crises, but much of it is applicable to other kinds of crisis.

1. Your own feelings

If you are in trouble, try not to allow your own feelings to complicate matters: much time and effort are lost during a crisis because of reactions such as, "Why is this happening to me?," "What will other people think?," or "How could they do this to me?"

Similarly, when someone needs help from you, don't indulge your own feelings or dwell on the way their problems are going to affect you. The priority is to deal with the crisis, not to waste time by dithering or agonizing.

2. Communicating anxiety

Whatever your role might be, try not to communicate anxiety when a crisis arises. When you are upset, your general demeanor, if you let it, can cause others to respond negatively. Try to stay calm, even if you do not feel it. If you add your own emotions and fears to the situation, you could accelerate the crisis.

Keep repeating to yourself, "What is the problem here?," "Calm down." Remember that just as others can "catch" anxiety from you, they can also "catch" calmness.

3. Using your intuition

When you are trying to sort out a crisis for someone else or if you are involved in a crisis that is not of your making, for example, as a parent, remember that intuition is a valuable source of information. Intuition may seem rather magical, but it is probably no more than a subconscious assessment of a situation based on experience that seems to enter the mind like a flash of inspiration.

A thought such as, "I have a feeling that my son has gone to his friend's house . . ." might be put down to intuition, but in fact is based on previous patterns of events or on clues picked up unconsciously from conversation.

In sorting out a crisis in which you are the "injured" person, it is also important to follow your intuition, despite possible criticism from others that you are giving in to your feelings. Your actions might not seem logical, but if your feeling is strong enough, follow it through.

4. What ought to be done

In a crisis, ignore what you think you *ought* to do to please other people or to conform with what society expects of you. All too often people are afraid of the opinions of others, and come to a conclusion that pleases them but does not help the person in difficulties.

If a child is abusing drugs or alcohol, parents often feel that one of their priorities is to make sure that other people do not find out—not in the interests of the child, but because it might reflect badly on the family. Parents of an anorexic child will often deny the anorexia, even to themselves, because they feel that it will cast a bad light on the way in which they have brought up the child.

If someone is in difficulties, it is important to realize that problems cause pain, and that this pain must be resolved. As a rule, it is impossible to cope successfully with a crisis, or sort out one on behalf of another person, and at the same time keep up appearances.

5. Gaining valuable insights

When you are the person who is trying to help resolve a crisis, always try to put yourself in the position of the sufferer. This will help to give you some insights as to why the crisis has occurred in the first place, and also ideas about how to set about achieving a solution.

The same is true if you are a passive recipient of trouble. If your child has run away from home, and you discover his or her whereabouts, there is little point in running angrily to haul back the miscreant. However great the temptation, try not to bombard the child with questions such as "How could you do this to us?," "Do you know what trouble you have caused everyone?," or "What will the neighbors think of all this fuss and commotion?" Such questions might seem important to you, but they are insignificant to the child. Indeed, they might simply make the child feel more wretched than ever and less likely to reveal why he or she ran off—which is the only thing that matters. Your negative questions might also make it more likely that incident will be repeated.

6. Dealing with resentment

If you get involved in a crisis because of another's actions, do not "punish" that person. It is all too human to take out your frustration, resentment, and anxiety on someone who, in your judgment, is responsible for causing a problem. Thus a child who has run away, or a partner who has left home, often comes back to an angry scene, not a joyful welcome. Imagine how you would feel in the circumstances and remember that recrimination solves nothing. Look to the long term and seek solutions that will minimize resentment on all sides.

Because people like to be in control of their lives in as many aspects as possible, they naturally resent persons and situations that interfere with this and force them to be problem-solvers. Similarly, resentment may be directed at those who are ill because their illness is inconvenient. Again, self-control is a valuable asset in coping with the crisis.

7. Talking and listening

Whatever your role in a crisis, it is worth talking through the situation with a neutral listener. You should also be prepared to listen to the advice of others and to understand what they are saying and why, even though their conclusions might contradict your own interests.

A parent, a partner, or a good friend might be able to provide the listening ear you need, but often it is better to talk to an outsider with no vested interest in the situation.

When others are offering you advice, it is important to decide whether the advice is worth following. In times of crisis, everyone becomes an "expert." You may be bombarded with the benefit of other people's vast experience. You urgently need to decide, however, whether they really do have your interests, or those of the person undergoing the crisis, at heart.

In such a situation, ask yourself do they *really* know? Why are they telling you this? Is their evidence anecdotal or factual? Is the situation being talked about really the same as yours? Have you good reason to have faith in their opinions and the advice they offer?

8. Where to get advice

If you wish to seek outside help in a crisis, whether for yourself or on behalf of someone else, try your doctor first. He will have access to many resources.

Social workers are other valuable sources of help. The social services have emergency facilities and can furnish you with immediate aid if necessary. A telephone call to an organization with some kind of "lifeline," such as the Samaritans, might also help. Merely talking about a crisis can often help you find a solution.

Psychiatrists and psychologists, many of whom are affiliated with hospitals, can also be of assistance. Psychiatrists are medically trained doctors who have undergone further training in psychiatry. Many people call themselves psychologists, but those who have been trained to help you with problems and difficulties are described as clinical or counseling psychologists. If you get in touch with a psychologist through your hospital, you can be sure that he is trained and qualified. Properly trained and qualified counselors are also available. A friend's recommendation of a qualified counselor would be a reliable aid to choosing; do not answer press advertisements, no matter how impressive people's qualifications appear.

9. Judging the "experts"

As well as judging the advice handed out to you by family, friends, and neighbors, it is also important to judge the advice given by outside experts—psychiatrists, psychologists, social workers, and counselors. Does their experience fit with yours? Do they really understand the position you are in? Does their advice sound as if it has come from a textbook, or is it based on experience and sensitivity?

If the advice you get does not sound or feel compatible with your own situation or responses, or those of the other people involved in the crisis, ask yourself why. It could be that the decisions you are making are based upon factors that are not sensible to, or understood by, outsiders. Or their advice might not take into account important factors that have led to your decisions. "Experts" do not know everything; but do not disregard their advice simply because they do not agree with you. Try to negotiate a rational solution with outsiders.

When you enter a long-term relationship, there is no way of knowing in advance how it will turn out. Although no relationship is perfect, there must be enough in it for both partners to view it as worthwhile, and to keep them together. But couples should be sensitive to the fact that during the course of time each partner's stake in the relationship can change.

There are no strict rules that guarantee the quality of relationships or ensure their survival. Nor are there any rules about when relationships should end. In assessing a relationship and its possible future, you can ask yourself certain questions. The most important of these are discussed in detail on these pages.

1. Should I continue?

The very fact that you are asking yourself this question means either that the relationship has considerable flaws or your expectations are too high. Your first step toward answering the question is to work out a balance sheet. What are the pros and cons of staying in and getting out? Make a list of each and see what keeps you in the relationship. Include all the factors and be totally honest with yourself. You may find that you are staying in a relationship because you are economically dependent, or are dependent because of disease or alcohol abuse, or because you are worried about how your family and friends will react. Any reason that is recognized and is important to you is valid.

The next step is to evaluate the items on your list. Again, it is important to consider what matters to you. Everyone has a unique personality and so rates matters differently. Many people feel, for example, that they have to sacrifice or compromise their own personal, intellectual, or career development for the sake of a permanent relationship. Others find that they cannot endure the frustration that results from such a situation, and will leave a relationship that does not allow them to fulfill their own potential.

For many people, especially those who have already been married and divorced, fear of further failure is given a high rating in assessing reasons for staying in any relationship.

Remember, however, that fear of hurting a partner is not the best reason for staying in a relationship in which there continues to be unhappiness for one or both partners.

2. How can I improve my relationship?

In seeking to improve their relationships, many couples fail to carry out the most obvious and important task—to find out what is actually wrong. Statements such as "He always criticizes me in public," or "She always nags me" are symptoms of the "disease," but not its cause. Being criticized, for instance, might be a result of the fact that your partner is threatened by your social performance. You might become a nag because your partner does not otherwise respond to you. Or both types of behavior might be a symptom of underlying unhappiness with your marriage or your partner.

Another reason for being wary of treating the symptoms of trouble is that the themes of most interpersonal difficulties emerge only after a period of time. It is no use selecting just the latest problem to work out what the root cause is. Think back over the other past events and actions (or lack of them) to decide the cause of your reactions and those of your partner.

3. What does my partner think?

Many couples attempt to outguess, outpredict, or simply describe what their partners are thinking. However, this is unreasonable since you will never be able to see the world as your partner does. Nor, more important, will you ever be able to see yourself as your partner sees you.

The best way of surmounting this problem is to discuss your relationship openly and frankly, and *not* to make mutual accusations. If you are not getting the discussion you want, do not blame your partner. If you are failing to get a discussion going, then you are using the wrong approach.

If you have tried one way of communicating in the past and it has failed, do not keep going on in the same way in the vain hope that somehow, this time, you will succeed. Instead, try another approach, taking your cues from your partner's responses to other people.

In any discussion about your relationship, you must create the sort of atmosphere that will encourage your partner to be more forthcoming. The reason for reticence might be fear of the consequences or of your reactions. Or one partner might feel that there is little point in discussion because the other partner always interrupts to defend his or her own position.

4. How can I discuss problems effectively?

Many people have discussions as if they were having debates. There is much point-scoring, and neither side will admit to being in the wrong. But when trying to sort out a relationship that has gone wrong, it is essential to realize that you are not in a battle to see who is right. Your aim is to resolve the problems and to improve the quality of the relationship.

If you do not allow yourself to be drawn into the attack-defend routine, then your partner will be less inclined to pursue that path. Make concessions freely and acknowledge your partner's point, even if the truth is hurtful. Do not allow a monologue to develop, but try to articulate and share your worries.

5. What are my expectations?

In an era when people are regularly exposed to the notion of "ideal" relationships on television, in the movies and theater, and in books, it is difficult to be realistic. If you feel that you are entitled to a perfect relationship and that nothing less is to be expected, then you are doomed to disappointment. Having accepted that life does not wave a magic wand over anyone, you must decide how far you can accept the discrepancy between expectation and reality.

Although you might feel disappointed, there is no reason why you cannot attempt to improve things. If improvement is impossible, then the choice between putting up with things as they are or getting out becomes a real one. But do not decide to get out of a relationship without making a concerted effort to improve it.

6. Is it my fault?

Finding fault or blame is not a constructive approach to solving problems. It is more useful to ask yourself, "Is there anything in my performance that might be producing some of the difficulties in the relationship?" If the answer is "yes," the next question is "How can I change it?" Follow up your answers with action.

You might be faced with a situation in which your partner is so selfish, self-absorbed, careless, or violent that changing your own performance is not possible or relevant. In this instance, you must ask yourself "Will, or can, my partner change?" If the answer to this is "no," then you have the choice of putting up with the situation or not. No

one should put up with violence of any kind. After that, most things are negotiable.

7. How important are sex/affection/fun/intellectual stimulation?

Each of these items is an important ingredient of a relationship. The difficulty arises when only one member of the partnership wants one or more of these elements.

It is up to every couple to work out what they want, and how and to what extent their needs are going to be met. Unfortunately, marriage is a situation in which most people start working out their needs after the contract has been signed. However, this does not mean that you cannot make it clear what you expect from your partner. When a couple marries young, the two members often mature differently and find that, as a result, they no longer have a workable relationship. In such a case it might be better for the partners to separate honestly and amicably.

8. Do I need a counselor?

There are some definite advantages in using the services of an outsider rather than trying to solve all the problems yourself. One is that it breaks the pattern; another is that an outsider can help to take the heat out of a situation. Also, an outsider can often present new alternatives.

You can turn to a marriage guidance counselor for help, or gain access to a marital therapist through your doctor. Some clinical psychologists and psychiatrists specialize in marital therapy.

9. Are gay relationships different?

The principles in all relationships are the same, and the same processes of negotiation and discussion apply. Most counselors will just as happily see homosexual as heterosexual couples.

10. What about children?

Children are remarkably adaptable, and it is the experience of many therapists that the upset is as great to the child whether warring parents divorce or not. If anything, the evidence is that children might be less upset by divorce than by being in a situation of constant tension and argument. Furthermore, children might grow up feeling guilty that the parents stayed together on their account. Above all, children should be kept in the picture and discouraged from taking sides.

The loss of a loved one is a crisis that has to be faced sooner or later. Grief and mourning are almost exclusively associated with death, but in fact you feel grief—and mourn your loss—whether you lose a job, a home, your ideals, a treasured possession, a much loved pet, a close friend, or a partner. In all such situations you have to make adjustments to new circumstances by means of mourning.

Helping yourself

In coming to terms with the loss—particularly the death—of a loved one, the people best able to cope could be those who come from cultures that have strict, formal, and intense mourning rituals. In modern society you are often expected to act as if nothing has happened, but research has shown that mourning is an essential part of coming to terms with a loss. Mourning occurs in three consecutive stages (see chart). But grief should not be used as an excuse for maintaining sympathy or for not changing your life. There comes a time—although its arrival is ill-defined—at which you have to give up some of your grief and rejoin the mainstream of life.

Mourning is also dangerous to physical and mental health if it does not progress properly through its various stages. Mourning that restarts after it has apparently finished, often accompanied by other signs of clinical depression (see pages 278–279), is another sign that professional psychological help is needed.

Grief is nothing to be ashamed of. It is not unseemly, undignified, or unnatural. Certainly those around you might think you are less attractive than usual, and sometimes it is important to try to keep up an appearance of "normality." However, it is not your duty to make life easier for those around you if you have sustained a loss. Equally, they should not feel that they have to avoid you because of embarrassment, but should be there to offer comfort during the stages of the mourning process. Do not think of yourself as an imposition on your friends, even if you are feeling wretched; there will be a time when they, too, will be in your position.

STAGES OF MOURNING			
Mourning, for whatever reason, takes place in three stages			
	Stage One	**Stage Two**	**Stage Three**
Characteristics	Shock and disbelief, a feeling of blank numbness. Inability to accept what has happened. Imagining that nothing has changed, such as expecting the arrival of a loved one at a certain time of day.	Realization that the loss has happened. Feelings of pain sweep over you. Recollection of old emotions and memories. Feelings of guilt. Odd behavior, difficulty in eating and sleeping. Depression.	Relief from the pain and negative feelings. Return of a positive approach. Acceptance of possible replacements, although you know they can never fully take the place of what has been lost. Acceptance of the loss. Seeking of alternatives.
Comments	It is important not to stay too long in this stage of mourning or your recovery will be delayed.	This stage can last weeks, months, or even years. Counseling is enormously helpful in this stage of mourning.	These show that your mourning has begun to be successful. You will not forget what you have lost, but you are coming to terms with reality.

If you are mourning, do not assume that you have to pull yourself together faster than you feel is necessary. There are no shortcuts to the resolution of grief. You will have to go through the mourning process at your own pace and be prepared to entertain thoughts and emotions that are alien and painful to you.

Following a bereavement, it takes many people about a year to come to terms with their loss. It is only if grief continues after such a period that you should question whether you are failing to get over that loss. It is at this stage that you might decide to seek outside help to give you that extra push you need to get going again.

Divorce and other types of loss

It is natural to grieve when a marriage ends in divorce, when you lose your job, or suffer a loss of similar proportions. In some ways, losses such as these are harder to cope with than death. With death, someone has gone from this earth and, although the loss is painful, after the numbness is over, you can, and must, start to come to terms with it and begin to create a new life.

With divorce, the "lost" partner is still alive, so beneath all the feelings that exist, there lurks the notion that the relationship might somehow be revived. You will probably have had friends in common who may tell you your expartner's latest news, and induce a feeling of nostalgia. For this reason, many people find it impossible to start mourning a divorce until long after it has occurred. Often it is the remarriage of one of the partners that finally spurs the other into proper, and necessary, mourning.

Also important in divorce is the sense of rejection with which it is associated. Although you might feel you could have improved the quality of a dead person's life, death is not usually surrounded by feelings of personal guilt. Divorce, on the other hand, is a situation in which guilt thrives, and this guilt—along with feelings of personal failure—complicates the logical steps of the mourning process.

After someone has died, you may cope with your feelings by building a memorial. This can be a physical thing, such as a gravestone or a collection of the dead person's prized possessions. You might also build a memorial psychologically, remembering all the good things about the person, and his or her actions, and forgetting the bad

ones. This cannot happen with divorce if the bitterness of the parting and intense awareness of the person's faults prevent it.

Losing a job has many features in common with divorce. The feelings of helplessness, rejection, and failure are paramount, yet people are usually discouraged from mourning. Friends might be sympathetic for a short while, but it is not long before they tell you to "pull yourself together," "stop looking back and start looking forward."

Helping others

There are many ways in which you can help someone who has been bereaved. Use the following guidelines to help you act sensibly:

● Let bereaved people give the lead. Do not make judgments on their behalf about whether they should be cheered up, or told to pull themselves together.

● Grieve with someone who is bereaved. This gives permission for grief and shows that you, too, valued the mourned person.

● Give practical help, especially during the early stages—before the funeral and for the first few weeks afterward—when the bereaved will not feel like doing day-to-day tasks.

● Remember that practical jobs can help bereaved people by distracting them. So if they show signs of wanting to accomplish practical tasks, always let them do so.

● Be there. Bereaved people often feel the need for help and support, even if they do not use them. Your support should not stop after the first few days of mourning, but will be needed for many months.

● Gently reassure the bereaved person that the feeling of grief will diminish, even though it may not seem that way.

● Do not encourage a bereaved person to take drugs, such as antidepressants or tranquilizers. It is better to work through the grief without them. But sleeping pills, taken on a short-term basis, can be useful.

● Be aware. If you are sensitive to a bereaved person, you will see when he or she is ready to be distracted from grief. When this time comes, seize the opportunity.

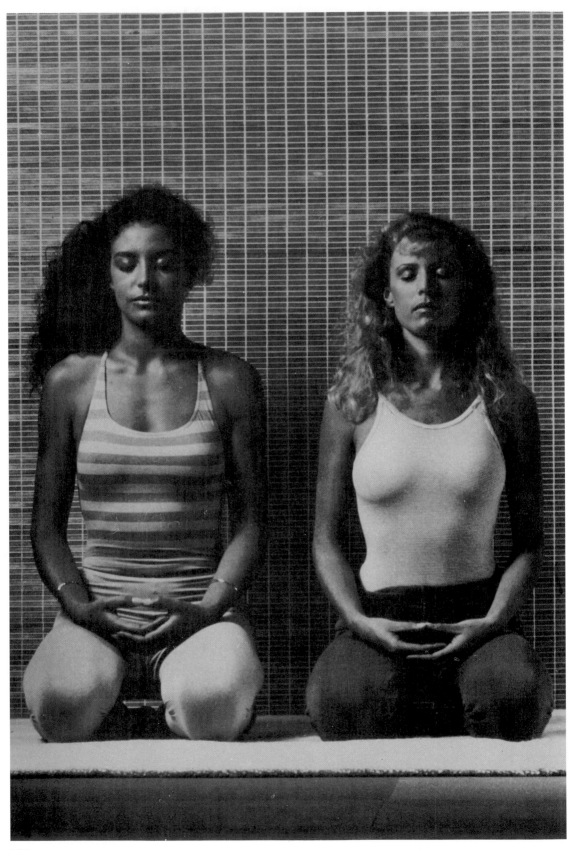

TREATMENTS AND THERAPIES

In their pursuit of fitness and well-being of body and mind, many people are turning to forms of treatment that sometimes fall outside conventional medical practice. Indeed, even the medical profession is beginning to accept many of these techniques as valuable alternatives or additions to more traditional forms of treatment. It is also becoming widely recognized that many physical ills do not have purely physical causes, and treatments that help people attain inner contentment and serenity relieve many troublesome and stress-related symptoms, such as migraine headaches and backache.

The emphasis throughout this chapter is on variety, safety, and self-help. Although there might be no sound medical basis for some of the treatments explored here, they often have their origins in ancient medicine. Furthermore, the placebo effect may play a role—that is, if you think a certain treatment is doing you good, then it probably is.

The options described in the pages that follow are readily available in most areas. Some, such as herbal remedies, can be self-administered. Others, however, demand the help of expert teachers, at least in the initial stages. These include meditation and the Alexander Technique. Still others, such as acupuncture and Rolfing, can be administered only by trained personnel. Yet many of these treatments can bring about an improved attitude that persists after the treatment itself is over. For example, with experience in biofeedback you should learn how to control your own automatic responses and so be affected less adversely by stress.

Changing attitudes and behavior are keys to improved health and happiness. For this reason, the chapter ends with examples of therapies that will help you alter the way you look at yourself. By reassessing your thoughts and adopting a holistic, or "whole person," approach to your problems, you should find that you are well on the way to finding solutions.

HEAT THERAPY

Warmth and water are two of the greatest sources of comfort to the human body. For many people the essence of relaxation is to lie on a beach, breathing the ozone-rich sea air, allowing tiredness and tension to dissolve between warm sand and a beneficial sun, and intermittently enjoying the most perfect exercise—a swim in salt water. It is no wonder that this neat package of heat, light, and hydrotherapy makes you feel good. Little wonder, too, that winterbound urban dwellers seek a substitute for a day at the beach in the form of whirlpools, saunas, sunbeds, plunge pools, and impulse showers at health clubs.

Yet warmth and water provide more than comfort; they re-create the conditions for life itself. Life on earth began in the ocean, a fetus lives in fluid, and the body is largely composed of water. Although, like all warm-blooded creatures, human beings can maintain their body temperature by means of internal regulators, these rely on the external temperature being conducive to life. At extremes of cold and heat, body processes, including temperature regulation, fail to function.

The uses of heat and hydrotherapies to promote fitness and well-being range from the simple hot bath to specific therapies for treating serious ailments. Although particular heat and hydrotherapies may be carried out separately, the two are often combined for dual benefit in the form of steam cabinets and whirlpool baths. After any heat therapy, which causes the heart rate to increase, it is wise to rest for about 30 minutes in order to allow the body to return to normal.

Therapies with dry heat

Dry-heat therapies act on the skin and circulation, and can bring relief from symptoms of musculo-skeletal problems, such as arthritis, rheumatism, respiratory problems, and sciatica. Therapies designed to induce sweating are useful in ridding the body of accumulated toxins. For example, sweat acts as a vehicle for the removal of lactic acid, the toxin that causes muscle pain during heavy exertion.

Therapies using dry heat induce a temporary condition called hyperemia (dilation of the blood vessels, combined with a local temperature rise and an abnormal increase in blood supply to the part of the body being treated). Hyperemia has positive effects, such as relieving congested blood

---

Benefits

Conditions that might be helped by one or more methods of heat therapy include:

● Rheumatism, arthritis, and a wide variety of the complaints involving the musculo-skeletal system.

● Sciatica and many other conditions affecting the nervous system.

● Some skin conditions. Treatments that mimic the radiation contained in sunlight are helpful in treating problems such as acne.

● Respiratory problems, including asthma and bronchitis.

● Success has also been reported in the relief of symptoms caused by inflammation of the kidneys and gallbladder.

Warnings

● Avoid heat treatments if you suffer from a heart condition or high blood pressure. After only seven minutes in a sauna, the heart rate almost doubles, imposing a dangerous strain on a weak heart.

● Never take a young baby for heat therapy, since the large surface area of his body in proportion to his weight will cause him to gain and lose heat extremely rapidly.

● Elderly people should use the cooler, lower sauna benches and limit exposure to extreme heat to 5 minutes.

● Overheating puts a strain on the heart, and subsequent cooling may result in a chill and respiratory problems.

● Never drink alcohol before heat treatments; you risk dehydration.

Other people at risk include:

● Expectant mothers.

● Diabetics.

● Those suffering from a heavy cold, flu, a heavy menstrual period, glandular obesity, or varicose veins.

● Those with low blood pressure.

● Those taking medication, who should first consult their doctor.

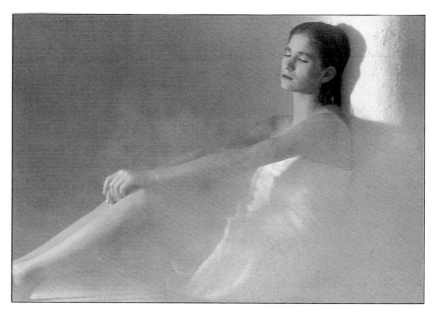

The Russian bath is essentially a steam-filled sauna. As with other types of sauna, the benefits are immediate; a glowing complexion, easier respiration, relaxed muscles, and a general sense of healthiness and well-being. In modern electric saunas, water ladled over hot stones produces steam to coax impurity-laden sweat out of the pores. The alternative to the traditional Finnish roll in the snow is a cold shower between bouts in the heat.

vessels or tissues, but should be followed by a brief cold shower, which speeds up the body's return to its normal condition.

The principal types of dry-heat treatment that are available include the following.

Infrared: Any invisible, heat-carrying wavelength of electromagnetic radiation beyond the red end of the visible light spectrum is infrared. Anything hot emits infrared, but it is effective only if it is emitted by a luminous or nonluminous source hotter than you are. General infrared treatment is helpful for rheumatic conditions, and local treatment can relieve lumbago and pain caused by injuries. Treatments last for about 15 minutes. Diabetics should avoid infrared therapy, and people with fair skins should protect themselves with an emollient before treatment.

Radiant heat: Musculo-skeletal pains and the pain of sciatica respond well to radiant heat. The patient sits or lies beneath a reflective surface lined with light bulbs. The head is kept well clear and cool during the body's exposure to temperatures of approximately 200°F. This treatment is not suitable for the very young, the elderly, or anyone with high blood pressure or heart disease.

Wax baths: The wax bath is used particularly to treat arthritis of the hands and wrists, but can also be used on other parts of the body. Paraffin wax with a melting point of 115°F is melted in a thermostatically controlled container. The affected part of the body is dipped into the melted wax about 10 times. Then it is wrapped in waxproof paper, placed in a plastic bag, and draped with a towel for about 20 to 30 minutes. Finally, the wax is painlessly removed, and the treated part is held under cold running water for 30 seconds to one minute.

Traditional Turkish bath: The popular misconception that steam is part of a traditional Turkish bath has arisen because steam facilities often are found on the same premises. What is commonly mistaken for a Turkish bath is a Russian bath, which is similar to a steam-filled sauna. In a Turkish bath the heat is supplied by dry hot air, not steam. The bather, wrapped in a towel, goes into the cool room, or *frigidarium*, to rest. Next he goes to the *tepidarium*, in which the heat is between 100°F and 112°F, and stays there until he begins to sweat. He then goes into a room of intense dry heat, the *caldarium*, where temperatures may reach 150°F. After approximately 30 minutes of profuse sweating, he is given a thorough massage, in which the skin is rubbed and brushed to remove dirt and impurities from the dilated pores. Finally, the bather takes a cooling shower or plunge to close the pores.

HOME SAUNA SAFETY

For many people, the dry heat of the sauna bath is the ultimate way to relax both the mind and the body. In some cultures it is also a place to meet for conversation. Once associated only with log cabins in Scandinavia, home saunas are growing in popularity. They can be installed in virtually any home that has a spare room or alcove, or space in a loft or under a staircase.

The cabin

The sauna cabin should be constructed of tongue-and-groove kiln-dried pine or spruce with a nominal thickness of at least half an inch, and must have a specially built door. One fresh-air vent should be located underneath the sauna heater, and a second vent should be positioned high up opposite the heater. This ensures that fresh air circulates continuously and an even temperature is maintained in the sauna.

Most saunas have slatted benches built into the walls around the room at two or three heights. Since hot air rises, the most intense heat is found at the level of the highest benches. A person can move gradually from one level to another—this is similar to moving through the different rooms in a Turkish bath (see pages 302–303).

The ideal operating temperature is between 190°F and 200°F, with a relative humidity between 10 and 15 percent. The heat is generated by a special sauna heater, which usually is electric, although gas- and wood-burning models are also available. The heater should be of a size capable of bringing the cabin to operating temperature within 30 minutes, and should have a deep stone bed, humidifier, and overheating protector built in. The heating casing should be designed and insulated so that you can safely put your hand on it without being burned. The temperature controls are usually on a wall outside the cabin.

The only other items of equipment you need are a thermometer and a timer, both of which should be mounted on the wall, and a bucket and ladle for the water to splash on the heater. Keep the illumination inside the cabin to a minimum; you will find that subdued lighting helps create a restful atmosphere.

Enjoying a sauna

To take a sauna bath properly and derive the most benefit from it, remove your clothing and any jewelry, and take a shower before entering the cabin. After about five minutes in the dry heat, you will begin to perspire. When you are perspiring freely, take a cold shower and then re-enter the sauna. Repeat this process two or three times until you feel completely relaxed. In your final period in the sauna, splash water onto the heater. This produces a wave of appreciably higher heat in the cabin, although in fact the temperature drops as the humidity suddenly increases. Take a final cool shower and rest for about half an hour while enjoying a cool, nonalcoholic drink.

The benefits

During the dry-heat phases in the sauna your pores dilate and you perspire profusely. This excretes wastes from the body and helps to cleanse the skin. The moist-heat phase tones your body, and many people find it is beneficial to the upper respiratory tract and eases the symptoms of arthritis and some skin ailments. The cold showers counteract the hyperemia induced by the dry heat and thus stimulate blood circulation.

Anyone suffering from high blood pressure, heart disease, diabetes, inflammation of the nose or eyes, or any disorder that might be aggravated by high heat should consult a doctor before using a sauna. You should not take a sauna after eating a heavy meal because this will cause a conflict in your body between your digestive system, which needs blood to digest the meal, and your heat regulating system, which has to increase the blood flow to your skin in order to counteract the effects of the heat. Taking a sauna after you have been drinking alcohol is not safe.

Some people seem to believe that the sauna is an endurance test and that the longer they can stay in, the tougher they have proved themselves to be. In fact, there is no physical advantage in prolonging your stay past the point when you are truly relaxed, and an overstay can give you a headache and make you feel ill.

Another common misconception is that using a sauna can help you to lose weight. Although you should perspire profusely during a sauna treatment, your body loses only a small amount of fluid, which is replaced as soon as you eat and drink.

*A **sauna** in your home will not take up very much space and provides a wonderful way to relax. Saunas like the one illustrated on the opposite page are available in do-it-yourself construction kits or can be installed by a dealer.*

HOME SAUNA CABIN

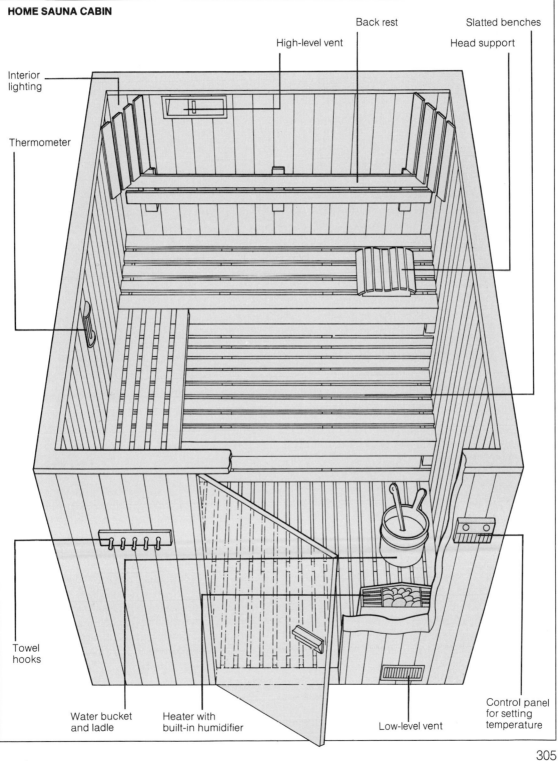

Back rest

Slatted benches

High-level vent

Head support

Interior lighting

Thermometer

Towel hooks

Water bucket and ladle

Heater with built-in humidifier

Low-level vent

Control panel for setting temperature

HYDROTHERAPY

The wide assortment of external and internal hydrotherapies are central to the "nature cures" offered in many modern health farms and spas. These therapies are based on the belief that a multitude of disorders, from chronic phlegm to cystitis, can be prevented and treated through deep cleansing of the body. To dedicated naturopaths, purification is tantamount to panacea; to others, a simple whirlpool bath is a balm to aching muscles and tired skin.

The practice of hydrotherapy dates back at least as far as the time of the Roman Empire and has been credited with curing everything from hangovers to insanity. Spas, now the generic word for health resorts where people "take the waters," declined in popularity with the advent of modern medicine and changing attitudes in the medical world. Today, however, hydros are making a well-deserved comeback.

Because it is possible to make fine adjustments to both the temperature and pressure of water, it is a highly adaptable treatment medium. Some hydrotherapy involves water in motion, either gently bubbled with air or, as in underwater massage, pumped powerfully by water jets.

Types of baths
In modern hydrotherapy the most elementary treatments are cold, hot, and alternating hot-and-cold baths. Changing water temperature induces reactions within the body. A cold bath, for a few minutes and at a temperature not less than 60°F, has a tonic effect. The small blood vessels in the skin contract during immersion and open up afterward, causing a noticeably warm feeling as the vessels dilate. Hot baths work in the opposite way, initially attracting the blood to the skin and stimulating the sweat glands, after which the body cools.

Alternate stimulation by hot and cold water causes the blood vessels to dilate and contract; this has a pumping effect on the blood that helps to reduce both congestion within the blood vessels and inflammation of the tissues. With this technique, hot sessions of a couple of minutes are interspersed with 30-second cold dips.

The sitz bath treatment offered in some hydrotherapy centers, uses hot and cold simultaneously. It consists of a chair portion containing enough water to cover the lower abdomen, and a smaller foot bath. The two sections are filled with water of

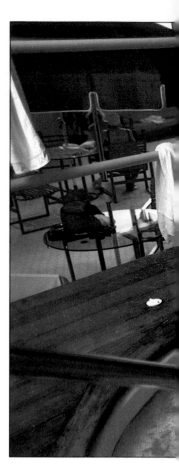

The whirlpool bath is a very popular form of pressure-movement hydrotherapy. Often located near the swimming pool in a health club, these smaller pools have strong underwater jets directed at different parts of the submerged body. Some whirlpools are designed for sitting in and others have individual frames on which to recline.

contrasting temperatures. You sit in hot water with your feet in cold for 10 minutes. The heat causes the blood vessels in the abdominal area to dilate. Then the water is changed so that your body is in cold water and your feet are in hot, your head and knees being kept clear at all times. The cold water around your abdomen now causes the blood vessels to contract. The treatment is prescribed for menstrual problems as well as for poor circulation.

A neutral bath, with water at almost exactly body temperature (98°F), is useful in treating tension, insomnia, and irritating skin conditions. The addition of special herbs, such as elderflower, horsetail, and peppermint, to the water enhances the effect of neutral baths, while the addition of Epsom salts (magnesium sulfate) encourages profuse sweating and is recommended for aching muscles. A warm shower should follow this treatment.

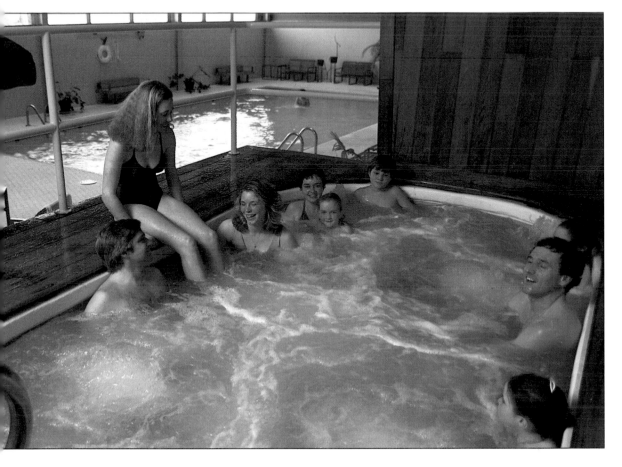

Pressure-movement treatments

Underwater massage is the most effective and widely used of the pressure-movement treatments. The water is circulated out of the bath, returning as a powerful jet, which can be directed to any part of the body. Since the body is nearly weightless in water and the muscles are relaxed, a more intense massage is possible, and it is important to lie down and rest for about 15 minutes afterward.

Whirlpool baths, with their gently swirling currents, are a standard part of physiotherapy for injuries to joints and connective tissue, and for some nervous conditions.

Aerated water, which occurs naturally in certain mineral springs but which can also be produced artificially, is a less powerful but still very effective form of underwater massage. It is used in physiotherapy and is a general tonic.

Douche refers to treatments with jets or sprays of water, from ordinary showers to high-pressure hot-and-cold alternating jets, fine needle sprays, and impulse showers. They are more effective than baths for localized treatment but are not advised for the very young.

Other treatments

Packs and cloth compresses soaked in hot water (to dilate the blood vessels) or cold water (to relieve congestion and swellings) can be applied to large or small areas.

Mineral water is often drunk for the reputed healing qualities of its mineral content. Sulfur and nitrogen, for example, are thought to help relieve rheumatism. Use bottled mineral waters during fasting—itself a purifying process.

Steam inhalation is used to treat mucous membrane inflammation and to relieve impaired breathing and wheezing caused by colds, asthma, or other respiratory disorders.

MASSAGE/1

Massage can be a natural tranquilizer. It has been used in virtually every culture throughout history to relieve aches and pains, unknot tense muscles, and help the body—and the mind—to relax. There are several types of massage, but the most popular are Oriental massage and Swedish massage. The chief difference between them is that some of the strokes in Swedish massage are designed to stimulate rather than to relax the body.

It is unfortunate that many people who might benefit from massage never try it, dismissing it as a specialized treatment for athletes or disabled people, or as an unjustifiable indulgence. If you think this way, you are missing out on something enjoyable. Anyone can learn to give massage; there is no mystique involved. It is a simple extension of warm human care and touch.

You can easily teach yourself a series of strokes that will help ease an aching neck, back, or head, or simply relieve tension at the end of an active day. Although there are parts of your body that you cannot possibly reach, you can nevertheless give yourself a relaxing massage.

Professional masseurs and masseuses offer the benefit of both skill and experience. They should be trained in anatomy and physiology so that they can identify muscles that are in spasm or painful knots that have built up by misuse of the body. Experienced professionals generally understand the requirements of the various body types and are able to choose the strokes that are beneficial for the individual. During a typical one-hour session the routine builds subtly in intensity and then subsides.

All massage is orchestrated in a series of basic strokes. *Effleurage*, traditionally used to begin or end a session, is a soothing, warm stroke. *Pétrissage* is useful for locating problem areas. Kneading is a deep massage movement applied between other strokes. Friction is the strongest stroke used in relaxation massage and is the crescendo, after which the massage is gradually wound down.

Although practice is better than theory, excellent books, workshops, and courses are available. To seek out the best of these, ask one of the professional organizations. To find a qualified masseur or masseuse who is licensed by the state, enquire at the local YMCA or health club, or ask your doctor or friends for recommendations.

THE BASIC TECHNIQUES

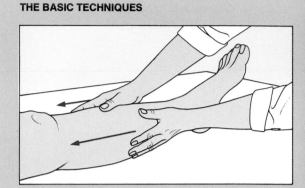

Effleurage
Use both hands and a moderately light touch. Sweep the full length of each leg, arm and the back. Use this stroke to apply oil or powder.

POINTS TO REMEMBER WHEN GIVING A MASSAGE

● Work in a warm, well-ventilated room. The temperature should be no lower than 70°F.

● Work at a comfortable height. The massage table can be a firm bed, or a mattress on a table or the floor. If you are working on the floor or a low bed, kneel beside it so that you can put your whole body into the massage.

● Remove all jewelry and be sure your fingernails have no rough edges.

● Before beginning, warm and loosen your hands by rubbing them together and shaking them.

● Put baby oil or powder on your hands to ensure that they move smoothly without dragging the skin.

● When you massage use your whole body.

● Really feel the body; don't merely touch it. A good massage flows smoothly from one stroke to the next.

● **Never massage**
The stomach of a pregnant woman. Yourself or anyone else right after eating. Varicose veins. Any part of the body you know to be weak or injured. Anyone with fever. Anyone with cardiac problems. Skin that is infected, inflamed, or bruised.

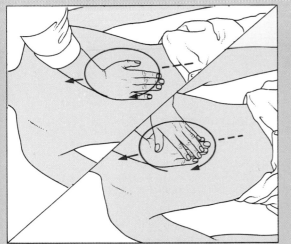

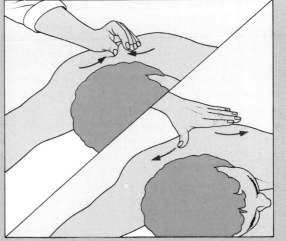

Pétrissage
This moderately deep circular stroke alternates pressure and relaxation. Work along a limb or from the buttocks to the neck. For the hand-on-hand method, move in clockwise circles up the area being massaged.

Kneading
Using the thumb and fingers of left and right hand in turn, work on the muscles as if they were dough, alternately grasping and lifting (but not pinching), then releasing the flesh in a smooth action.

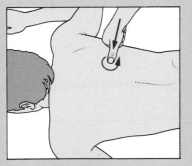

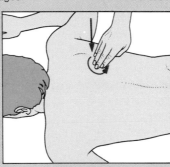

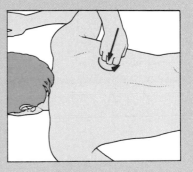

Friction
Using the thumbs, apply deep pressure in small, tight circles.

For finger friction, use the tips of the fingers instead of the thumbs.

For knuckle friction, use the finger joints as shown.

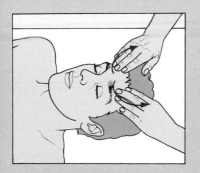

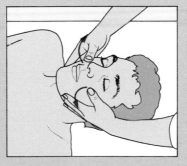

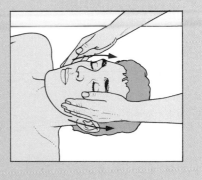

FACIAL MASSAGE
1. Smooth upward and outward over the brows with your fingertips.

2. Ease along the cheekbones with your thumbs.

3. Smooth upward over the sides of the face from chin to forehead.

Massage is one of the most pleasurable agents of well-being. It improves circulation, relieves pain and fatigue, enhances body awareness, and promotes relaxation, but it cannot reduce weight or reverse the aging process, nor can it improve muscle tone.

The sequence for a complete body massage is a matter of choice, but it is usual to start with the back and finish with the feet. Begin with the person who is to be massaged lying in a face-down position. Massage the back, shoulders, neck, buttocks, thighs, and legs. Then ask the person to turn over and continue with the arms, hands, head and face, the front of the shoulders, the stomach (with the person's knees bent), the legs and ankles, and finally the feet.

The Swedish massage strokes, generally classified as *tapotement*, include hacking, clapping, slapping, and pummeling. As an amateur, you should use these strokes very cautiously. Remember that they are designed to stimulate and should not make the person tense up his muscles in self-defense.

For self-massage, your own hands are the best aids, but appliances can also be effective. Among those that are fun to try and can do no harm are: wooden rollers, on frames for the feet and on bands for the back; vibrating appliances; and rubber-spiked massage sandals.

THE FULL BACK MASSAGE

For a beginner in the art of massage, the back is an ideal learning area since it is large and flat. Follow the steps illustrated on these pages to give a full back massage, which should last 20 to 30 minutes. Make sure that you are calm and relaxed before you begin, and that your fingernails are short so that they will not dig into the person. Remember to remove any jewelry that might interfere with the massage. As you work, try to be aware of tense areas in the person's body. Apply the strokes evenly—you will develop your own rhythm as you become more adept. For more information about the strokes, see pages 308–309.

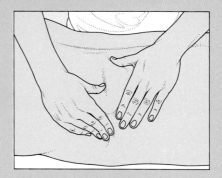

3. Turn sideways to the person. Starting at one side of the lower back, make kneading movements all the way up each side of the back. Seek out tense areas of muscle.

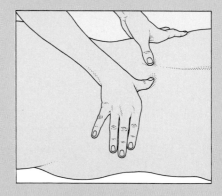

6. With your thumbs on each side of the spine, apply friction. Work up in small, deep circles, searching out knotty areas. Broaden the strokes at the shoulders.

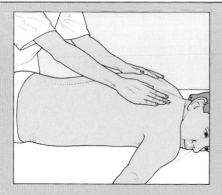

1. Pour a little oil into warmed hands and spread it over the back. Make smooth *effleurage* strokes starting at the top of the buttocks and sweeping up each side of the spine.

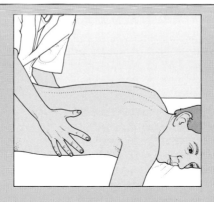

2. Continue on up to the neck. Run back down both sides of the body, then repeat steps (1) and (2) about a dozen times, gradually increasing the pressure as you do so.

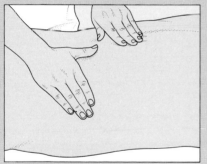

4. Make alternate inward- and outward-moving *pétrissage* circles all the way up the back to the shoulders. Repeat for the sides of the body.

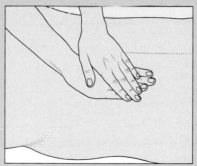

5. Using the hand-on-hand method, make *pétrissage* strokes all the way up the back, working on each side of the spine. Adjust the pressure to suit the person.

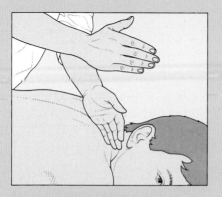

7. Hacking strokes, borrowed from the repertoire of Swedish massage, may be applied to areas such as the shoulders and sides if the person wishes.

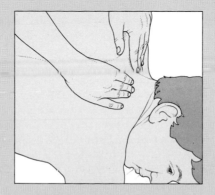

8. Wind down by applying more medium-pressure strokes to tense areas. End with a series of flowing *effleurage* strokes. Leave the person warmly covered to rest.

Points to remember

● Cover all areas of the body that are not being worked on.

● Always work equally on both sides and stroke in the direction of the heart—upward on arms and legs.

● To use the two-handed method, make simultaneous clockwise circles with one hand and counterclockwise circles with the other.

● To use the hand-on-hand method, place one hand on top of the other and move in clockwise circles up the left side of the part being massaged, and in counterclockwise circles up the right side.

● Exhale to reinforce the outward stroke.

Mistakes to avoid

● Never pour oil directly from the bottle onto the person. Do not use cream or lotions absorbed by the upper layers of skin, but keep to plant or mineral oils.

● Do not talk, except to exchange relevant observations, and avoid playing music with any rhythm. Relaxing environmental recordings, such as the sounds of the seashore, can be enjoyable and therapeutic.

● Do not continue for more than an hour.

● Do not press too heavily on bony areas, and avoid massaging directly over the spine.

OSTEOPATHY AND CHIROPRACTIC

The back is the mysterious side of every body; you need two mirrors to see it comfortably. Yet it has attracted its fair share of attention. The prevalence of back pain has led to a variety of manipulative therapies with wide applications.

Manipulation has been used to heal disorders of the musculo-skeletal system in countless cultures throughout history. Derived from the Latin word for handful, "manipulation" simply means the use of the hands to examine or treat a patient. It is one of the most ancient forms of therapy, dating at least as far back as the ancient Egyptians.

Osteopathy and chiropractic are distinct but related manipulative treatments for dealing with disorders of the spine. Both methods had their beginnings in the late nineteenth century in the heartland of America, at a time when the practice of medicine was far less sophisticated than it is today.

Techniques of osteopathy

Osteopathy was evolved by Dr. Andrew Taylor Still (1828–1917), a Missouri physician. Still emphasized the role of the musculo-skeletal system—that is, the bones, muscles and joints, particularly those of the spine—in health and disease and advocated the use of spinal manipulation as a treatment of many ills. His new philosophy of health care was introduced in 1874, and he opened the first school of osteopathy in 1892, in Kirksville, Missouri.

The name osteopathy, from the Greek words for bone disease, is misleading, since it is not connected with bone disease but with conditions arising from disturbances of the bones and joints, and of the spine in particular. Still's central concept was what he called an osteopathic lesion, a structural abnormality that could cause functional or organic disease.

Osteopathy teaches that the musculo-skeletal system, which makes up more than 60 percent of body mass, plays a central role in overall health. It holds that all body systems are interdependent and that a disturbance in one causes altered function in other systems of the body. This interrelationship of body systems is effected through the nervous and circulatory systems. The emphasis on the re-lationship between body structure and organic functioning gives a broader base for the treatment of the patient as a unit. These concepts require a thorough understanding of anatomy as well as the development of special skills in recognizing and treating structural problems through manipulative therapy.

Osteopathic physicians are fully trained and licensed physicians. In addition to providing manipulative therapy, they offer a wide range of treatments for all human ailments and diseases, including the use of drugs, radiology and surgery.

Techniques of chiropractic

Chiropractic is a widely recognized form of alternative medicine, and more than 10 million Americans are currently receiving treatment. Chiropractors do not use drugs or surgical procedures.

Named for the Greek words meaning "done by hand," chiropractic was developed by Daniel David Palmer, who introduced the theory in Davenport, Iowa, in 1895. Palmer placed great emphasis on the nervous system and on the way mechanical disorders of the joints interfere with it. He proposed that mechanical dysfunction was best corrected by mechanical means. He referred to slight displacements or deviations of bony parts, notably the vertebrae, as "subluxations." Correcting such displacements by manipulation, he believed, might eliminate a variety of symptoms, including not only back pains but also headaches and indigestion.

Chiropractic diagnosis makes use of X-rays and other conventional medical tests that determine a person's general health. Typically, treatment involves the manipulation of the spine, called spinal adjustment, and is performed on an adjustment table. Studies of patients have shown that treatments by trained, registered chiropractors have helped them find relief from back pain.

However, manipulation should not be expected to cure advanced illnesses, such as severe arthritis resulting from tissue damage. Nor can it correct a structural deformity of the spine. Manipulation could increase the pain of a slipped disk, and it could crush a vertebra weakened by osteoporosis.

VISITING AN OSTEOPATH FOR BACK PAIN

On a first visit to an osteopath, the practitioner takes a full case history and performs a thorough physical examination. Next, the osteopath manipulates each joint through its range of movement to assess how the body rates mechanically; the joints and soft tissues are then felt and may provide diagnostic clues. Where movement is restricted, the osteopath manipulates to open the joint and restore alignment—usually between two vertebrae. If the bones slip back into place, relief is immediate.

Examination of the lower, or lumbar, region of the spine is an important part of the osteopath's work. This is a part of the body that is particularly prone to trouble. Backache is prevalent because of the upright posture but is also related to stress. The osteopath will check for any indication of muscle spasm, of limited joint movement, or of bone disease.

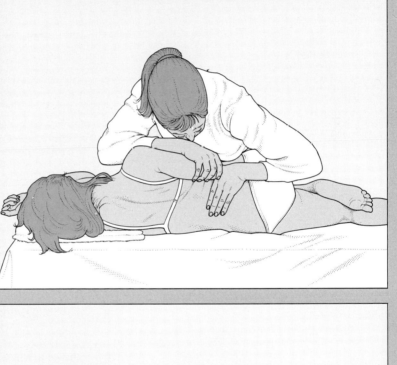

An osteopath will encourage patients to take care of all parts of the body but especially the spine. Positions such as this one mimic the actions of many animals as they yawn and stretch on waking. They allow the bones of the vertebral column to mesh into their correct alignment and exercise the surrounding muscles beneficially. Such actions also alleviate the strain that is put on the spine during daily routines.

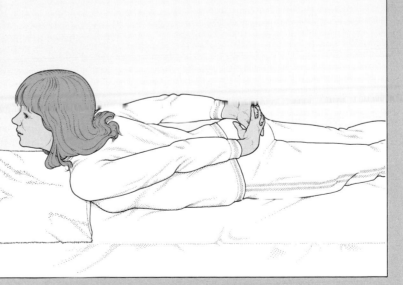

ALEXANDER TECHNIQUE

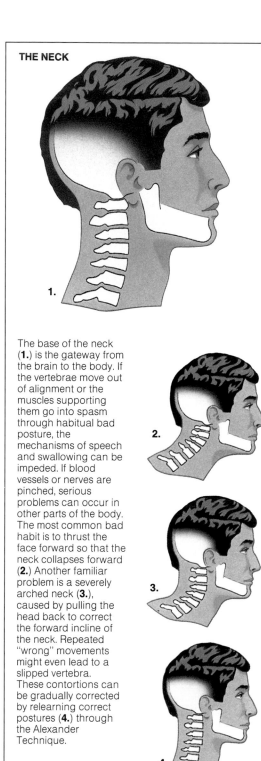

THE NECK

1.

The base of the neck
(**1.**) is the gateway from
the brain to the body. If
the vertebrae move out
of alignment or the
muscles supporting
them go into spasm
through habitual bad
posture, the
mechanisms of speech
and swallowing can be
impeded. If blood
vessels or nerves are
pinched, serious
problems can occur in
other parts of the body.
The most common bad
habit is to thrust the
face forward so that the
neck collapses forward
(**2.**) Another familiar
problem is a severely
arched neck (**3.**),
caused by pulling the
head back to correct
the forward incline of
the neck. Repeated
"wrong" movements
might even lead to a
slipped vertebra.
These contortions can
be gradually corrected
by relearning correct
postures (**4.**) through
the Alexander
Technique.

The Alexander Technique, or Principle, aims to correct habitual bad posture, which could be affecting your mental and physical efficiency.

An Australian actor, F. Matthias Alexander (1869–1955), developed the Technique late in the nineteenth century when he set about discovering what was making him lose his voice and potentially his career. By investigating every nuance of his physical behavior, he established that he shut off his own voice because of the way he drew his head backward and downward. Beginning with this realization, he pursued a meticulous study of how the human mechanism is designed to operate and of how modern man frequently interferes with the smooth running of his own machine.

Alexander agreed with the views of osteopaths and chiropractors (see pages 312–313) on the central role of the spine to fitness and well-being. But, unlike them, he attributed maladjustment directly to habitual misuse. He also perceived a relationship between physiological and psychological attitudes; that is, a slumping mind or spirit is the likely tenant of a slumping body, and muscular tension may reflect emotional unease. In this respect his approach is holistic.

Many people slouch because it comes naturally, but the aggregate product of years of slouching is a misshapen, poorly functioning spine. The greatest challenge raised by the Alexander Technique is to unlearn old habits.

Demonstration and learning

The Alexander Technique does not consist of exercises nor can it be learned from a book alone. It must be demonstrated by a qualified teacher, who adapts the instruction to suit the individual pupil. The teacher demonstrates the correct use of the body by arranging the pupil's body in the correct position so that he or she can feel what is right. Many people are initially confused because postures that feel comfortable through habit are wrong.

The Alexander Technique can be taught privately or in group sessions supplemented by private sessions, which are essential. The theory alone makes fascinating listening, and many people feel fired with optimism and exhilaration at the end of a class. A typical class might involve a re-enactment of postural evolution, with class members imitating primitive species or babies.

The aim is to return people to the state they were in before they began making postural mistakes—induced by tension, trauma, too-soft furniture, and habitual laziness.

In private sessions the pupil's body is subtly manipulated into the deceptively tricky postures of sitting, standing, walking, and lying down. Particular emphasis is placed on the transitions between each position. Through painless manipulation, the pupil has the sensation of growing.

The gradual re-education of the body involves visualizing yourself moving correctly while lengthening the body at the same time. The head has a key role. It is described as a locomotive pulling the body train, or as suspended from a hook, allowing every part of the body to fall into correct alignment.

Many people have found using the Alexander Technique an enlightening experience. Aldous Huxley, who was one of its most articulate devotees, described it as an ideal form of true physical education, leading to heightened consciousness at all levels "and a way to prevent the body from slipping back under the influence of greedy 'end-gaining' into its old habits." Actors, singers, and musicians have also claimed that practicing the Technique leads to improved, less stressful performance.

The therapy is infinitely subtle and sophisticated and requires perseverance to obtain lasting benefits. Teachers train for three to four years, and most pupils need about 30 sessions.

On a physical level, the Technique, which involves neither risk nor exertion, claims to reduce the side effects of stress and help relieve back pain, neuralgia, asthma, indigestion, migraine headaches, and high blood pressure, although none of these is scientifically verified.

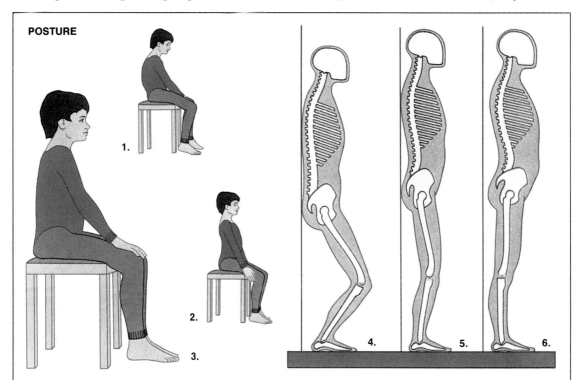

POSTURE

Most people slouch (**1.**) when they think they are sitting in a relaxed way and overarch their backs (**2.**) when they think they are sitting correctly. In fact, sitting with a straight back, eyes level, feet firmly on the floor, and weight evenly spread (**3.**) demands less effort than either of these postures and is more beneficial.

Use this exercise to help you practice the Alexander Technique. Stand with your lower back against a wall, knees bent, head slightly inclined forward (**4.**). If you find your back tires rapidly, you need to correct your posture. Slowly straighten your knees (**5.** and **6.**) and feel how your stance has changed.

ROLFING

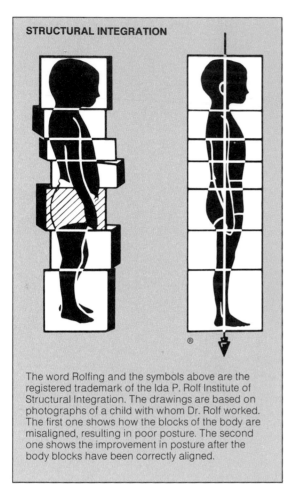

STRUCTURAL INTEGRATION

The word Rolfing and the symbols above are the registered trademark of the Ida P. Rolf Institute of Structural Integration. The drawings are based on photographs of a child with whom Dr. Rolf worked. The first one shows how the blocks of the body are misaligned, resulting in poor posture. The second one shows the improvement in posture after the body blocks have been correctly aligned.

The Rolf Method of Structural Integration is a form of physical re-education aimed at returning the body to its optimum balance. It was developed by the American biochemist Dr. Ida P. Rolf (1896–1979), who began her work in the 1930's and drew her principles from many sources, including osteopathy (see pages 312–313), yoga (see pages 148–153), and the theories of Wilhelm Reich and F.M. Alexander (see pages 314–315).

Like Alexander, Rolf realized that posture affects a person's general health. A slouched posture, for example, can interfere with breathing, circulation, and digestion. It can lead to pain or restriction of movement as the muscles of the back, chest, and shoulders tighten and gradually "set" the posture. It can even affect your attitude toward life and the way you respond to other people. She noticed that many people have areas of chronic tension and restricted movement, which, she believed, reflect the body's struggle with the force of gravity.

Rolf observed that through the progressive stages of rolling, sitting, and crawling, the human animal uncurls into its upright position to walk. But many events can interfere with the achievement and maintenance of an easy upright posture. Imitating other people, physical injury, and even emotional attitudes shape posture and movement, giving it a characteristic pattern that friends can recognize even from a distance. For example, if a boy sprains his ankle, he walks with more weight on his other leg while the injury heals. Even after the ankle has stopped hurting, he might unconsciously not trust it completely and continue to put more of his weight on his "good" leg. Gradually, the sinewy network of connective tissues in his hips and torso knits itself differently to accommodate this new pattern. His whole body subtly alters to adjust to the slight shift in strain. Over a period of years this small but fundamental change can lead to weakened muscles and pain in his back and neck.

The treatment

The purpose of Rolfing is to alleviate chronic tension, lengthen the body, and balance it in gravity, so that you use minimum energy in standing up, and the muscles and joints work as they are designed to do. This is achieved by using stretching and movement techniques to loosen and lengthen the connective tissues, or fascia— the tendons, ligaments, muscles, nerves, and other tissues that hold the skeleton together— that have thickened and shortened under continued tension and strain.

Rolfing usually requires a series of sessions, each one tailored to the individual's needs. On your first visit the Rolfer will take your detailed history and will take photographs of you in your underwear as both an aid in analyzing your standing posture and a record of what you looked like before you received any treatment. He or she will take more photographs of you during and at the end of the course of treatment to chart your progress, which should also be evident in the way you feel and move.

During the treatment you lie on a table or sit on a bench. The Rolfer uses his hands, knuckles, and even an occasional elbow to slowly and deeply

ASSESSING YOUR OWN STRUCTURE

1. Stand in a relaxed way on both feet facing a full-length mirror, preferably in your underwear. Drop an imaginary plumb line down your middle. Looking carefully from head to toe, can you see any differences between your right and left sides?

2. Draw an imaginary line across your waist and consider your top and bottom halves. Do they match or are they out of proportion with each other?

Turn to the side and look at yourself out of the corner of your eye. Draw another imaginary line down through your body. Are your major centers of weight—head, rib cage, and pelvis—lined up over one another or do you zigzag your way to the ground?

To the degree that you are out of balance, you are spending your energy in holding yourself up through muscular effort. If you improve your balance, you will release that energy for other things.

3. Face yourself again in the mirror and look for your body's prevailing attitude. If you saw yourself at a party or at work, what would your impression be of that person? Does your outside appearance match your inner feeling?

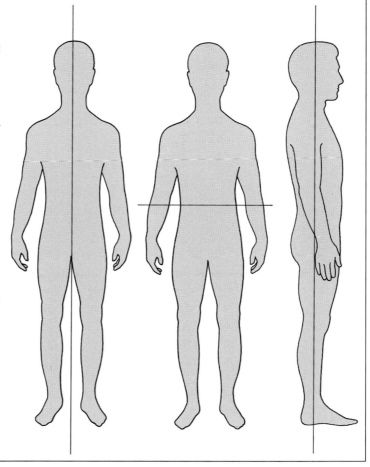

release tensed and distorted tissues. You help this process by relaxing and making small movements in response to his directions. The work can be uncomfortable at times, especially where you have an old injury or if you are very tense. However, the Rolfer works with you sensitively to open up these painful areas and restore them to their full range of movement and resilience.

The results of Rolfing vary from person to person. Because it works on structure, structural problems such as flat feet, chronic body pain due to tension or imbalance, some breathing difficulties, and excessive spinal curvatures and slouches are the most obvious areas of improvement. Most people experience a relief from pain, a lessening of fatigue, and a greater sense of lightness, ease, and energy.

Doctors know that tension, posture, and emo-

tional distress are linked; people who are chronically afraid or depressed, for example, express this through their posture, walking with their heads down and shoulders rounded. Just as psychotherapy and analysis can have an effect on physical health, Rolfing can have an effect on the mind. Rolfers believe that by changing the structural relation between parts of your body, they can often produce an opening and thereby help improve your underlying attitudes toward life and other people.

Rolfing has a wide application physically for athletes, dancers, and musicians; as an adjunct to psychotherapy; and for the average person who simply wishes to get the best from himself by improving his mental and physical integration. Because it is concerned with how you move, it is compatible with almost any form of exercise.

ACUPUNCTURE AND REFLEXOLOGY

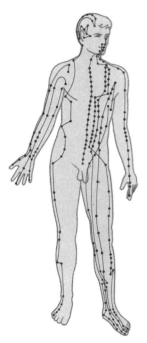

*When the acupuncture
points relating to a particular
organ or system are joined up
in a connect-the-dots style, they
form meridians. The chi
energy is said to flow along
these 12 paths so that a
needle in the foot, for
instance, benefits a migraine
headache. The main
meridians in the front of the
body include circulation, sex,
lungs, heart, stomach, liver,
kidneys, spleen, and large
intestines.*

Acupuncture is a traditional Chinese therapy used to maintain optimum health, and to diagnose and treat a wide range of disorders. In the West it has attracted notice as a drugless analgesic, as an anesthetic, and, less widely, as a treatment for the withdrawal symptoms of drug addiction.

The practice of acupuncture is based on the belief that the body flows with a vital energy, termed *chi*, which must be kept in balance to maintain good health. Western medicine has long been skeptical, since the existence of *chi* has not yet been identified in the same way as, for example, the nervous impulse. Nevertheless, in recent years acupuncture techniques have been more generally accepted in medical circles as a means of pain control. The theoretical basis for this is that if a sensory nerve is blocked by simple stimuli, other more serious signals are impeded. Additionally, this nerve stimulation induces the pituitary gland to produce endorphins: substances that control pain in the body.

The flow of energy

According to the ancient theory, when *chi* becomes blocked or stagnates, it must be stimulated to flow freely. This is done by inserting ultrafine needles into the skin at designated points—hence *acu*, Latin for "with a needle" and "puncture." The acupuncturist may simply leave the needles in place or may stimulate certain points either by gently rotating or pumping the needles or, sometimes, by passing a low-frequency electric current through them. Some conventional medical practitioners still find the remote character of the therapy hard to accept, for it treats internal complaints by external means, often using skin areas that are at a puzzling distance from the organ or system undergoing treatment. However, the action of the endorphins may explain how acupuncture has successfully produced anesthesia.

Another alien feature of acupuncture is the preliminary taking of 12 pulses—six in each wrist—compared with just one in Western medicine. These are the acupuncturist's chief diagnostic tool and are an invaluable early warning system for any serious ailments that might be developing. The practitioner palpates the radial artery in the wrist to detect fullness, hardness, and the degree of activity, and from these and other observations decides which points to use and painlessly inserts a sterilized needle.

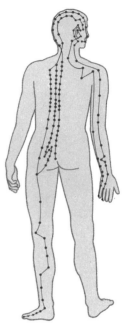

*The main meridians at the
back of the body include the
bladder, gallbladder, small
intestine, large intestine, and
triple warmer (a regulating/
distributing function). Many
acupuncturists advise that you
visit them four times a year,
at each change of season, for
a general health tune-up.
This ensures your systems
are all working well and any
unsuspected problems can be
discovered and treated.*

Moxibustion

Moxibustion is a form of acupuncture that uses heat. A cone of dried herbs, or moxa, is placed round the head of each needle and ignited. When you feel the heat, the acupuncturist quickly removes the cone. Sometimes the moxa is in the form of a cigarlike stick, which he holds close to your skin until you feel the heat. Another method employs a special needle with a cup at one end. The needle is inserted into the skin in the usual way, then the moxa is placed in the cup and lit, and the heat passes down the needle.

The practice of reflexology

Reflexology, also called zone therapy, works on the principle that the entire body is mapped in the feet and that deep massage of the appropriate areas brings relief to corresponding organs and systems. Reflexology also refers to meridians. There are ten of them, all terminating in the toes.

When there are ailments or problems in specific parts of the body, tiny crystalline deposits may form in the related position in the foot, making it too tender to touch. Reflexologists first diagnose any illness by touching the different parts of the feet, judging the severity of the ailment by the degree of tenderness. Then they use their fingers and thumbs to massage the appropriate areas of the feet to relieve tension, break down the crystalline deposits, and stimulate blood circulation. When the feet cannot be massaged for any reason, reflexologists massage the hands in the same way. Although the feet might be sensitive during treatment, the relief obtained can be dramatic.

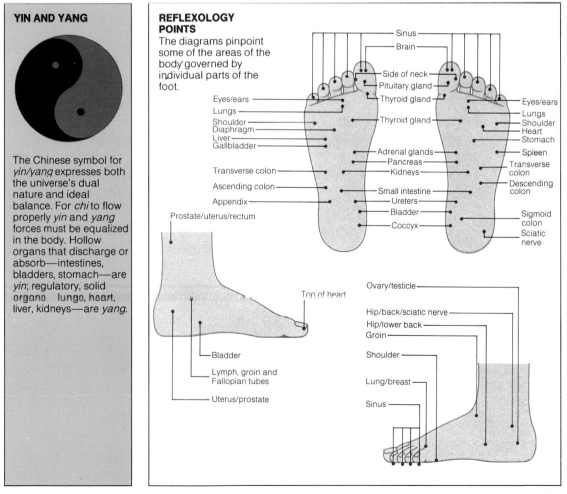

YIN AND YANG

The Chinese symbol for *yin/yang* expresses both the universe's dual nature and ideal balance. For *chi* to flow properly *yin* and *yang* forces must be equalized in the body. Hollow organs that discharge or absorb—intestines, bladders, stomach—are *yin*; regulatory, solid organs—lungs, heart, liver, kidneys—are *yang*.

REFLEXOLOGY POINTS
The diagrams pinpoint some of the areas of the body governed by individual parts of the foot.

Sinus
Brain
Side of neck
Pituitary gland
Thyroid gland
Thyroid gland
Eyes/ears
Lungs
Shoulder
Diaphragm
Liver
Gallbladder
Adrenal glands
Pancreas
Kidneys
Transverse colon
Ascending colon
Appendix
Small intestine
Ureters
Bladder
Coccyx
Prostate/uterus/rectum

Eyes/ears
Lungs
Shoulder
Heart
Stomach
Spleen
Transverse colon
Descending colon
Sigmoid colon
Sciatic nerve

Top of head
Bladder
Lymph, groin and Fallopian tubes
Uterus/prostate

Ovary/testicle
Hip/back/sciatic nerve
Hip/lower back
Groin
Shoulder
Lung/breast
Sinus

SHIATSU MASSAGE

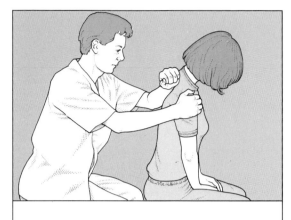

Applying a deep, holding pressure with the elbow
relaxes the muscles and reduces their resistance.

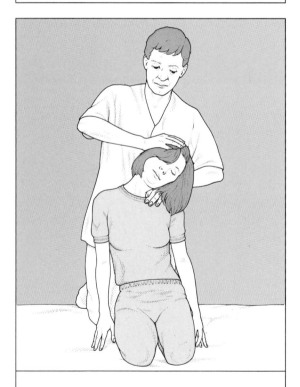

The degree of pressure exerted in stretching the
neck can be adjusted by changing the angle of the
elbow.

*The illustrations here and on the opposite page are
examples of some of the many shiatsu techniques.*

Shiatsu is a Japanese version of therapeutic
massage, commonly known as "acupressure." It
has been practiced in different forms throughout
the Far East for centuries and is growing in
popularity in the West. It is based on the same
system of medicine as acupuncture (see pages
318–319), and many people believe that some
form of touch therapy might have preceded the
use of needles.

Like acupuncture, shiatsu is based on the belief
that a vital energy, called *ki* in Japanese, flows
through the body along paths called meridians or
channels. Ten of the 14 main channels are named
after and related to vital body organs, such as the
heart, kidneys, and lungs. However, they have a
wider meaning too, encompassing a person's
complete physical and emotional functioning.
When the flow of *ki* is excessive, deficient, or
obstructed—perhaps by injury—the person becomes ill in the related part of his being.

The aim of shiatsu is to restore the balanced
free flow of *ki* along the channels. Like any form of
massage, it is particularly suitable for treating
stress-related conditions, such as tension headaches and insomnia. It is also used to treat
digestive ailments, stomach ulcers, menstrual
disorders, asthma, migraine headaches, and an
infinite variety of musculo-skeletal problems
from tennis elbow to lower back pain. Regular
shiatsu practiced in conjunction with other basic
good health habits is a form of preventive
medicine, maintaining the body's balanced state
and enabling it to cope with the stresses of life.

Diagnosis

Diagnosis and treatment take place on a mat on
the floor. First the practitioner assesses your
condition without touching you. Because shiatsu
is concerned with the whole person, everything
about you can help him in forming the diagnosis,
so he will check your facial color and characteristics, your posture and body structure, the condition of your tongue, the sound of your voice, and
even your characteristic smell.

Next the practitioner performs a *hara*, or
abdominal, diagnosis. He palpates the reflex
areas in your abdomen—these correspond to
each of the channels and are believed to be where
the body's principal energies reside—to find out
which ones are *jitsu*, or overenergized, and which
are *kyo*, or deficient. The purpose of the shiatsu

treatment is to disperse energy from the *jitsu* meridians and supply it to the *kyo* ones, thus rebalancing and harmonizing the *ki*.

Techniques of treatment

No oil is used in shiatsu and the treatment is performed through your clothing, which should be loose and made of natural fibers. You can be treated in different positions—lying face down or on your side, or sitting up. The shiatsu practitioner works on the entire length of the meridians, stretching and massaging them, as well as on the acupuncture points. One of the most characteristic shiatsu techniques is pressure, which he applies with his hands, thumbs, knees, elbows, and feet. He uses his whole body to press, support, and stretch yours to influence the flow of energy. He treats the *kyo* meridians with gentle but deep holding pressure and stretches, and the *jitsu* ones with more forceful, dispersing techniques such as shaking, slapping, or vibrating. Some practitioners perform adjustments as in osteopathy (see pages 312–313), but often a bone will click into place by itself when a spasm in the surrounding muscle is released.

In Japan shiatsu tends to be strong. Pleasure verging on pain is a characteristic sensation, which many people describe as a "good hurt." In the West shiatsu tends to be gentler. In both cases the recipients feel a great release of tension, becoming deeply relaxed and filled with energy.

Shiatsu treatment is considered a constant process of diagnosis, with the giver sensing your energy through his hands and projecting his energy through his body. Shiatsu practitioners use exercises similar to those taught in the martial arts to develop mental and physical power and are also trained in self-awareness and meditation to achieve a quiet and focused state.

However, the practice of shiatsu is not restricted to professional therapists. In Japan, for example, shiatsu is practiced in the home without complicated techniques or training. Many people consider it a useful way to help to ease family tensions and bring people closer together as well as an effective means of dealing with minor ailments.

There are various forms of self-shiatsu, the best known of which is *do-in*. This is a combination of shiatsu techniques and stretching exercises that many people find invigorating.

SHIATSU TECHNIQUES

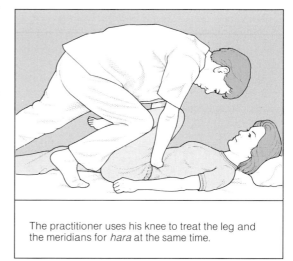

The practitioner uses his knee to treat the leg and the meridians for *hara* at the same time.

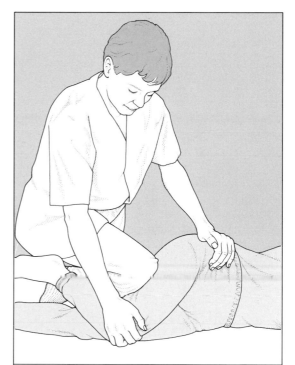

The knee is used to apply pressure down the sciatic nerve while the subject lies on one side.

HERBALISM AND AROMATHERAPY

Herbalism is the internal and external use of plant-based remedies to treat virtually any human ailment. Herbalists claim that their remedies also keep the body's systems healthy and help to maintain its natural resistance to disease. Skeptics might respond that the efficacy of herbalism is due to the placebo effect, which means that if you think a preparation is doing you good, then your condition improves.

Herbalism makes use not only of aromatic culinary herbs but also ferns, trees, lichens, seaweed and other plants. The particular part of the plant—leaf, stem, root or seed—is used whole, as opposed to conventional drugs based on isolated and synthesized "active ingredients." The plant parts will usually be prepared either to be taken internally, as a medicine, or to be applied externally, as an ointment.

The history of herbalism is as old as the human race or older, for many animals have always instinctively sought the plants that would cure their ills. All ancient civilizations probably practiced herbal medicine—largely because there were no alternatives. A plant was so closely identified with its healing properties that later these properties became the basis for official taxonomic classification. The advent of printing brought forth the great herbals such as Gerard's (1636) and Culpeper's (1653), both still regularly consulted by herbalists today.

Herbal remedies are inexpensive and, if taken in moderation, free from toxic side effects—reasons

Herbal remedies are usually prescribed as fluid extracts, tinctures, or syrups, but may also be supplied dried, to be taken as infusions or decoctions, or in powdered form as tablets or capsules. External applications can be made with ointments, lotions, or poultices.

SOME COMMON HERBAL REMEDIES		
Ailment	**Herb**	**Preparation**
Cough, colds, and sore throat	Chamomile	Tea of flowers
	Sage	Tea of dried leaves; infusion as gargle
	Eucalyptus	Dried leaves or oil in infusion As inhalant
	Rose	Infusion of leaves and petals as gargle
	Garlic	Juice
	Peppermint	Tea
Headache	Lavender	Weak tea of dried flowers
	Rosemary	Weak tea of dried leaves
	Lime tree	Infusion of powdered leaves or flowers
Diarrhea	Raspberry	Infusion of leaves
	Oak tree	Decoction of bark
	Blackberry	Infusion of leaves or root
	Strawberry	Infusion of leaves
Constipation	Basil	Leaves mixed with oil
	Honeysuckle	Infusion of leaves
	Walnut	Infusion of powdered bark
	Mulberry	Decoction of bark; syrup of berries
Flatulence and indigestion	Parsley	Tea
	Black or white pepper	Powder
	Marjoram	Infusion of leaves
	Tarragon	Infusion of leaves
	Caraway	Powdered seeds or oil of seeds
Insomnia	Dill	Seeds boiled in wine
	Violet	Tea of leaves and flower
	Bergamot	Tea
	Peppermint	Tea
	Valerian	Tea

for their popularity with people disillusioned with modern drug treatments. Plants contain substances that naturally buffer and enhance their main ingredient, so safeguarding against the harm caused by using strong constituents in isolation.

The huge range of herbal preparations now widely available can be used both for preventive health care and for helping to treat all manner of everyday ills. Try herbal preparations in place of coffee and tea to reduce your caffeine intake (see pages 282–283). Herbal remedies have succeeded in relieving many common conditions, including migraine headaches and chronic mucous membrane inflammation.

Unless you are expert in identifying plants and trained in their use you should not try to make your own herbal remedies. To derive the most benefit, especially for more serious or long-standing complaints, consult a qualified herbalist. Herbalists are trained to treat the whole individual, not just a disease or its symptoms. Two patients suffering from the same symptoms might require different restorative remedies.

Aromatherapy

The practice of aromatherapy was given its name by the French cosmetic chemist René Maurice Gattefosse, whose book, the first on the subject, was published in 1928. The therapy is similar to herbalism in that it uses plant substances. Unlike herbalism, however, it uses highly concentrated, volatile, and expensive aromatic essential oils extracted from plants. These are most often massaged into the skin, or inhaled or added to bath water. Sometimes they may be prescribed for internal use. Aromatherapy is used to treat a wide range of circulatory, respiratory, digestive, and neuromuscular complaints, and remedies are always tailored to the patient. The influence of smell on the mind is such that the remedies aim to treat mental as well as physical ills.

Versions of aromatherapy have been known since before Biblical times. The modern practice ranges from self-help to services offered by specialist practitioners.

For both baths and inhalations, a few drops of essential oil are mixed in the water. For massage, the pure oils are diluted considerably and penetrate the skin within minutes. Dosage is critical, since the same oil can act as a sedative or as a stimulant.

Bach Flower Remedies

Edward Bach (1880–1936), a fully qualified medical practitioner, pathologist, and bacteriologist, became convinced that human illness arose from imbalances caused by negative states of mind. His credo was "treat the patient, not the disease." He abandoned London and conventional medicine for the Welsh countryside and an intuitive approach to therapy. He found the cures he sought in 38 species of wild flower, whose vital forces he captured by steeping the flower heads in sun-warmed spring water.

The seven categories of Bach remedies are:

Fear Rock rose (terror/panic), Mimulus (shyness) Cherry plum (fear of mental collapse), Aspen (fear of the unknown), Red chestnut (fear/anxiety for others).

Uncertainty Cerato (self-distrust), Scleranthus (indecision), Gentian (depression), Gorse (despair), Hornbeam (inability to cope, tiredness), Wild oat (dissatisfaction, lack of direction).

Lack of interest in the present Clematis (daydreaming), Honeysuckle (clinging nostalgia), Wild rose (resignation, apathy), Olive (post-stress exhaustion), White chestnut (persistent worries, mental arguments), Mustard (depression for no apparent reason), Chestnut bud (slow learner of life's lessons, repeated mistakes).

Despondency and despair Larch (inaction through fear of failure); Pine (guilt); Elm (temporary despair), Sweet chestnut (extreme anguish), Star of Bethlehem (all forms of shock and sorrow), Willow (resentment, bitterness), Oak (despondency through lack of progress), Crab-apple (feeling unclean, self-dislike).

Loneliness Water violet (pride, aloofness), Impatiens (impatience), Heather (dislike of being alone, self-concern, poor listener).

Oversensitivity to influences and ideas Agrimony (mental torment hidden behind a brave face), Centaury (weak will, exploited easily), Walnut (major life changes such as puberty/menopause), Holly (jealousy, hatred).

Over-concern for the welfare of others Chicory (possessiveness), Vervain (stress caused by over-enthusiasm), Vine (domination, inflexibility), Beech (intolerance, arrogance), Rock water (self-denial).

SPORTS PSYCHOLOGY

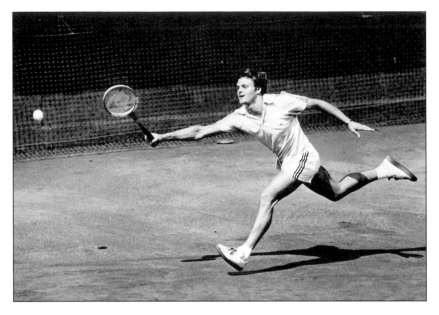

Sustained confidence, control, and sharpened reactions are essential qualities for winning at sports. Autogenic training helps you block out distractions and improve coordination so that body follows mind in perfect harmony.

Over the last 20 years there has been a growing awareness that although physical conditioning and practice are important, they alone will not maximize success in sports. Surprising Soviet and East German successes in the 1972 and 1976 Olympics focused attention on a new approach to sports. It was found that autogenic techniques emphasizing mental preparation were used to facilitate superior physical performance. Developed into a program of sports psychology, these techniques have now been incorporated in many sports training programs at both the collegiate and professional level in the United States.

Techniques of autogenics

Autogenics, or self-generation, uses the power of self-suggestion to alter the body's responses and achieve concentrated relaxation. The method was developed in the 1920's by a German neurologist, Dr. J.K. Schulz, who had been using hypnosis to treat his patients. Many of them derived great benefit from the relaxation produced by the hypnotic process, so Dr. Schulz experimented to see if they would fall into deep relaxation without hypnosis. He found that teaching verbal suggestion was highly effective.

Autogenic exercises have been used to combat stress headaches, high blood pressure, ulcers, and many psychosomatic problems. The aim is to try to focus on a specific part of the body and to

control experiences within it. You can learn to make parts of your body light or heavy, warm or cool, calm or tense. For example, you might begin by saying to yourself: "My fingers and hands feel warm and heavy." You repeat this several times before moving on to the other parts of the body until your whole body feels warm and relaxed.

Autogenic exercises might also include suggestions that help to slow breathing and heart rate and thus deepen the state of relaxation. Mental alertness is assisted during the process with suggestions such as "My forehead is cool and relaxed," which prevent you from becoming too drowsy.

Constant practice usually leads to an automatic response when a phrase is repeated. You can use this effectively during times of stress. For example, saying to yourself "My shoulders feel warm and heavy," may be sufficient to reduce tension if you are sitting in a traffic jam worrying about being late for an appointment.

During deep relaxation, long-standing physical aches and pains might surface temporarily because the muscle tissue becomes more sensitive. You may also feel tired, as muscular tension uses a great deal of energy and the muscles feel fatigued when they eventually relax.

Realizing your potential

You have probably noticed that when you play

your favorite sport you have good days and bad days. Sometimes you're just off your game and you can't seem to get it together. You probably also know one or two people who don't play quite as well as you but are hard to beat. These hard-to-beat people make the most of what abilities they have. They don't make as many mistakes or seem to lose concentration or hesitate as much as more talented players and thus seem to win more often than they should.

Sports psychology uses autogenic techniques to help you play up to your potential more often. You can still have bad days, certainly, but they should be less and less frequent. You'll still feel your concentration slipping away, but you'll be able to get it back more often.

How it works

Pressure is the most destructive force an athlete faces. If you play tennis, you know that hitting well in the warm-up is easier than hitting well at set point. Golfers who have been banging the ball out 200 yards on the driving range start hooking and slicing when they get on the course. Yet when you watch the top professionals in a sudden death play-off or match-point rally, you might see play of astounding force and accuracy. How do the great players play so well under pressure?

They don't. No one does anything well under great pressure. What the great players do is to avoid the feeling of pressure. When you are feeling relaxed and confident, you don't feel pressure—it's not there. But when certain thoughts, usually about winning and losing, come into your head, you turn on the pressure machine. You do it in order to help yourself but it doesn't work, so you simply have to learn to turn it off.

Preparation and rehearsal

In order to prepare yourself you can use the relaxation techniques described on page 273 or, alternatively, simply tense and relax each of the major muscle groups in the body sequentially while sitting down. For example, to the count of four tense your right leg, make it tenser, then relax. Then do the same with your left leg, right arm, left arm, abdomen, chest, jaw, and the muscles of the face and eyes.

After this, concentrate one at a time on pressure reducing thoughts (see box in next column). Use them to enhance your feeling of

relaxation. Then mentally rehearse one or more key motions of your game. For example, if you are a tennis player, you might rehearse your forehand. Make it as real as possible. See yourself hitting the forehand in slow motion, first from above, then from the front, then from the side. Feel the breeze and the sun. See the ball come into the strings and see the deformation of the strings and hear the sound they make when you hit it. If you are a weightlifter, visualize yourself in the gymnasium in the process of doing a lift. Feel the smooth, cool metal, hear the clink of the weights and the exhalation of breath.

Controlling pressure

Pressure producers
1. I've got to win.
2. If I don't win, people will think less of me.
3. If I just try harder, I'll win.
4. The wind is driving me crazy, these line calls are making me furious, this sun is impossible, etc.

Pressure reducers
1. I'm here because I want to be. Of all the places in the world I could be right now I choose to be here.
2. I'm here to have fun. This is exhilarating and wonderful.
3. I feel the breeze on my face and the sun on my arms, and I see the ball as big as the moon.
4. I don't know who'll win. I'm curious, but it is impossible to control outcomes, so I'll just have to wait and see. Meanwhile I'm going to watch this fascinating ball (or feel those smooth weights, etc.) and let my body take over.

You may also want to do the relaxation exercises and then just focus on the ball (or weights, etc.) in your mind for a minute or two. This visualization will help your attention to the ball in a match.

Through repeated rehearsal the body learns to function smoothly on its own, and is relaxed and efficient. Your performance will improve and you will enjoy it more. If you feel your concentration slipping away during a game, give yourself cues. Take a second while walking back to the service line or up to the tee to tense and relax your abdomen or your jaw. Your body will remember the relaxation exercises you have been doing and the rehearsing of your swing. Staring at the ball for a second or two will also help reduce tension by reminding your body of the visualization exercise practiced in moments of complete calm.

BIOFEEDBACK

Biofeedback is based on the idea that by feeding information back to a subject, he can learn to control his own physiological responses. As he does so, anxiety, pain, and tension can be remarkably modified. A calibrated machine feeds information about factors such as blood pressure, localized muscular tension, and skin resistance and temperature back to the individual in the form of light or sound signals. As he learns to relax and his body responds to that relaxation by changes in physiology, he is gradually able to eliminate the signal from the machine.

In the middle of the nineteenth century various people studying hypnosis, among them Carl Jung (see pages 332–333), discovered that states of anxiety in their subjects caused a marked rise in the electrical resistance of the skin. From the 1930's onward, this and other measurements related to involuntary changes in body physiology were chiefly used in polygraph, or lie detector, tests.

It was not until the 1960's that researchers began to realize the potential of such measurements in the detection and control of stress. As a result of extensive work on both humans and laboratory animals, several devices were developed that, with modifications, are used for biofeedback treatments today.

The benefits

Biofeedback is one of the few medically accepted techniques to demonstrate that the imagination can influence the body. Internal processes such as pulse rate and skin temperature, which were formerly considered beyond voluntary control, are particularly responsive. The debilitating effects of stress, which can take the form of headaches, indigestion, tension, insomnia, and other ailments, can be self-regulated. For this reason, biofeedback instruments are now used in some hospitals and clinics to treat a wide range of medical problems caused by anxiety. This approach has also been used, though less widely, to investigate altered states of consciousness, including meditation and hypnosis.

Messages from the skin

The relaxometer is a typical biofeedback machine that measures levels of arousal by recording the electrical conductivity of the skin through electrodes placed on the fingers. When the body is

aroused or stressed, sweating increases; as the skin becomes moist, it conducts more electricity. The stronger current flowing through the electrodes to the machine increases a light or sound signal, which in turn alerts the user to his level of arousal. When the body relaxes, sweating decreases. The skin becomes drier and conducts less electrical current to the machine. As a result, the displayed signal decreases, thereby informing the user that he is more relaxed. As he learns to reduce the signal by relaxing, the individual does indeed learn to control the sweat glands.

Another biofeedback instrument is the temperature meter, which registers the amount of warmth in the skin. When you are under stress, the fight or flight response of your autonomic nervous system (see pages 268–269) causes the blood vessels to contract and to draw blood away from the surface of the skin. As a result, the skin temperature drops. When you relax, the blood flows back to the surface of the skin. The machine indicates the changes in temperature. Many people find that by simply imagining themselves in a warm situation, such as sitting in front of a fire, their hands actually warm up. Yet if you try to use willpower rather than imagination to increase skin temperature, the hands are likely to remain cold because willpower cannot activate the fight or flight response which is governed by the autonomic nervous system.

Learning to relax

Biofeedback devices do not induce relaxation in themselves but can be used to learn the knack. You are encouraged to allow yourself to become receptive to messages of tension or relaxation, or warmth or coldness, given out by your body, usually by imagining a warm and relaxing situation. Subjects report suddenly discovering they can do it but cannot explain how. With practice, many also learn to relax without the instrument, through autosuggestion.

Messages from the brain

The electroencephalogram (EEG), which is used for research into the various levels of brainwave activity, is one of the best-known biofeedback monitors. Specific wave frequencies have been found to be associated with different states of mind: *beta*, the most common brainwave in a

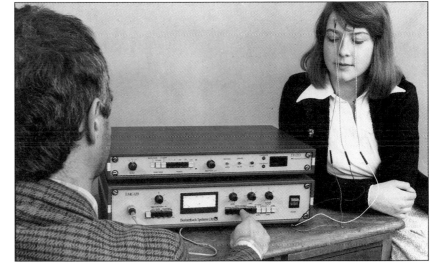

The electrical activity of the brain, which is measured with a type of electroencephalogram (EEG), indicates to the trained operator the state of consciousness of the subject. The aim of biofeedback is to teach the subject to control aspects of body physiology that normally occur involuntarily and, in so doing, reduce stress and its associated ills.

normally active mind, represents the fastest level of electrical activity and is associated with active concentration, as when solving a practical problem. *Alpha* is a slower rhythm, usually described as being pleasantly relaxed. The second slowest is *theta*, which many people experience between waking and falling asleep, and it is often associated with creative or disturbing images. The slowest brainwave rhythm is *delta*, which occurs during sleep.

The biofeedback machine gives feedback about the *alpha* waves and is a simpler version of the EEG found in hospitals. The object of the training is to help a person relax into the *alpha* state, which creates a feeling of well-being. More sophisticated practice can help the individual reach higher states of awareness and, conversely, deeper states of relaxation, which might otherwise take years of meditation to achieve.

Reducing hypertension

Biofeedback has proved effective in easing hypertension—a major cause of heart attacks. The alarm response of the autonomic nervous system increases blood pressure and mobilizes the whole body into a state of arousal. Many people are unaware of living in a semipermanent state of tension. Through biofeedback and relaxation exercises an individual can learn to rebound from a state of arousal to a state of calmness. This involves normalizing the heartbeat and pulsation of blood, and modifying the digestion and muscular tension. Although this process takes longer than, for example, treatment with antihypertensive or tranquilizing drugs, it can reduce the risk of drug dependency and allow for a healthier way of life.

Placebos

The effect of placebos suggests how the mind can influence the body. A placebo is an innocuous substance that the individual believes to be a genuine drug prescribed for a specific condition. A variety of research studies has shown that the blood pressure of hypertensive patients was reduced equally well whether they were given hypertensive drugs or placebos. The belief that the pill will help solve a problem often brings about a temporary "cure," which reflects people's powerful physical response to a conviction.

Although biofeedback instruments are useful in the treatment of physical and psychological problems, they are not essential for the development of self-awareness. If you choose to be attentive, internal and external environments supply continuous feedback about your state of health. A mirror indicates clearly if you are tired, tense, overweight, or simply looking out of condition. Trusted friends can give valuable feedback as to how you behave or look to them. Most important of all, however, is your ability to listen to your own internal messages, for they are the most accurate prompters, advising you whether you should be active or should rest.

ZEN AND MEDITATION

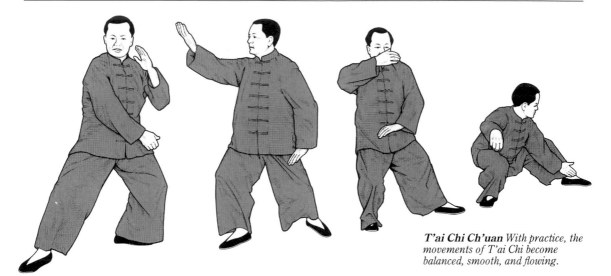

T'ai Chi Ch'uan *With practice, the movements of T'ai Chi become balanced, smooth, and flowing.*

The aim of meditation is to relax the body and mind and to create a focused awareness in which the "chatter" within your head gives way to stillness and inner peace. Regular periods of meditation carried out in quiet, peaceful surroundings can provide you with a respite from the hustle and bustle of daily life. They also allow you to find inner peace and reduce stress.

Meditation has been practiced for centuries in both the East and the West. In the West it has traditionally been identified with prayer and direct communication with God; in the East its aim has been to free the mind from excessive thought. Simplified forms of many meditation techniques have in recent times been incorporated into holistic approaches to health.

The means of meditation
One approach common to all forms of meditation is one-pointedness. This means that all your attention is directed to one feature of experience to the exclusion of all else. In Zen meditation you focus on the inward and outward flow of breath. When your thoughts begin to stray, you merely return your attention to your breathing. In transcendental meditation, the meditator repeats one word, a mantra, over and over again in silence.

A typical meditation involves sitting comfortably but erect and focusing on a mantra, on breathing, or on an object such as a picture or a candle flame. By gradually becoming more adept at letting go of conscious thoughts and feelings, the meditator discovers a fresh way of being at the center of his own experience.

Zen Buddhism is a spiritual tradition that practices a form of seated meditation. It emphasizes the need for "emptiness," so that by emptying your mind of all its prejudices and preoccupations you get closer to the true nature of reality. In Zen there is also considerable emphasis on trusting in the natural course of life. From the rhythms and processes of nature, its practitioners argue, you find continual wisdom and simplicity.

All meditative approaches, if performed with full awareness and over a considerable period of time, can have a profound influence on your ordinary life and fitness. By learning how to let go, to enter states of deep relaxation, and to develop peace of mind, you can become mentally and physically revitalized. Many people report that they are more sensitive to their surroundings as a result of regular meditation.

Recent research on the brain has provided some understanding of the effects of meditation. Neurophysiologists have discovered that in most people the left hemisphere of the brain is dominant over the right. The left hemisphere is concerned with logical thoughts and ideas, speech, and mathematical concepts and similar matters. Its dominance is believed to be due in a large part to a cultural bias toward rationality.

The right hemisphere of the brain deals with artistic appreciation, nonlogical thought and images, and intuitive methods of understanding. In meditation it has been found that there is a shift in activity away from the dominant left hemisphere and toward the right. This shift of emphasis enables the meditator to attain a higher level of receptivity and awareness than is ordinarily possible in the Western world today.

T'ai Chi Ch'uan

The ancient art of T'ai Chi (illustrated left) is a form of meditation in motion, with a superficial resemblance to the martial arts. It has a variety of aims and benefits, none of which is concerned with self-defense. These include:

● To experience a sense of balance, grace, and meaning that is inherent in movement.

● To deepen the breathing and clear the mind.

● To effect a complete fusion between movement and thought.

● To make you, by being in contact with the ground, more rooted and secure.

● To create a harmonious unity between body, mind, and spirit.

Other research into the physiological effects of meditation has shown a marked decrease in the fight or flight responses (see pages 268–269) when people start to meditate. Pulse rate, skin conductivity, and muscle tension all show marked decreases during meditation. And a person can learn how to maintain these benefits so that they become permanent. This has obvious value in the treatment of a wide variety of psychosomatic and stress-related disorders, such as high blood pressure, migraine headaches, some digestive disorders, and insomnia. It is also one of the reasons why the value of meditation is beginning to be appreciated by the medical profession as part of a holistic approach to health.

Meditation and spirituality

Many people use meditation as an opportunity to communicate with God or to think about the essence of life. They find that meditation quiets the mind and allows them to listen to God or let the spirit of life enter them. Some people say that listening for the word of God does not mean waiting for some extraordinary revelation, for what they hear or know through meditation is something basic to life that is already known, such as, "Be more accepting."

Meditation, prayer, contemplation, and faith can give you a vital sense of transcendence, of being connected to something larger than yourself. On a practical level, they can be enormously useful in helping you to cope with the crises of life and to come to terms with shattering concepts, such as your own death. People often speak of "going" beyond their own minor worries when they meditate or pray, to a sense of being unified with others and with the universe.

Peak experiences—those moments at which people are filled with revelation, insight, or deep feeling—can also be brought about by physical activity or sport. One woman described recurrent experiences of religious faith while jogging: "I feel more inspired when I'm jogging than I ever did in church. Sometimes I just have the sense of going beyond myself and being aware of and part of everything around me."

Meditation can deepen faith, of which trust and love are necessary components. There can be no doubt that in a troubled world any way of reaching a deeper recognition of the value of life and the universe must be important.

Meditation: the benefits

● Relieves stress and stress-related disorders.

● Helps you become more in touch with the nature of reality.

● Dispels negative thoughts and self-doubts.

● Encourages a heightened sense of worth.

● Deepens faith.

● Enhances your happiness.

● Increases your awareness of your surroundings.

Meditation: the method

The following instructions are guides to a simple form of meditation.

1. Sit quietly in a comfortable position and close your eyes.

2. Deeply relax all your muscles and keep them relaxed.

3. Breathe through your nose and become aware of your breathing. As you breathe out say the word "one" quietly to yourself

4. When distracting thoughts arise, repeat the word "one."

5. Continue for 10 to 20 minutes. When you have finished, sit quietly for several minutes, first with your eyes closed, then with them open.

HYPNOSIS

Hypnosis is an altered state of consciousness, into which a person enters voluntarily. Usually accompanied by feelings of deep relaxation, it can create physical and psychological changes. These are produced by altering a person's emotions, sensations, and imaginings. For many people, hypnosis is a useful means of reducing stress and the behavior associated with it, and of coming to terms with deep-seated problems. It can also be valuable in the relief of pain.

The nature of hypnosis

Hypnosis is essentially a "consent" state. To be susceptible to hypnosis (and most people are), a subject must have a certain degree of trust in the practitioner and a willingness to put aside any resistance. The hypnotist acts primarily as a guide to the subject, giving simple instructions, which, when followed, lead the subject gradually into a trance.

A popular image of the hypnotist at work has the subject looking at a pendulum or a swinging watch, or gazing into the hypnotist's eyes. These techniques and others have been used in the past and may still be in use. What is important about any method is that it should focus the attention and exclude distractions.

Most modern hypnotists use a wide variety of methods. For example, the subject might be asked to count backward from, say, 300 or to gaze at a fixed spot on the ceiling. Often, however, it is sufficient for the subject to sit and listen to the hypnotist's suggestions. By following these suggestions, the subject allows himself to be guided into an altered state of intense but narrow concentration.

A popular myth is that hypnosis is a form of sleep induced by a longwinded hypnotist counting at length in a boring tone of voice. In fact, EEG studies show that the hypnotic state is not a form of sleep at all. It is a form of focused alertness, with increased attention in one area and decreased or absent focus on other events. People who lose themselves in a movie, a book, or a daydream are probably experiencing a mild form of self-hypnosis. Hypnosis is perhaps best described as a daydream so intense that one temporarily believes one is in it, and is oblivious to anything else going on in the surroundings.

When the mind and body are calm and relaxed, the suggestions given by the hypnotist pass

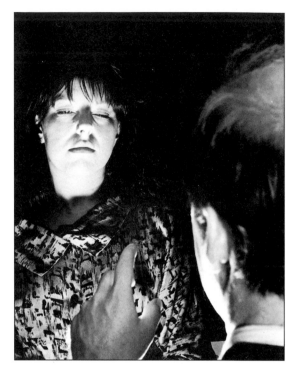

The hypnotist *is holding a small glass object in his hand. The woman he is hypnotizing is focusing her attention on this object to keep her mind free of distractions and open to his suggestions.*

directly into the subject's consciousness and are much more likely to be accepted. For this reason, there must be a prior agreement between the subject and the therapist about the nature of the suggestions to be given. It is particularly important that the instructions are given in a calming, reassuring and positive way, because in some instances unpleasant and unsettling memories and feelings might be brought to the surface of the mind in the course of treatment.

It is often much easier to explore disturbing aspects of your life in hypnosis than in the normal waking state because the resistance, or "critical censor," which the mind normally imposes on such material is in abeyance. In such hypnoanalysis, the therapist must have considerable skill, sensitivity, and knowledge to be able to conduct safe and effective treatment.

Practical hypnosis

Once their fears have been dispelled with proper explanation and reassurance, most people can be hypnotized, at least into a light trance. It might take a person many sessions to achieve a state of deep trance. However, it is not always necessary to enter a deep trance for hypnotherapy to be effective. A wide range of problems can be treated with the use of systematic relaxation and suggestion, both of which are important aspects of hypnosis. Eating disorders, smoking, nail-biting, and other problems can all be dealt with through hypnosis. In general, anything that can be accomplished with hypnosis can also be accomplished without it, but, particularly in addictions such as smoking, hypnosis may achieve quicker results.

In solving people's problems, the hypnotist might use one or a combination of strategies. Ego-strengthening is an effective way of building up a person's confidence in his ability to overcome his difficulties. It involves the use of positive suggestion to reinforce motivation and a sense of self-esteem. With some addictive problems, such as smoking, overeating, or the use and abuse of alcohol or other drugs, a type of aversion therapy might be used that emphasizes the unpleasant or damaging aspects of the habit.

Alternatively, or in addition, the therapist might stress the positive aspects of breaking the addiction so that new associations are gradually established and begin to assert themselves in the normal, waking state. For many people, the light trance state may be sufficient for the mind to be receptive to the new associations and for the problem to be surmounted.

As a rule, the greater the ability of a subject to create imaginative ideas or fantasies, the greater the likelihood of success. People who have difficulty in visualizing, or creating internally, sensory perceptions such as smell, taste, sound, and touch, are those most likely to prove more resistant to this approach.

Pain relief

Hypnosis can be used successfully to relieve pain during childbirth and dentistry. This use of hypnosis involves the generation of relaxation and local anesthesia to reduce or eliminate painful sensations in a particular area. For it to be successful, the subject must be adequately trained beforehand so that the hypnotic state can be achieved reasonably quickly when required. Classes in self-hypnosis for childbirth are carried out at some hospitals and by some doctors who find this a valuable approach to drug-free labor.

With this technique, the subject is taught that under hypnosis a particular part of the body will become numb. So, for example, the suggestion is given that no pain or sensation will be perceived in the hand. After sufficient repetition of the suggestion, the hand is tested with a small pinprick, which should produce no pain response. The subject is then told that he or she is able to transfer this lack of sensation to any area of the body as required, such as the mouth in the case of dentistry, or the lower back region in the case of labor.

Many practitioners believe that in using hypnosis for pain relief it is most important to concentrate on the positive aspects of desensitization by avoiding direct references to pain, which might generate anxiety. Instead, they refer to contractions or to numbness, both of which are more neutral terms.

Many people find that, with practice, they can teach themselves a type of self- or autohypnosis. This is related to autogenics (see pages 324–325) and can be a useful tool in helping people to cope with and find relief from a wide variety of stress-related symptoms.

Myths about hypnosis

● The subject is unconscious in the hypnotic state.

● Removing symptoms by hypnosis will lead to substitution of other symptoms.

● Your mind can be taken over or dominated by the hypnotist so that you behave in a way that is unacceptable.

● You do not return to a normal waking state at the end of a session.

Truths about hypnosis

● Hypnosis involves the full cooperation and participation of the subject.

● The subject actually hypnotizes himself under the guidance of the hypnotist.

● The subject is aware of what is happening during the session and can, if he wishes, bring himself out of the trance at any time.

● The subject is to some extent suspending critical judgment and thus could be vulnerable to a limited degree of exploitation in an unprofessional setting.

● It is impossible for the subject not to return to the normal waking state. At worst, he will fall asleep naturally if not aroused by the hypnotist.

PSYCHOANALYSIS

The method of solving problems by psychoanalysis was pioneered by the Austrian physician Sigmund Freud (1856–1939) at the end of the nineteenth century. Freud, who was working with people who had nervous disorders, theorized that human behavior and emotions are largely influenced by unconscious wishes. Emotional problems, he argued, originate in the developmental needs and frustrations of childhood. In most people these feelings remain subconscious because they are linked with sexual longings that are frightening or shameful.

Exploring the mind

Freud described the mind as having three parts. The ego includes that part of the mind of which a person is generally conscious, the part that perceives, remembers, and feels, the part that is used to figure out what to do today, tomorrow, and next week.

The other two parts of the mind, the superego and the id, Freud maintained, are largely unconscious. The superego includes parental, social, and moral injunctions, and tells people when they are good and when they are bad. When it is in conflict with something you have done or something you want, you might feel discomfort, shame, or anxiety.

The id contains many of your desires, cravings, and wishes, and can be in direct conflict with the superego. The ego referees between the desires of the id and the prohibitions of the superego, and the things that you say and don't say, do and don't do are considered to be the product of this constant and unconscious process.

Psychoanalytic techniques

Psychoanalysts believe that problems experienced during childhood surface in adult life in the form of marital discord, overeating, alcohol dependence, and other problems. Psychoanalysis, unlike many other therapies, is not primarily concerned with the relief of such symptoms, but with gradually uncovering the underlying cause, which is hidden in repressed memories. Unless the original conflict is revealed, psychoanalysts assert, the relief of one symptom, such as excessive drinking, will merely be replaced by another—increased anxiety or overeating, for example.

The analytic approach to problem solving involves certain fundamental methods by which the analyst attempts to help the individual to reach into his unconscious mind. In classical analysis a person visits the analyst frequently, usually four or five times a week. At each session, which usually lasts between 45 and 50 minutes, he lies down on a couch, with the analyst sitting to one side or behind him out of direct view. The person is asked to free associate, that is, to say whatever comes into his mind, without censorship. These spontaneous associations are thought to initiate an unraveling process in the mind. Thus the person's most intimate and influential attitudes and memories begin to come to the surface.

Repressed needs and conflicts are uncovered through the relationship between the subject and the analyst. On the whole, the analyst remains aloof, making interpretations designed to break through the individual's resistance to recognizing and dealing with buried emotions and memories. Gradually, in theory, the positive and negative feelings that the person has repressed begin to manifest themselves in his developing relationship with the analyst.

Through such a manifestation, commonly known as transference, the individual may feel emotions such as love, anger, and hate toward the analyst, which are considered to be re-enactments of feelings he held earlier about other important people in his life. By separating the reality of these feelings from their fantasy content, and by uncovering their antecedents, the analyst helps the person to separate the real from projected feelings, the past from the present, and to integrate these emotions into his consciousness.

The interpretation of dreams is another method the analyst uses to delve into the unconscious, a method for which Freud is famous. Critics of Freudian theory point out that his interpretation of dream symbols and events are primarily sexual and reflect Freud's belief that the sexual desires of the child are at the heart of internal human conflict. Dream interpretation remains central to many types of psychoanalysis.

Suitable subjects

Psychoanalysis is most useful for someone who desires a long-term quest for self-knowledge, and for anyone with a character disorder. The latter is usually a person who is content with his situation, but seeks treatment and sincerely wants to change because someone in close contact with him, such as a partner or employer, has expressed dissatisfaction with him.

Psychotherapies

When considering ways of solving problems it is important not to confuse psychoanalysis with psychotherapy. Psychoanalytic psychotherapy is a talking therapy in which the individual and the therapist, who maintains a fundamental belief in unconscious processes, meet usually once or twice a week and sit facing each other. The therapy continues for as long as it takes to resolve the problems to the satisfaction of the subject, which may be a matter of months or, more usually, years.

Brief therapies are usually recommended for people who are functioning well and develop a specific isolated problem, which is the product of a "core conflict"—a past mal-adaptive reaction or behavior. They have a time-limited approach, generally between six and 20 sessions. The task of this kind of therapy is to bring the core conflict to consciousness, analyze it and it alone, and to resolve it.

Finding a therapist

The relationship between the subject and the analyst is an important element in the success of the therapy, so it is important to find a reputable therapist with whom you can establish a rapport and in whom you have confidence. Your local teaching hospital can recommend a therapist, or you may learn of one through a friend, your family doctor, or a social worker.

Other analytic movements

All the analytic therapies available today are descended from Freudian psychoanalysis, and most of the famous names of psychoanalysis were early members of Freud's circle.

Carl Gustav Jung (1875–1961) was a psychiatrist and younger colleague of Freud, and parted from Freud because he believed that there are other dimensions to the individual unconscious than the sexual desires of childhood. Much of Jung's work was based on his extensive knowledge of the religions, myths, and philosophies of many different cultures, whose contents were, he felt, evident in people's dreams and fantasies.

Jung based his analytic theory on his belief in a universal unconsciousness with common themes, which he called archetypes. An example of a Jungian archetype is the duality of the masculine (*animus*) and feminine (*anima*) sides of the personality. Jung emphasized that within every individual there are healthy "masculine" and "feminine" dimensions, and that if they are not acknowledged, imbalance and difficulties with relationships might result. Thus a woman who is out of touch with her *animus* might be drawn to have a series of unsuccessful relationships with overtly masculine men, who eventually prove too harsh. By getting in touch with the masculine side of herself, through analysis, she may have less need of this type of man and develop a relationship with someone gentler and less dominant.

Jung believed that his approach to therapy is best used by people in their middle years who need perspective and meaning in their lives. He also felt that it was important to pay attention to the particular phase of life that a person is in, and to the seven-year cycles that, in Jung's view, are common to human experience.

Alfred Adler (1870–1937) worked with many children, and was impressed with the degree to which a child who was doing poorly in one area, such as school, would overcompensate and do very well in another, such as sports, or become a bully. He developed the theory of an inferiority complex and a counter-balancing superiority complex.

Otto Rank (1884–1939), who was not medically trained, was mainly concerned with the cause of anxiety. He believed, as Freud did, that all problems were caused by earlier events. He proposed the theory of birth trauma, believing that all anxieties stem from that original anxiety. Thus he saw the fears of intimacy, sexual involvement, dying, and separation, for example, as fears of departure from the womb, of change, and ending. In his therapy he focused on endings, tending to set time limits on treatment, and to discuss the ending and inevitable leave-taking from the beginning In this way, he was the father of modern brief therapy.

Harry Stack Sullivan (1890–1949) was the first great American psychiatrist. He had a great understanding of unconscious processes, but believed that there were no unconscious structures. He built his theory around interpersonal relations. He felt that human behavior was motivated by strivings for satisfaction and often conflicting strivings for security, that people relate to each other well or badly, and can learn to relate in a more satisfactory manner. In many ways he was the antecedent of many brief, behavioristic therapies.

BEHAVIOR THERAPY

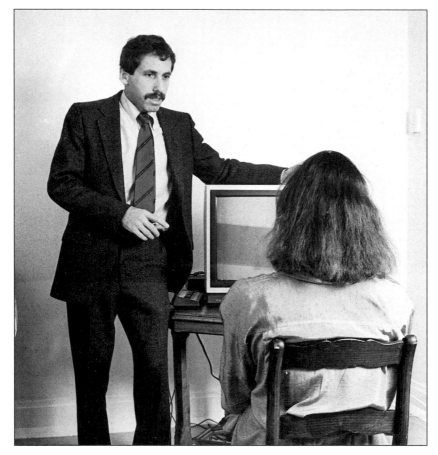

This woman is receiving behavior therapy for a fear of heights. In the early stages the therapist shows her a film of scenes photographed from heights.

In treating emotional problems, behavior therapy is an extreme reaction against psychoanalysis. Psychoanalysis is based on the premise that all human behavior is the end product of an internal struggle between desires, or drives, and prohibitions, and that behavior can be improved only when those conflicts are revealed, understood, and resolved. Behavior therapy is concerned with a person's current behavior, not with internal drives and defenses, past traumas and experiences. It is based on the premise that you can modify problem behavior through a series of behavioral exercises.

The effects of a phobia

The greatest success of behavior therapy is in the treatment of anxiety disorders, such as phobias, obsessive or irrational fears, which can have far-reaching effects on your life. The following is a good example of a phobia.

Alice is a successful young woman, but whenever she sees a cat her heart pounds, she breaks into a sweat, she feels terrified, becomes light-headed, and thinks she is about to faint or even die. Alice avoids cats, of course, but the problem gets worse; it *generalizes*. This means that if Alice sees a cat on Main Street, she subsequently links Main Street with her fear and begins to avoid it in the same way that she avoids cats. Soon she has seen cats at various locations in town and will not leave her house.

Anxiety disorders like this probably afflict about 15 million Americans. Many people consider their fears a weakness and are ashamed to discuss them. At first family, friends, and colleagues might attribute their decreased social activity to shyness or other causes, but if they reach the stage where they are afraid to leave the house it becomes obvious that help is needed. Behavior therapy can cure phobias.

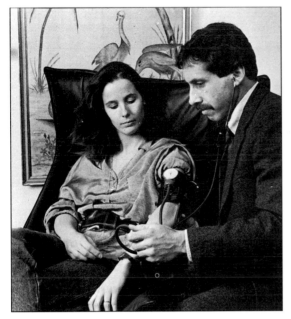

After anxiety has been induced, the woman performs relaxation exercises while the therapist monitors her heart rate and blood pressure.

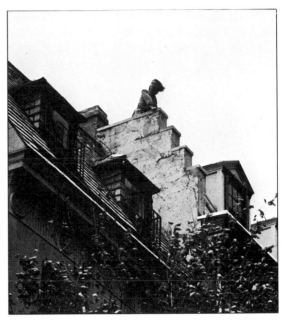

Eventually the woman is exposed to a situation that used to make her panic, but now she is able to overcome her anxiety.

Treating phobias

The treatment involves progressive exposure to the phobic stimulus—the cause of the fear—in this case, cats. Here is a somewhat simplified explanation of how the treatment works. On the first day the therapist might show Alice a picture of a cat and make her sit with it for an hour. At first her heart will pound and she will be anxious. After about 40 to 80 minutes her anxiety will subside, perhaps with the aid of relaxation techniques. Each time Alice endures the anxiety, the phobia is weakened.

When Alice can remain calm at the sight of a picture of a cat, the therapist might show her a cat across the street. Alice's anxiety will mount and, as before, gradually subside. When Alice can remain calm at the sight of a cat across the street, the therapist might show her a cat on the other side of a room. Alice will become anxious and then calm. Finally, Alice will hold the cat.

She will experience some anxiety, which will also subside. Once she has held the cat and had her anxiety go away, Alice will no longer be afraid of cats. She must be careful, however, not to avoid cats in the future or her phobia might return.

Behavior therapy is not a self-help technique. It must be carefully and skillfully directed by a professional to make sure that the treatment is always tolerable to the individual.

Psychoanalysts were highly critical of behavior therapy in its early days. They maintained that curing the symptoms did not cure the illness, which had to be done by finding out what caused the initial fear. Otherwise if a person was cured of a cat phobia, it would be replaced by, say, a dog phobia. However, studies of people with phobias have shown that in most cases no reason for the phobia can be found, and when they have been cured of their phobia, no other phobia replaces it.

Behavior therapy has been shown to be effective in treating various other disorders that involve a particular isolated problematic behavior, but it is not particularly successful in treating more general problems.

Everyone encounters a variety of problems throughout life. Many of them can be solved or resolved by using self-help techniques. However, it is important to recognize that there may be times when such treatments are inappropriate and you need professional help. If you feel that you would benefit from such help, ask your doctor or local hospital to recommend a therapist.

335

COGNITIVE THERAPY

Cognitive therapy is a brief psychotherapy (see pages 332–333) that involves a personal reassessment of fixed, often self-defeating attitudes. It is based on the rationale that your actions are determined by your view of the world and the way you interpret experiences. Cognitions, or the impressions formed of events, develop into an automatic pattern of understanding, which you come to regard as infallible, even though it is not true. Because these habitual thought processes are believable and their validity rarely questioned, many people spend their entire lives laboring under long-held, sometimes damaging, misconceptions about themselves and others. Cognitive therapy does not deal with the source of these attitudes but with the logic of the thoughts.

Changing your thinking

Take the case of a woman who was recently divorced from a man she had relied on to take care of practical household repairs, family finances, and disciplining the children. Not long after the divorce, she realized that she felt depressed and lacked confidence in her ability to manage the household alone. She sought cognitive therapy, and when she began to analyze her feelings, she realized that the underlying thought that triggered her depressed mood was "I've never been good at anything in my life." Gradually, she identified the illogic in her thinking, which was of an all-or-nothing nature: "I don't know how to

manage my finances" automatically became "I've never been good at anything." She began to look at herself more realistically and changed the negative statement to "I have some abilities, but I need help in learning how to cope with money, with my children, and with loneliness." Over a period, this reassessment boosted her confidence and resolved her depression.

This example illustrates a common pattern of thinking that can lead to emotional and behavioral problems. Troublesome thoughts are often simple statements representing absolute beliefs that are never questioned. In contrast to this primitive approach, cognitive therapy teaches people to think maturely, to examine their thoughts logically, in order to confront situations from different perspectives.

Cognitive therapeutic methods can be used with people of all ages. An eight-year-old boy, for example, became excessively anxious whenever his parents had a difference of opinion, however amicable. The underlying thought that sparked his fear was found to be: "If Mommy and Daddy disagree, they will get divorced." Using cognitive therapy, the boy was encouraged to test the reality of his belief by talking to the mailman, a teacher, and his parents. After learning that a mere disagreement did not automatically lead to divorce, the boy changed his view and stopped becoming upset by his parents' differences.

Children, even more so than adults, are inclined

TYPES OF THINKING		
Your thoughts about yourself and your own behavior may be unnecessarily harsh and condemning. Repetition of these negative thoughts over the years may cause significant under-achievement in the long term, unless you realize that the human personality is dynamic and capable of considerable adaption and change in response to more positive thinking. If you find yourself thinking negatively about your character, try to take a more objective view.	**Primitive thinking** **Global:** "I'm a bitter person." **Judgmental:** "I'm a nasty sort." **Inflexible:** "I always have been and always will be angry." **Character judgment:** "I have a defect in my character." **Unchangeable:** "There's nothing that can be done about it."	**Mature thinking** **Many faceted:** "I'm moderately bitter, generous, and fairly intelligent." **Non-judgmental:** "I can be more harsh than most people I know." **Flexible:** "My irritations vary in intensity from situation to situation." **Behavioral judgment:** "I react too assertively in certain situations." **Changeable:** "I can learn to respond in other ways."

to see things in black and white. Lacking a varied vocabulary, a child thinks about his feelings in terms of polarities such as happy and sad. If a child is not happy, he might conclude that he is sad. Cognitive therapy aims to open up the many levels of feeling between extremes. If a child's emotional vocabulary can be expanded in this way, he will gain measurably in security.

Unrealistic expectations

Fixed concepts of masculinity and femininity emphasize how unrealistic the expectations absorbed from the mass media, parents, and peers can be. Many unemployed men, for example, have to suffer the pain of re-evaluating their identities: "I'm not a man unless I go out to work and earn money." For many years women obeyed the myth that they should not be assertive or career-minded, and men believed that it was unmanly to show tenderness or tears.

From an early age people are taught to have expectations about relationships and life. Many of them come from television, films, magazines, books, and "experts" who try to tell people what relationships *ought* to be like. Many close relationships break down because the partners cannot measure up to these unquestioned, unrealistic, and often unexpressed expectations. If a couple is experiencing problems, it can help to clarify what each person expects of the other.

Mature people frequently fall prey to misconceptions too. One woman, who had enjoyed an active, satisfying life up to the age of 65, suddenly became inactive and depressed. After analyzing her state, it became clear that she was disturbed by her conviction that life held nothing after retirement except death. After testing her belief by visiting some organizations run by and for senior citizens (see pages 246–247), she became more positive about the future.

If you want to change something that troubles you, try the following approach.
1. Take 15 minutes to write down what you believe your problem is.
2. Identify when an automatic negative thought surfaces.
3. Notice how this thought influences your feelings and actions; try to put it into words.
4. Try talking to other people to see if your belief is really accurate.
5. Check your belief and reword it so that it fits a more realistic and positive perspective.
6. Repeat the newer and more mature thought frequently, particularly when you are in a situation that stimulates the older, habitual thinking.
7. If your negative thought fits the situation accurately, you might need to explore its importance in your life. Suppose, for example, that you are not loved by somebody close to you. You may have to face that this is the reality and that other people who love you can help to compensate.

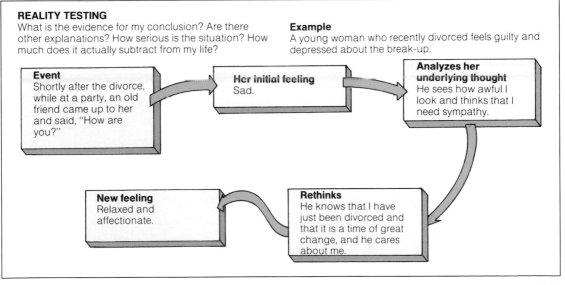

REALITY TESTING
What is the evidence for my conclusion? Are there other explanations? How serious is the situation? How much does it actually subtract from my life?

Example
A young woman who recently divorced feels guilty and depressed about the break-up.

Event
Shortly after the divorce, while at a party, an old friend came up to her and said, "How are you?"

Her initial feeling
Sad.

Analyzes her underlying thought
He sees how awful I look and thinks that I need sympathy.

Rethinks
He knows that I have just been divorced and that it is a time of great change, and he cares about me.

New feeling
Relaxed and affectionate.

Use these charts to help plan your healthy diet. With a few exceptions, you can eat as many raw fruits and vegetables as you wish. Remember, however, that as soon as any food is cooked with added ingredients such as sugar or fat, the calorie count may dramatically increase.

The approximate measure of each food is given in ounces, cups, or another measure that is appropriate for a particular food, such as slices of bread or the number of pieces of fruit. The approximate weight of each item in grams is also given. (1 ounce = 28.35 grams.)

MEAT, MEAT PRODUCTS, POULTRY	Portion	Weight (grams)	Calories	Protein (grams)	Fat (grams)	Carbohydrate (grams)
Bacon, **bd, f**	2 slices	15	85	4	8	Tr
Beef						
corned						
hash, **c**	1 cup	220	400	19	25	24
meat, **c**	3 oz	85	185	22	10	0
cuts						
L/F, st	3 oz	85	245	23	16	0
LO, st	2.5 oz	72	140	22	5	0
ground, lean, **bd**	1 patty	85	185	23	10	0
roast						
rib, **L/F**	3 oz	85	375	17	33	0
rib, **LO**	1.8 oz	51	125	14	7	0
round, **L/F**	3 oz	85	165	25	7	0
round, **LO**	2.8 oz	78	125	24	3	0
steak						
sirloin, **L/F, bd**	3 oz	85	330	20	27	0
sirloin, **LO, bd**	2 oz	56	115	18	4	0
round, **L/F, bd**	3 oz	85	220	24	13	0
round, **LO, bd**	2.4 oz	68	130	21	4	0
Chicken						
breast, **W/B, f**	3.3 oz	94	160	26	5	1
drumstick, **W/B, f**	2 oz	56	90	12	4	Tr
half broiler, **W/B, bd**	10.4 oz	176	240	42	7	0
roast, **MO**	3.5 oz	100	148	25	5	0
roast, **M/S**	3.5 oz	100	216	23	14	0
Duck						
breast **MO, rst**	3.5 oz	100	189	25	10	0
breast **M/S, rst**	3.5 oz	100	339	20	29	0
Lamb						
chop, **L/F, bd**	3.1 oz	89	360	18	32	0
chop, **LO, bd**	2 oz	57	120	16	6	0
leg, **L/F, rst**	3 oz	85	235	22	16	0
leg, **LO, rst**	2.5 oz	71	130	20	5	0
shoulder, **L/F, rst**	3 oz	85	285	18	23	0
shoulder, **LO, rst**	2.3 oz	64	130	17	6	0
Liver, beef, **f**	3 oz	85	195	22	9	5

	Portion	Weight (grams)	Calories	Protein (grams)	Fat (grams)	Carbohydrate (grams)
Pork, cured						
ham, **L/F, rst**	3 oz	85	245	18	19	0
ham, **L/F, bd**	1 oz	28	175	9	15	1
Pork, fresh						
chop, **L/F, bd**	2.7 oz	78	305	19	25	0
chop, **LO, bd**	2 oz	56	150	17	9	0
roast, **L/F**	3 oz	85	310	21	24	0
roast, **LO**	2.4 oz	68	175	20	10	0
Sausage						
bologna	1 slice	28	85	3	8	Tr
brown and serve	1 link	17	70	3	6	Tr
frankfurter	1	56	170	7	15	1
pork	1 link	13	60	2	6	Tr
salami, dry	1 slice	10	45	2	4	Tr
salami, cooked	1 slice	28	90	5	7	Tr
Turkey						
dark meat, **MO, rst**	3 oz	85	175	26	7	0
light meat, **MO, rst**	3 oz	85	150	28	3	0
Veal						
cutlet, **bd**	3 oz	85	185	23	9	0
rib, **rst**	3 oz	85	230	23	14	0

FISH AND SHELLFISH	Portion	Weight (grams)	Calories	Protein (grams)	Fat (grams)	Carbohydrate (grams)
Bluefish, **ba**	3 oz	85	135	22	4	0
Clams						
raw, **MO**	3 oz	85	65	11	1	2
canned, **M/L**	3 oz	85	45	7	1	2
Crab						
fresh, **W/S, b**	3.5 oz	100	25	4	1	0
canned	1 cup	135	135	24	3	1
Fish sticks, **br, fn**	1 stick	28	50	5	3	2
Haddock, **br, f**	3 oz	85	140	17	5	5
Ocean perch, **br, f**	1 fillet	85	195	16	11	6
Oysters, **r**	1 cup	240	160	20	4	8
Salmon						
pink, **c, M/L**	3 oz	85	120	17	5	0

KEY

b	boiled	**fn**	frozen	**p**	poached	**Tr**	trace
ba	baked	**Fr**	fresh	**P**	peeled	**unsw**	unsweetened
bd	broiled	**L**	liquid	**pr**	pressurized	**unw**	unwhipped
br	breaded	**L/F**	lean and fat	**pwd**	powdered	**v**	vegetable shortening
c	canned	**LO**	lean only	**r**	raw	**Wh**	whole
cr	creamed	**M/L**	meat and liquid	**rst**	roast	**W/B**	weighed with bones
D	dried	**MO**	meat only	**sd**	shelled	**W/S**	weighed in shells
d	diluted	**M/S**	meat and skin	**sr**	stone/pit removed		
dr	drained	**nmsa**	no milk solids added	**st**	stewed		
f	fried	**o**	oil	**sw**	sweetened		

	Portion	Weight (grams)	Calories	Protein (grams)	Fat (grams)	Carbohydrate (grams)
fresh, **p, W/B**	3.5 oz	100	160	16	11	0
smoked	3.5 oz	100	142	25	5	0
Sardines, **c, o, dr**	3 oz	85	175	20	9	0
Scallops, **br, fn, f**	6	90	175	16	8	9
Shrimp						
fresh, **br, f**	3 oz	85	190	17	9	9
canned	3 oz	85	100	21	1	1
Tuna, **c, o, dr**	3 oz	85	170	24	7	0

DAIRY PRODUCTS

	Portion	Weight (grams)	Calories	Protein (grams)	Fat (grams)	Carbohydrate (grams)
Butter						
regular	1 stick	113	815	1	92	Tr
regular	1 tbsp	14	100	Tr	12	Tr
regular	1 pat	5	35	Tr	4	Tr
whipped	1 stick	76	540	1	61	Tr
whipped	1 tbsp	9	65	Tr	8	Tr
whipped	1 pat	4	25	Tr	3	Tr
Cheese						
American	1 oz	28	105	6	9	Tr
blue	1 oz	28	100	6	8	1
Camembert	1.3 oz	38	115	8	9	Tr
Cheddar	1 oz	28	115	7	9	Tr
cottage, large curd, **cr**	1 cup	225	235	28	10	6
cottage, small curd, **cr**	1 cup	210	220	26	9	6
cottage, 2% fat	1 cup	226	205	31	4	8
cottage, 1% fat	1 cup	226	165	28	2	6
cottage, dry curd	1 cup	145	125	25	1	3
cream	1 oz	28	100	2	10	1
Edam	3.5 oz	100	304	24	23	0
Mozzarella, whole milk	1 oz	28	90	6	7	1
Parmesan, grated	1 tbsp	5	25	2	2	Tr
Provolone	1 oz	28	100	7	8	1
Ricotta, whole milk	1 cup	246	430	28	32	7
Swiss	1 oz	28	105	8	8	1
Cream						
coffee, light, or table	1 tbsp	15	30	Tr	3	1
half-and-half	1 tbsp	15	20	Tr	2	1
sour	1 tbsp	12	25	Tr	3	1
whipping, light, **unw**	1 cup	239	700	5	74	7
whipping, heavy, **unw**	1 cup	230	820	5	88	7
Cream products, imitation						
creamer, sweet, **fn, L**	1 tbsp	15	20	Tr	1	2
creamer, sweet, **pwd**	1 tsp	2	10	Tr	1	1
sour dressing	1 tbsp	12	20	Tr	2	1
whipped topping, **fn**	1 cup	75	240	1	19	17
whipped topping, **pr**	1 cup	70	185	1	16	11
Eggs						
white, **r**	1	33	15	3	Tr	Tr
whole, **r, sd**	1	50	80	6	6	1
whole, **f**	1	46	85	5	6	1
whole, hard-cooked, **sd**	1	50	80	6	6	1
whole, **p**	1	50	80	6	6	1
whole, scrambled with milk	1	64	95	6	7	1
yolk, **r**	1	17	65	3	6	Tr
Milk, fresh						
buttermilk	1 cup	245	100	8	2	12

	Portion	Weight (grams)	Calories	Protein (grams)	Fat (grams)	Carbohydrate (grams)
2% fat, **nmsa**	1 cup	244	120	8	5	12
1% fat, **nmsa**	1 cup	244	100	8	3	12
skim (nonfat), **nmsa**	1 cup	245	85	8	Tr	12
whole (3.3% fat)	1 cup	244	150	8	8	11
Milk, canned						
condensed, **sw**	1 cup	306	980	24	27	166
evaporated, skim, **unsw**	1 cup	255	200	19	1	29
evaporated, whole, **unsw**	1 cup	252	340	17	19	25
Milk desserts						
custard, **ba**	1 cup	265	305	14	15	29
ice cream, hard, **fn**	1 cup	133	270	5	14	32
ice cream, soft, **fn**	1 cup	173	375	7	23	38
ice milk, hard, **fn**	1 cup	131	185	5	6	29
ice milk, soft, **fn**	1 cup	175	225	8	5	38
pudding, homemade, chocolate	1 cup	260	385	8	12	67
pudding, mix, cooked	1 cup	260	320	9	8	59
pudding, mix, instant	1 cup	260	325	8	7	63
sherbet, **fn**	1 cup	193	270	2	4	59
Yogurt						
skim milk, plain	8 oz	227	125	13	Tr	17
whole milk, plain, **nmsa**	8 oz	227	140	8	7	11

FRUITS AND FRUIT PRODUCTS

	Portion	Weight (grams)	Calories	Protein (grams)	Fat (grams)	Carbohydrate (grams)
Apples, **Fr, Wh**	1	138	80	Tr	1	20
Apple juice, **c**	1 cup	248	120	Tr	Tr	30
Applesauce, **c, sw**	1 cup	255	230	1	Tr	61
Applesauce, **c, unsw**	1 cup	244	100	Tr	Tr	26
Apricots, heavy syrup, **c**	1 cup	258	220	2	Tr	57
Apricots, **D, r**	1 cup	130	340	7	1	86
Apricot nectar, **c**	1 cup	251	145	1	Tr	37
Avocados, **Fr, P, sr**	1 small	216	370	5	37	13
Bananas	1	119	100	1	Tr	26
Blackberries, **Fr**	1 cup	144	85	2	1	19
Blueberries, **Fr**	1 cup	145	90	1	1	22
Cherries, **Fr, sr**	10	68	45	1	Tr	12
Cranberry juice, **c, sw**	1 cup	253	165	Tr	Tr	42
Cranberry sauce, **c, sw**	1 cup	277	405	Tr	1	104
Dates, **Wh, sr**	10	80	220	2	Tr	58
Grapefruit, pink, **Fr**	$\frac{1}{2}$	241	50	1	Tr	13
Grapefruit, white, **Fr**	$\frac{1}{2}$	241	45	1	Tr	12
Grapefruit, syrup, **c**	1 cup	254	180	2	Tr	45
Grapefruit juice, **Fr**	1 cup	246	95	1	Tr	23
Grapefruit juice, **c, sw**	1 cup	250	135	1	Tr	32
Grapefruit juice, **c, unsw**	1 cup	247	100	1	Tr	24
Grapefruit juice, **fn, unsw, d**	1 cup	247	100	1	Tr	24
Grapes	10	50	35	Tr	Tr	9
Grape juice, **c**	1 cup	253	165	1	Tr	42
Grape juice, **fn, sw, d**	1 cup	250	135	1	Tr	33
Lemons, **P, sr**	1	74	20	1	Tr	6
Lemonade, **fn, d**	1 cup	248	105	Tr	Tr	28
Melons						
cantaloupe	$\frac{1}{2}$	477	80	2	Tr	20
honeydew	$\frac{1}{10}$	226	50	1	Tr	11
watermelon	1 wedge	926	110	2	1	27

CALORIE CHARTS/2

	Portion	Weight (grams)	Calories	Protein (grams)	Fat (grams)	Carbohydrate (grams)
Oranges, **Wh**, **P**, **sr**	1	131	65	1	Tr	16
Peaches, **Fr**, **Wh**, **P**, **sr**	1	100	40	1	Tr	10
Peaches, syrup, **c**	1 cup	256	200	1	Tr	51
Peaches, water-pack, **c**	1 cup	244	75	1	Tr	20
Peaches, **D**, **r**	1 cup	160	420	5	1	109
Pears, **Fr**	1	164	100	1	1	25
Pears, heavy syrup, **c**	1 cup	255	195	1	1	50
Pineapple, diced, **Fr**	1 cup	155	80	1	Tr	21
Pineapple, heavy syrup, **c**	1 slice	58	45	Tr	Tr	11
Pineapple juice, **c**, **unsw**	1 cup	250	140	1	Tr	34
Plums, **Fr**, **sr**	1	66	30	Tr	Tr	8
Plums, heavy syrup, **c**	1 cup	272	215	1	Tr	56
Prunes, **D**, **r**	5	49	110	1	Tr	29
Prune juice, **c**	1 cup	256	195	1	Tr	49
Raisins, seedless	1 cup	145	420	4	Tr	112
Raspberries, **Fr**	1 cup	123	70	1	1	17
Raspberries, **fn**, **sw**	10 oz	284	280	2	1	70
Strawberries, **Fr**	1 cup	149	55	1	1	13
Strawberries, **fn**, **sw**	10 oz	284	310	1	1	79
Tangerines, **Fr**, **P**	1	86	40	1	Tr	10

VEGETABLES AND VEGETABLE PRODUCTS

	Portion	Weight (grams)	Calories	Protein (grams)	Fat (grams)	Carbohydrate (grams)
Asparagus, spears, **Fr**	4	60	10	1	Tr	2
Asparagus, spears, **fn**	4	60	15	2	Tr	2
Asparagus, spears, **c**	4	80	15	2	Tr	3
Beans						
baby lima, **fn**, **b**	1 cup	180	210	13	Tr	40
fordhook lima, **fn**, **b**	1 cup	170	170	10	Tr	32
green snap, **Fr**, **b**	1 cup	125	30	2	Tr	7
green snap, **fn**, **b**	1 cup	130	35	2	Tr	8
green snap, **c**	1 cup	135	30	2	Tr	7
kidney, **c**	1 cup	255	230	15	1	42
yellow or wax, **Fr**, **b**	1 cup	125	30	2	Tr	6
yellow or wax, **fn**, **b**	1 cup	135	35	2	Tr	8
yellow or wax, **c**	1 cup	135	30	2	Tr	7
Bean sprouts, **r**	1 cup	105	35	4	Tr	7
Beets, **Fr**, **P**, **b**, **Wh**	2	100	30	1	Tr	7
Beets, diced, **c**	1 cup	170	65	2	Tr	15
Black-eyed peas, **Fr**, **c**, **dr**	1 cup	165	180	13	1	30
Broccoli, **Fr**, **b**	1 stalk	180	45	6	1	8
Broccoli, chopped, **fn**	1 cup	185	50	5	1	9
Brussels sprouts, **Fr**, **b**	1 cup	155	55	7	1	10
Brussels sprouts, **fn**, **b**	1 cup	155	50	5	Tr	10

	Portion	Weight (grams)	Calories	Protein (grams)	Fat (grams)	Carbohydrate (grams)
Cabbage, shredded, **r**	1 cup	70	15	1	Tr	4
Cabbage, **b**	1 cup	145	30	2	Tr	6
Cabbage, red, shredded, **r**	1 cup	70	20	1	Tr	5
Carrots, **Fr**, **r**, **Wh**	1	72	30	1	Tr	7
Carrots, **Fr**, **b**	1 cup	155	50	1	Tr	11
Carrots, **c**	1 cup	155	45	1	Tr	10
Cauliflower, chopped, **Fr**, **r**	1 cup	115	31	3	Tr	6
Cauliflower, **Fr**, **b**	1 cup	125	30	3	Tr	5
Cauliflower, **fn**, **b**	1 cup	180	30	3	Tr	6
Celery, **Fr**, **r**	1 stalk	40	5	Tr	Tr	2
Collards, **Fr**, **b**	1 cup	190	65	7	1	10
Collards, **fn**, **b**	1 cup	170	50	5	1	10
Corn, **Fr**, **b**	1 ear	140	70	2	1	16
Corn, **fn**, **b**	1 ear	229	120	4	1	27
Corn, kernels, **fn**	1 cup	165	130	5	1	31
Corn, **c**, **cr**	1 cup	256	210	5	2	51
Cucumber	8 slices	28	5	Tr	Tr	1
Lentils, **b**	1 cup	200	210	16	Tr	39
Lettuce						
butterhead	1 head	220	25	2	Tr	4
crisphead	1 head	567	70	5	1	16
leaf, chopped	1 cup	55	10	1	Tr	2
Mushrooms, chopped, **r**	1 cup	70	20	2	Tr	3
Onions,						
green	6	30	15	Tr	Tr	3
white, chopped, **r**	1 cup	170	65	3	Tr	15
white, cooked	1 cup	210	60	3	Tr	14
Peas, **c**	1 cup	170	150	8	1	29
Peas, **fn**, **b**	1 cup	160	110	8	Tr	19
Potatoes, **ba**, **P**	1	156	145	4	Tr	33
Potatoes, **b**, **P**	1	135	90	3	Tr	20
Potatoes, french-fried	10 strips	50	135	2	7	18
Spinach, chopped, **Fr**, **r**	1 cup	55	15	2	Tr	2
Spinach, chopped, **Fr**, **b**	1 cup	180	40	5	1	6
Spinach, chopped, **fn**, **b**	1 cup	205	45	6	1	8
Sweet potatoes, **ba**, **P**	1	114	160	2	1	37
Sweet potatoes, candied	1 piece	105	175	1	3	36
Tomatoes, **Fr**	1	135	25	1	Tr	6
Tomatoes, **c**	1 cup	241	50	2	Tr	10
Tomato juice, **c**	1 cup	243	45	2	Tr	10
Turnips, chopped, **b**	1 cup	155	35	1	Tr	8

KEY

b	boiled	**fn**	frozen	**rst**	roast
ba	baked	**Fr**	fresh	**sd**	shelled
bd	broiled	**L**	liquid	**sr**	stone/pit removed
br	breaded	**nmsa**	no milk solids added	**st**	stewed
c	canned	**o**	oil	**sw**	sweetened
cr	creamed	**p**	poached	**Tr**	trace
D	dried	**P**	peeled	**unsw**	unsweetened
d	diluted	**pr**	pressurized	**unw**	unwhipped
dr	drained	**pwd**	powdered	**v**	vegetable shortening
f	fried	**r**	raw	**Wh**	whole

CEREAL AND GRAIN PRODUCTS	Portion	Weight (grams)	Calories	Protein (grams)	Fat (grams)	Carbohydrate (grams)
Bread						
cracked wheat	1 slice	25	65	2	1	13
French, enriched	1 slice	35	100	3	1	19
pumpernickel	1 slice	32	80	3	Tr	17
raisin, enriched	1 slice	25	65	2	1	13
rye, light	1 slice	25	60	2	Tr	13
white, enriched	1 slice	23	65	2	1	12
whole-wheat	1 slice	25	60	3	1	12
Breakfast cereals						
bran flakes, **sw**	1 cup	35	105	4	1	28
corn flakes, **unsw**	1 cup	25	95	2	Tr	21
corn flakes, **sw**	1 cup	40	155	2	Tr	37
oats, puffed, **sw**	1 cup	25	100	3	1	19
oatmeal	1 cup	240	130	5	2	23
rice, puffed, **unsw**	1 cup	15	60	1	Tr	13
rice, puffed, **sw**	1 cup	28	115	1	0	26
wheat flakes, **sw**	1 cup	30	105	3	Tr	24
wheat, shredded	1 biscuit	25	90	2	1	20
Crackers						
graham	2	14	55	1	1	10
rye	2	13	45	2	Tr	10
saltines	4	11	50	1	1	8
Flour						
all-purpose, sifted	1 cup	115	420	12	1	88
whole-wheat	1 cup	120	400	16	2	85
Pancakes						
buckwheat	1	27	55	2	2	6
plain	1	27	60	2	2	9
Pasta, **b**	1 cup	140	155	5	1	32
Rice						
white, ready-to-serve	1 cup	165	180	4	Tr	40
white, long grain, **b**	1 cup	205	225	4	Tr	50
Rolls, commercial						
brown and serve	1	26	85	2	2	14
cloverleaf	1	28	85	2	2	15
hot dog, hamburger						
bun	1	40	120	3	2	21
hard	1	50	155	5	2	30
Waffles	1	75	205	7	8	27

NUTS AND SEEDS	Portion	Weight (grams)	Calories	Protein (grams)	Fat (grams)	Carbohydrate (grams)
Almonds, chopped, **sd**	1 cup	130	775	24	70	25
Brazil nuts, **sd**	1 oz	28	185	4	19	3
Cashews, **rst**, **o**	1 cup	140	785	24	64	41
Filberts/hazelnuts, chopped	1 cup	115	730	14	72	19
Peanuts, chopped, **rst**, **o**	1 cup	144	840	37	72	27
Peanut butter	1 tbsp	16	95	4	8	3
Pecans	1 cup	118	810	11	84	17
Sunflower seeds, hulled, **D**	1 cup	145	810	35	69	29
Walnuts, English, chopped	1 cup	120	780	18	77	19

CAKES, COOKIES, PASTRIES, AND SWEETS	Portion	Weight (grams)	Calories	Protein (grams)	Fat (grams)	Carbohydrate (grams)
Cakes, from mixes						
angel food	1 piece	53	135	3	Tr	32
coffee cake	1 piece	72	230	5	7	38
cupcakes, chocolate icing	1	36	130	2	5	21
devil's food, chocolate	1 piece	69	235	3	8	40
gingerbread	1 piece	63	175	2	4	32
white, chocolate icing	1 piece	71	250	3	8	45
yellow, chocolate icing	1 piece	69	235	3	8	40
Candy						
caramels	1 oz	28	115	1	3	22
chocolate, milk	1 oz	28	145	2	9	16
fudge, chocolate	1 oz	28	115	1	3	21
hard	1 oz	28	110	1	Tr	23
Cookies						
brownies, with nuts	1	20	95	1	6	10
chocolate chip	4	42	200	2	9	29
fig bars	4	56	200	2	3	42
gingersnaps	4	28	90	2	2	22
oatmeal	4	52	235	3	8	38
vanilla wafers	10	40	185	2	6	30
Danish pastry, plain	1	65	275	5	15	30
Doughnut, plain	1	25	100	1	5	13
Honey	1 tbsp	21	65	Tr	0	17
Jams and preserves	1 tbsp	20	55	Tr	Tr	14
Pies						
apple	1 piece	135	345	3	15	51
banana cream	1 piece	130	285	6	12	40
blueberry	1 piece	135	325	3	15	47
cherry	1 piece	135	350	4	15	52
lemon meringue	1 piece	120	305	4	12	45
pecan	1 piece	118	495	6	27	61
pumpkin	1 piece	130	275	5	15	32
Sugar						
brown	1 cup	220	820	0	0	212
white, granulated	1 cup	200	770	0	0	199

INDEX

Note: Numbers in **boldface** refer to principal entries. Numbers in *italic* refer to illustrations, charts, or diagrams and their captions.

A

Abdomen, 218–219
  and aging, 239
Abdominal muscles, 119–122, 126–127, 132–134, 138, 140, **142–143**
  See also Abdomen; Strengthening.
Abortion, 197
  See also Miscarriage.
Accident prevention, 103, 257
  aids for the elderly, **256–257**
  safety tips, 103, 257
Achilles tendon, 127
  injury to, 137
Acne, 31, 162, 164, 302
Acquired Immune Deficiency Syndrome (AIDS), 192–193
Acupuncture, 229, **318–319**
Adenosine triphosphate (ATP), 70–71
Adler, Alfred, 333
Adolescence
  discovering sexuality in, 188–189
  health screening in, 31
  hero worshiping in, *189*
  homosexuality and, 192
  masturbation in, 188–189
  menstruation and, 187–188
  mental and emotional changes in, 188
  promiscuity in, 189
  rebellion in, 265
  sexual fantasies in, 189
  social pressures and, 188
  sport and, *186*
  voice change in, 187
Adrenal glands, 268, *268*
Adrenalin, 158
Adults, life goals in
  men, **32–33, 36–37, 40–41, 44–45, 48, 51**
  women, **34–35, 38–39, 42–43, 46–51**
Aerobic exercise, 12, 15, 35, 78, 95, **98–99**, 100, 102–103, 120, 122, 134, 158, 203, 222, 232
  dance program, *121*
  effects on the heart, 12, 97
  for the elderly, 254–255
  and health clubs, **104–105**
  oxygen usage and, 102
  warm-up and cool-down exercises, **106–107**
  water exercises, 118
AFP (serum alpha fetoprotein), 219
Aging
  accident prevention, **256–257**
  celebrating birthdays, *259*
  exercise routines, 252, *254–255*
  fitness and, **250–255**
  generation gap, *238*
  health problems of, 250, *251*
  maintaining good health, **252–253**
  mental attitude to, **238–239**

mental fitness, **258–259**
physical process of, 239, 250, 251
retirement and, 239, **240–249**
sexual relations, 249
  See also Elderly people; Retirement.
Agoraphobia, 279
Al Anon, 292
  See also Alcohol.
Alateen, 292
  See also Alcohol.
Alcohol, **289–293**
  abstinence from, **292–293**
  blood alcohol level (BAL), 290
  body absorbtion rate, 290–291
  calories and, 56, 68
  cirrhosis of the liver, 289, 291
  defining drinking problems, **291**
  dependence on, 292
  hangover, 291
  and men, 32, 37, 40–41, 44, *290*, 291
  overconsumption of, **292–293**
  pregnancy and, 218, 220
  reducing intake, 293
  stress and, 269
  and vitamins, 59
  and women, 34, 38, 43, 47, *289*
  and young people, 30, 292–293
Alcoholics, 292
  detoxification centers for, 292
Alcoholics Anonymous (AA), 292
Alcoholism, **292–293**
  See also Alcohol; Alcoholics.
Alexander, F. Matthias, 314
Alexander Technique, **314–315**
  back pain and, 139
  neck and, *314*
  posture and, *315*
Ali, Muhammad, *33*
Allergen, 92
Allergies
  of children, 93
  to eggs, 93
  to gluten, 92
  to lactose, 92–93
  to milk, 93
  to peanuts, 93
  skin, 163
  to wheat, 93
Alternative medicine, 312
Amblyopia ("lazy eye"), 173
Amenorrhea, 205
American Association of Retired Persons (AARP), 242
American Cancer Society, 63–64, 72
American Diabetes Association, 63
American Diabetic Association, 63
American Heart Association, 54–55, 63–64
Amino acids, 54, 88
Amniocentesis, 217, 219
Amphetamines, 282–283
Amundsen, Roald, *40*
Amygdalin, 59
Anaerobic activity, 71
Anaerobic exertion, 98
Analytic movements, **332–333**
Androgens, 170, 187
Angina pectoris, 96
Ankle weights, 98, 122

Anorexia nervosa, 294
Anti-D globulin, 218
Antihistamines, 280
Antinausea medication (pregnancy), 220
Anxiety, 266
  communication of, 294
  tranquilizers and, 281
  See also Stress; Crises.
Appetite
  control of, 66
  suppressants, 77
Arm exercises, 122, **146–147**
Armstrong, Neil, *41*
Aromatherapy, **323**
Arterial plaque, 250
Arteries, 96, 239, 250
Arthritis, 72, 251, 278, 302
Artificial insemination, 216
Ascorbate, 64
Aspirin, 282
Asthma, 278, 302, 307
Astigmatism, 173
Astor, Nancy, *42*
Atavan, 280
Atheroma, 96–97
Atherosclerosis, 14
Athletes
  fluid loss in, 90
  See also Jogging; Running.
Athlete's foot, 183
Autogenics, **324–325**
  and hypnosis, 331
  and sports training, *324*

B

Baby
  birth of, 228
  bottle-feeding, 230
  breast-feeding, 230
  breathing, 229
  cramps, *234*
  exercises with, **234–235**
    ankle rotating, *235*
    "crunches", *235*
    "escapes", *235*
    leg press, *235*
    leg stretch, *235*
    "push-off", *235*
  heart beat and blood pressure, 229
  and heat therapy, 302
  mobiles and toys 234
  sleep patterns, *230*
  swimming, *234*
  See also Labor; Postnatal well-being; Preconception; Pregnancy.
Bach, Edward, 323
Bach Flower Remedies, *323*
Back, **138–139**
  exercises for **140–141**
  furniture and the, 139
  pain, remedies, *139*
  posture, *138*
  strengthening muscles, 140
  stretch, yoga, *151*
  See also Alexander Technique; Chiropractic; Osteopathy; Rolfing.
Barnard, Christiaan, *41*
Basal metabolic rate (BMR), 71, 112
Bat ears, 177

Behavior
  monitoring, *334–335*
  patterns, 44, **264–265**
  therapy, **334–335**
Bell, Alexander Graham, *37*
Bench press, 135
  See also Strengthening.
Bereavement, 258–259, **299**
Best, Charles, *33*
Beta blockers, 281
Bicycle riding, 108, **110–111**
  for children, 28, *155*
  effect of wind on, *110*
  exercise bicycles, *110*, 120, 122
  programs, *111*, 120
  special stretch programs, 128–129, **131**
Bile acids, 55
Biofeedback, 263, **326–327**
  reducing hypertension, 327
  relaxometer, 326
Biotin, 58
Birth. *See* Childbirth; Labor.
Birth control. *See* Contraception.
Bladder, 284
Blepharoplasty, 165
Blood alcohol level (BAL), 290
Blood cholesterol, 24, 41
  and contraception, 196
Blood pressure, 32, 34, 37, 39, 41, 43, 45–46, 49–50, *97*, 98, 100, 278
  aerobic training and, 97
  contraception and, 196
  diastolic, 97
  females and, 204
  heat therapy and, 302–304
  obesity and, 72
  pregnancy and, 218
  stress and, 268–269, 278
  systolic, 97
Blood tests
  in pregnancy, 217–218
Body
  cells, *91*
  how it works, **161–183**
  odor, 163
  reactions to stress, *268*, 269
Body mass index (BMI), 30, 45, 72, *73*
Bottle-feeding, 230
Bowels
  during pregnancy, 220
  and stress, 268
Braille, Louis, *31*
Brain
  and aging, 239
  effect of smoking on, *284*
Bread, 56
Breast-feeding, 230
  preparing for, 221
Breasts
  benign tumors, 206
  cancer of, 24, *206*, **206–207**
  cysts, 206
  development of, 186
  examination of, 31, 35, 39, 42, 46–47, 49, 51, 204, *206–207*
  mastitis, 206
  in pregnancy, 206, 217, 221
  self-examination, *207*

Breathing
  baby's, 229
  the elderly and, 254
  jogging and running, 115
  pregnancy and, 221, *225*
  and relaxation, 148
Breech birth, 229
Bronchi, 98, *284*
Bronchitis, 302
Brontë, Charlotte, *39*
Bumbry, Grace, 35
Bunions, 183
Burroughs, Edgar Rice, *49*
Buttocks, 127–128, 130–131, 141, *144*

C
Caesarean delivery, 229
  See also Childbirth.
Caffeine, 220, 282
Cakes and cookies, calorie chart, *341*
Calcium
  in foods, 56, 60
  in nails, 181
  needs in pregnancy, 221
Calisthenics, 99
Calories
  charts, **338–341**
  controlling consumption of, 31, 40, 46, 80–81
  diets and, 76–77
  energy and, *68–69*
  in foods, 43, *68–69*
  meal planning and, 80–83
  needs, 56, *69*
  weight and, 68, 78
Cancer
  and the aging, 251
  breast, 204, 206–207
  cervical, 34, 38, 42, 196, 204, *205*
  cigarette smoking and, 285–287
  contraceptive pill and, 196–198
  ovarian, 208
Candidiasis (Monilia or Thrush), 193
Carbohydrates
  as calories, 68
  diets and, 70, 76
  energy supplied by, 54, 70
Carbon dioxide, 98, *99*
Cardiac output, 97
Cardiopulmonary resuscitation (CPR), 104
Cardiovascular system, 12, 98, 100, 102, 112, 118, 250
Career goals 34–37, 39, 43–44, 46
Caries, 178
  See also Teeth and gums.
Carson, Rachel, *46*
Carter, Howard, *44*
Cataract, 173
Cather, Willa, *47*
Catheter, 229
Cerebral cortex, *280*
Cervical (Pap) smear test, 34, 38, 42, 196, 204, *205*, 231
Chanel, Gabrielle "Coco", *42*
Chaplin, Charlie, *29*
Check-ups. *See* Health screening.
Chemabrasion, 164
Chest expanders, 122

Chichester, Francis *253*
Childbirth, 213, **228–229**
  birthing chair, *229*
  breech birth, 229
  Caesarean delivery, 229
  See also Labor.
Children
  anorexia nervosa in, 294
  and cigarette smoking, 285–286
  and conformity, *264*, **265**
  and crises, 297
  dental care, 28, 31, 178
  drugs and, 283
  eye tests, 29, 31
  fitness, 154–155, *155*
  food allergies, 93
  footwear, 182
  goals, growing up, **28–29**, 30–31
  hearing tests, 29, 176–177
  menstruation, 187–188
  and money, 31
  nail biting, 180
  overweight, 74, *74*
  personality traits, 262–263
  relationships with parents, 29–30, 33, 35–36, 200, 265
  sex education, 188
  sexual development, **186–187**
  sunshine, effects on, 167
  swimming, 29
Chinning bar, 122
Chin-ups, *133*
Chiropractic, 312
Chloride, in foods, 60
Cholesterol
  diet and, 55
  fatty acids and, 54
  heart disease and, *55*, 96
  hyperlipidemia, 24
  levels of, 37, *55*
Chromosomes, 216
Churchill, Winston, *50*
Cigarette smoking, **284–289**
  antismoking publicity, *286*
  children and, 285–286
  dangers of, *25*, *73*, *284*, 285–287
  effect on placenta, 215
  giving up, 32, 34, 36, 103, 286–287, *288*
  obesity and, 72, *73*
  pregnancy and, 215, 220
  reasons for, 285
  smoker's diary, *287*
  withdrawal symptoms, 288
Cirrhosis, 289, 291
Claustrophobia, 279
Clitoris, 190, 191
Cobalt, in foods, 60
Cocaine, 282
Cochlea, 175, 177
Coffee, decaffeinated, 282
Cognitive therapy, **336–337**
Coitus interruptus, 198–199, 231
  See also Contraception.
Colette, *50*
Collagen fibers, 162, 164–165
Color blindness, 173
Colostrum, 230
Comaneci, Nadia, *30*

Competition, in sport, **158–159**
Condom, 196, 198–199, 231
  See also Contraception.
Conformity, **264–265**
Conjunctivitis, 173
Connolly, Maureen "Little Mo", *35*
Constipation, 63, 220, 230, 278
Contact lenses, *174*
Contraception, 34, 37, 39, 43, **196–199**
  health risks and, 196–197
  menopause and, 208
  postnatal, 199, **231**
  research into, 196
Contraceptive methods, **198–199**
  coitus interruptus, *198–199*, 231
  condom, 196, *198–199*, 214
  diaphragm, 196, *198–199*, 214
  future developments, 197
  hysterectomy, 197
  injections, *198–199*
  intrauterine device (IUD), *198–199*, 231
  pill, 43, 196, *198–199*, 204, 214, 231
    minipill, *198–199*
  rhythm, *198–199*, 231
  spermicides, *198–199*
  sponge, *198–199*
  sterilization, 196–197
  vasectomy, 41, 190, 197
Cool-down exercises, **106–107**, 113, 140
Copper, in foods, 60
Corns, 183
Coronary artery, 96
  disease, 55
Cosmetics, 163
Cramps, easing in babies, 234
Cramps, leg, 221
Crises, **294–299**
  assessing situations 46, 294–295
  bereavement, **298–299**
  divorce, **299**
  effect on children, 297
  effect on relationships, **296–297**
  job loss, 299
Curie, Marie, *42*
Cystic fibrosis, 24
Cystitis, 306
Cysts, breast, 206
Cytotest, 204
Cytotoxic test, 92

D

Dairy products
  calorie charts, *339*
  as protein, 56
Dandruff, 170
  See also Hair.
Deafness. *See* Ears; Hearing tests.
Death, 51, 103, **298–299**
Defoe, Daniel, *44*
Dehydration, 91, 158
Delirium tremens, 292
Demerol, 229
Dental care, *179*
  and hypnosis, 331
  in old age, 253
  in pregnancy, 221
  See also Teeth and gums.

Dental problems, 57, 65
  See also Teeth and gums.
Department of Agriculture, 62
Department of Health and Human
  Services, 62
Depression
  alcohol and, 289
  endogenous, 279
  exogenous, 278–279
  menopause and, 209
  old age and, 258
  stress and, 278–279
  treatment of, 103, 336
Dermabrasion, 164
Dextrose, 64
Diabetes, 24, 210, 215, 218
  glucose and, 70
  heat treatments and, 302, 304
  obesity and, 72
Diaphragm, contraceptive 196, 198–199
  See also Contraception.
Diarrhea, 278
Diastolic pressure. *See* Blood pressure.
Didrikson, Mildred "Babe", *38*
Diet
  after childbirth, 230
  balanced, 30, 48, 56, 63
  calories and, 76–77
  carbohydrates in, 76
  children and, 16, 28, 31
  choice of, 76
  "crash", 35, 91, 214
  and digestion, *57*
  fiber in, *63*
  fluid balance and, 90
  healthy, 54, **62–65**
  high-fat, 77
  high-fiber, *84*
  low-calorie, reducing, *80–83*
  low-sodium, **85**
  medically supervised, 76
  pills, 77
  preconception, *214*
  during pregnancy, 218, 220–221
  teeth and, 178
  vegetarian, **86–89**
Dietary Guidelines for Americans, 62–63
Digestive system, 56, *57*, 70
  problems, *57*
  stress and the, 268–269, 278
Digestive tract, 57, 63
Dilation and curettage (D & C), 205, 216
Diseases, hereditary, 24, 59
Disks (spinal), 138–139
Disney, Walt, *37*
Diuretics, 91
Divorce, 201, **299**
Dodgson, Charles, *36*
Down's syndrome, 215, 219
Dreams, 332
Drugs
  addiction to, 44, 282–283
  aging and, 251
  amphetamines, 282–283
  antidepressant, 210, 279–281
  beta blockers, 281
  the brain and, *280*, *283*
  caffeine, 282–283

  children and, 31, 283
  cigarettes, 285
  cocaine, 282–283
  dependence on, 281, 283
  glue, 283
  hallucinogenic, 283
  heroin, 282–283
  lysergic acid diethylamide (LSD), 282–283
  morphine, 283
  nonprescribed, **282–283**
  pregnancy and, 39, 215, 220
  prescribed, 41, 47, **280–281**
  sex and, 210–211
  side effects of, 281
  stress and, 280–281
  tranquilizers, 280–281
  withdrawal symptoms, 281, 283
Duodenum, 57

E

Eardrum, *175*, 176
  perforation of, 176
Earhart, Amelia, 38
Ears **175–177**
  bat, 177
  care of, 175
  in children, 29, 176
  effects of air travel on, 175
  in elderly people, 176
  how they work, *175*
  infections, 175
  noise levels and, *176*
  piercing, 177
  wax, 175
  See also Hearing.
Eating habits **16–17**, 28–29, 33–43, 45–48, 50–51, **66–67**
  to avoid, 66
  to cultivate, 66
  healthy, **52–93**
Eczema, 170, 278
Eddy, Mary Baker, *47*
Edison, Thomas Alva, *28*
Edward VIII, King of England, *41*
Eggs, 56
Ego, 332
Eiffel, Alexandre, *45*
Ejaculation, 191, 195
Elderly people
  and accident prevention, **256–257**
  body weight in, 74, *74*
  claims of, 240
  cognitive therapy and, 337
  diet for, 252
  drugs and, 281
  energy and calories, 49, 51, **68–69**
  exercise routines for, 252, *254–255*
    ankle stretch, *254*
    breathing, *254*
    finger stretch, *253*
    shoulder lifts, *255*
    shoulder rolls, *255*
    sitting jog, *255*
    wrist stretch, *255*
  eye tests for, 49, 51
  fitness and, **250–255**
  hearing tests and, 48, 51, 176, 253
  heat treatment and, 302

motivation of, *240*
as percentage of population, *241*
physical activity and, *250*
responses to, 238
and retirement, 239, **240–249**
roles of, 234
sexual relations, 249
skin care for, 164–165
sleep and, 48, 51
treatment of, 239
See also Aging; Retirement.
Electrocardiogram (EKG), *97*, 100, *101*
Electroencephalogram (EEG), *276*, 326–327
hypnosis and, 330
Electrolysis, 171
Elimination diet, 92
Emotional health, personal tests, **19–21**
Emphysema, 72
Energy sources
calories, 51, **68–69**
carbohydrates 70–71
glycogen 70 71
Krebs cycle, 70–71
Epidermis, 162
Epididymis, 190
Epidural anesthetic, 229
Epilepsy, 215
Erogenous zones, 191
Esophagus, 57, *284*
Estrogen, 186, 202, 208–209
Eustachian tube, **175**, 176
Evening primrose oil, 203
Exercise
aerobic. *See* Aerobic exercise.
benefits and risks of, 42, 103, 158–159
for children, 29
choosing a program, **108–109**
for elderly people, 48–49, 51, 252, *254–255*
groups and organizations, *78*
middle age and, 44, *211*
postnatal, 230
pregnancy and, 215, 218, 220–221, **222–227**
for stamina, 140
stress and, 103, 272–273, 277
See also Aerobic exercise; Exercise programs; Jogging; Running; Sports.
Exercise programs and routines
for abdominals, **142–143**
aerobic dance, **123**
for back, **140–141**
bicycling, **110–111**, 120
for children, **154–155**
choosing, **108–109**
for hips and thighs, **144–145**
home gym, **124–125**
indoor, **120–121**
jogging, 35, **112–115**, 122–123
maintaining, 156
postnatal, 34, 230, **232–233**
prenatal, 222–227
rowing machine, **122**
running, **114–115**
skipping rope, **123**

strengthening, **132–135**
stretching, **126–131**
swimming, **116–118**
for upper body, **146–147**
walking, **109**
warm-up, cool-down, **106–107**, 128
water, **118–19**
yoga, **148–153**
Exercises
alternate knee bend, *126*
alternate leg stretch, *142*
alternating crunch (obliques), *143*
ankle circles, *107*
body circles, *106*
body twists, *107*
cat stretch, *127*
chest lift exercise, *147*
chin-ups, *133*
curb-stretch, *128*
curl-back, *141*
curling against a wall, *141*
curl-up, *142*
deep lunge, *129*
diagonal crunch, *140*
dips, *133*
double knee roll, *127*
face-down leg lifts, *145*
figure 8 arms toner, *118*
four-part open and close, *145*
head roll, *126*
hip circles, *131*
hip shift, *106*
inner thigh lift, *145*
inner thigh stretch. *127*
jumping jacks, *118*
knee and hip flex, *106*
knee hugs, *107*, *141*
leg rock, *131*
leg stretch, *127*
leg up stretch, *129*
lunge stretch, *127*
outer thigh lift, *144*
quad lift, *144*
quad stretch, *127*
reach-up, *143*
rock and roll, *131*
roll backs against wall, *142*
shoulder stretch, *130*
side bend, *126*
side leg lifts, *143*
side slide, *140*
side stretch, *119*
sit-ups, *98*, *132*
skier's squat, *131*
standing knee hug, *128*
standing swing, *128*
swing through, *107*
tabletop stretch, *131*
thigh toner, *135*
total body stretch, *119*
towel stretch, *130*
upper body stretch, *129*
waist toner, *119*
wall stretch, *106*
windmill, *128*
Exfoliation, 164
Exhaustion, and stress, 269
Extramarital affairs, 201
Eyeglasses, 174

Eyes **172–174**
amblyopia ("lazy eye"), 173
astigmatism, 173
cataract, 173
color blindness, 173
conjunctivitis, 173
contact lenses, 32, 35, 37, 39, *174*
glaucoma, 172
how they work, *172*
hypermetropia (farsightedness), 173
iris, 172
myopia (nearsightedness), 173
problems, 173
protection of, 117
pupils, 172, 268
retina, 172
strain, 173, *174*
styes, 173
tears, 172
tests, 29, 31–32, 35, 37, 39, 41, 43, 45, 47, 49, 51, 172

F
Face
exercises, *165*
facelift, 165
make-up, 163
See also Skin.
Fallopian tubes, 197, 208, 216
Family fitness, **154–155**
Farsightedness (hypermetropia), 173
Fartlek, 99
Fast foods, 31, 67
Fats
animal, 55
as calories, 68
in diet, **16–17**, 54, 65
reducing intake of, 65
vegetable, 55
vitamins in, 54
Fatty acids, 54
Feeding babies
bottle, 230
breast, 230
See also Baby.
Feet, **182–183**,
exercises, 183
footwear, 182
old age, and, 49, 253
preventing problems, *183*
running shoes, 112, *182*
treatments, 183
Fertility, 214, 216
drugs, 216
Fertilization (conception), 215
artificial insemination, 216
Fetal alcohol syndrome, 215
Fetal deformity, 219
Fetal heart rate, 214–215
Fetus, effect of drugs on, 214–215
Fiber, in foods, 56, 63
Fibroid tumors, 208, 216
Field, Marshall, *45*
"Fight or flight" response, 158, **268–269**, 270–272
See also Stress.
Financial matters
adults, 32, 35–36, 39, 41, 45, 47, 49
children, 29, 31

Fischer, Robert (Bobby), *30*
Fish
  calorie charts, *338–339*
  as protein, 56
Fitness, **95–159**
  aerobics, **98–99**
  in children, 154–155, *155*
  definition of, **96–97**
  family, **154–155**
  goals, **102–103**
  health clubs, **104–105**
  indoor, **120–123, 124–125**
  maintaining programs, **156**
  in old age, **250–255**
  personal tests, **12–15**
  in pregnancy, **220–227**
  record, **156**
  safety, 100–101
  testing, **100–101**
    treadmill, *101*
  whole-life programs, **27–51**
  yoga, **148–153**
  See also Exercise programs and
    routines.
Fitzgerald, F. Scott, *32*
Flossing, 178, *179*
Fluids, 29, 51, 90–91
Fluoride
  effects of, 178
  in foods, 60
Folic acid, 58–59, 217
  for alcoholics, 59
  in foods, 56
  in pregnancy, 59, 214
Food
  additives, 93
  allergies, **92–93**, *See also* Allergies.
  aversions, 92–93
  calorie content, *68*
  groups, **56–57**, 62
  intolerance, 92–93
  nutrients, **54–55**
  packaging labels, 64
Ford, Henry, *44*
Frame size, *75*
Framingham Study, *55*
Frank, Anne, *28*
Franklin, Benjamin, *50*
Freud, Sigmund, 332
Friedman, Mayer 263
Fructose, 64
Fruits
  calorie charts, *339–340*
  vitamin content, 56

G
Gallbladder, 14, 24, *57*, 302
Gallstones, 57
Gammalinolenic acid, 203
Garland, Judy, *31*
Gastrointestinal tract, 88, 230
Gattefosse, René Maurice, 323
Genetic counseling, 215
Genital herpes, 192–193
Gestation period, 219
Gestring, Marjorie, *28*
Glaucoma, 172
Glenn, John, *37*
Glucose, 54, 64, 70, 98, 103

Glue-sniffing, 282
Gluten, 92
Glycogen, 70–71, 98, 103
Goggles (protective), 117–118, 174
Golf, special stretch program,
  128–131
Gonadotrophins, 187
Gonorrhea, 193
Gout, 72
Graham, Florence, *39*
Graham, Katharine, *47*
Grains, 56
  calorie charts, *341*
Grandparents, role of, 45, 47–48, 51,
  236–239
Grief, **298–299**
Grip developers, 122
Gums, **178–179**
  See also Teeth and Gums.
Gym, home, **124–125**
Gynecological check-up, 34, 38, 46

H
Hair, 162, **168–171**
  aging and, 239
  baldness, *170*
  body distribution, *171*
  care, *168–169*, 171
  growth, 168
  lice, 171
  problems, 170–171
  structure and types, 168
  toupees, 171
  transplants, 171
  unwanted, 171
  wigs, 171
Hallucinogenic drugs, 282, *283*
Hamstring
  exercises, 129, 140, *141*, 154, 225
  injury to, 137
Hands and nails, **180–181**
  cuticle care, *181*
  discoloration of nails, 181
  exercises for hands and wrists, 181
  hand weights, 122
  nail biting, 180
  nail care, 180–181
  nail problems, 181
  protection of hands, *180*
Hangover, 291
  See also Alcohol.
Hatha yoga, 149
Headaches, allergic reactions and, 93
  See also Migraine headaches.
Health clubs, **104–105**
Health farms, 78, *79*
Health screening (female), 34, 42, 46,
  204–207
  blood pressure, *204*
  breast examination 204
  cervical smear (Pap) test, *205*
  checklists, 205, 209
  children, 29
  gynecological examination, 204–205
  range of tests, 204
  routine checks for elderly, 253
Health screening (male), 37, 40,
  210–211
  children, 29, 31

range of tests, 210
  routine checks for elderly, 253
Healthy diet, **62–65**
Hearing, **175–177**
  impaired, 176, 177
  tests for children, 29, 176–177
  tests for elderly, 48, 51, 176, 253
  See also Ears.
Heart, *96*
  cardiac output, 12–13, 97
  exercise and, 96–97
  rate, 12–13, 100
Heart disease
  atheroma, 96–97
  cholesterol and, 54, *55*, 72, 100
  cigarette smoking and, 97, *284*
  coronary, 55
  in the elderly, 239
  fitness and, 100
  overweight and, 14, 72
  thrombosis, 196
Heat exhaustion, 158
Heat therapy, **302–303**
  Russian bath, *303*
Hemoglobin, 98
Hemophilia, 24
Hemorrhoids, 63
Henry VIII, King of England, *31*
Herbalism, **322–323**
  Bach Flower Remedies, *323*
  herbal remedies, *322*
Hereditary disease, 24, 59
Heroin, 282
Herpes (genital), 229
High-density lipoprotein (HDL), *55*
High-fiber diet, *82*, 220, 230
Hiking, exercise program, *109*
Hillary, Edmund, *36*
Hips and thighs, exercises for, *144–145*
Home gyms, 122
Homosexuality, 192, 297
Hormone replacement therapy (HRT),
  209
Hormones 55
  epinephrine, 158
  female, 186
  human chorionic gonadotrophin
    (HCG), 217
  male, 187, 190
  production of, 215
  prostaglandin, 203
  synthetic, 197
Hormone shots, 77
Hydrotherapy, **306–307**
  sitz bath, 306
  whirlpool bath, *306*
Hyperemia, 302
Hypermetropia (farsightedness), 173
Hypertension, 216, 327
Hypnosis, **330–331**
  and pain relief, 229, 331
Hypoallergenic products, 163
Hypochondria, 278
Hypothalamus, 268, *283*

I
Illness
  cigarette smoking and, 286
  stress and, **278–279**

Immune system, stress and the, 268, 278
Immunization, 214
Immunological tests, 92
Incontinence, 251
Indigestion, 278
Indoor fitness, **120–123**
Infertility
  causes of, 216
  See also Fertility.
Infrared therapy, 303
Injuries
  in old age, 256
  preventing sports, **136–137**, 159
Insomnia, 209–210, 276–278, 306
Interval training, 99
Intestines, *57*
Intrauterine device (IUD), 231
Iodine, in foods, 60
Iron
  deficiency anemia, 214
  in foods, 56, 60
  during pregnancy, 214, 217
  for vegetarians, 88
Isokinetic exertion, 98, 122
Isometric exertion, 98, 122
Isotonic exertion, 98

J
Jet lag, 270, *271*
  See also Travel.
Job loss, 299
  See also Stress.
Jogging, 35, **112–115**, 122–123
  pregnancy and, 222
  special stretch program, **128–131**
Joyce, James, *40*
Jung, Carl Gustav, 326, 333

K
Keller, Helen, *34*
Kennedy, John F., *41*
Keratin, 162, 168, 181
Ketones, 70
Kidneys, 90–91, 302
  pregnancy and, 218
  stress and, 268
Kilocalorie, 68
Kilojoules (KJ), 68
King, Martin Luther Jr., *37*
Knee, injury to, *137*
Krebs cycle, *70–71*

L
Labor (childbirth), **228–229**
  Caesarean delivery, 229
  epidural anesthetic, 229
  hypnosis in, 331
  induction of, 229
  methods, 228–229
  painkillers, 229
  premature, 215
  signs of, 228–229
Lactic acid, 71, 302
Lactose, 64
Laetrile, 59
Lange, Dorothea, *43*
Latissimus station, *134*

See also Strengthening.
Leg and arm stretcher, 122, *123*
Legumes, 89
Leisure and physical activities, 13, 15, 19, 33, 35–38, 42, 45–47
Lentigos, 164
Lewis, Carl, *113*
Life expectancy, personal tests, **24–25**
Lifestyle, personal tests, **18–19**
Limbic system, *280*
Lindbergh, Charles, *33*
Lipids, 55
Lipoproteins, 55
Liszt, Franz, *29*
Liver, stress, 268
Low-density lipoprotein (LDL), *55*
Low-sodium diet, *85*
Luce, Henry, *33*
Lungs, 95–97, 239
  effects of cigarette smoking on, *284*
  tests, 14, 100
Lysergic acid diethylamide (LSD), 282, *283*

M
Macrominerals, 60
Macronutrients, defined, 54
Magnesium, in foods, 56, 60
Make-up (facial), 163
Maltose, 64
Mammography, 196, *206*, 207
  See also Breasts.
Manganese, in foods, 60
Marathon, *113*, 158
Marijuana, 282
Massage, **308–311**
  effleurage, 308
  facial, *309*
  friction, *309*
  full-back, *310–311*
  kneading, *309*
  pétrissage, 309
  stress and, 272
  teeth and gum, 178, *179*
  tapotement, 310
Mastitis, 206
Masturbation, 188–189
McClintock, Barbara, *51*
Meal planning, **80–89**
Meat
  calorie charts, **338**
  in diet, 54
  protein in, 54, 56
Meditation, 203, 263, 272, **328–329**
  and spirituality, 329
Megajoules (MJ), 68
Meir, Golda, *48*
Melanin, 162, 167
Melanocytes, 162
Memory, in aging, 251
Menarche. *See* Menstruation.
Menopause, 46–47, 197, 205–206, **208–209**
  contraception and, 208
  definition of, 208
  problems, 208–209
  sexual intercourse and, 209
  surgical, 208
Menorrhagia, 205

Menstruation, **186–188**
  adolescence and, 187
  menarche, 186–187
  menopause and, 208
  menstrual cycle, 191, 206, *215*
  pregnancy and, 216–217
  problems of, 204, 306
Mental fitness, **258–259**
Menus, **80–89**
  high-fiber, **84**
  low-calorie, **81–83**
  low-sodium, **85**
  vegetarian, **86–89**
Metabolism, 40, **70–71**
Metrorrhagia, 205
Midlife transition
  men, **210–211**
  women, **208–209**
Migraine headaches, 93
  alcohol and, 293
  stress and, 267, 278
Milk and milk products
  calorie charts, 339
  protein in, 56
Minerals, **60–61**
  essential, *60*
  pregnancy and, 61
  RDA, 60, *61*
  sources and role of, *61*
  See also specific minerals.
Minoxidil, 171
Miscarriage (spontaneous abortion), 204, **216**, 219
  causes, 215
Mitchell, Margaret, *43*
Moisturizer, 163
Molybdenum, in foods, 60
Monet, Charles, *51*
Mongolism. *See* Down's Syndrome.
Monilia (Candidiasis or Thrush), 193, 204
Monosaccharides, 54
Monosodium glutamate (MSG), 64
Morphine, 282
Morse, Samuel, *45*
Moses, Grandma, *51*
Mourning, 259, 299
  stages of, *298*
Mouth and digestive system, *57*
Moxibustion, 319
Muscles
  abdominal 119–123, 126–127, 132–134, 138, 140, **142–143**
  aerobics and, 98, 103
  aging and, 239
  arm, 122–123
  back, 122–123, 134, 138, 140, 143
  fibers, slow-twitch, 99, 102–103
  fueling of, 70
  heart, 96
  hip and thighs, 144–145
  injuries to, **136–137**
  leg, 119–123
  papillary, *96*
  pectoral, *135*, 138, 146–147
  pelvic, 138
  performance of, 102–103, 107
  quadriceps, 135, 144
  shoulder, 122, 135

strength of, 15, 98, 132
strengthening, 119, **134–135**
stress and, 268–269
stretching, **126–127**
vaginal, 195
Myopia (nearsightedness), 173

N

Nails. *See* Hands and Nails.
National Academy of Sciences, 54
National Cancer Institute, 63–64
National Health and Nutrition
    Examination Survey, 72
"Natural" childbirth, 229
Nausea, during pregnancy, 220
Nearsightedness (myopia), 173
Neck, exercises for, 146–147
    muscles, 138
Needle biopsy, 206
Nervous system, 302
    and aging, 239
    autonomic, 312, 326
Niacin (nicotinic acid), 56
Nicotine, 282, 284–285
    chewing gum, 288
Nightmares, 277
Nipples, 221, 230
Noise levels, *176*
    decibels, 177
Nonspecific urethritis (NSU), 193
"Nun's Prayer", 258
Nureyev, Rudolph, *32*
Nutrients
    for children, 32, 59
    essential, 56–57
    foods and, **54–55**
    for vegetarians, 88–89
Nuts and seeds, calorie charts, *341*

O

Obesity, 14, 66, **77–73**, 81
    in children, 74
    cigarette smoking and, 72, *73*
    diabetes and, 14, 72
    glandular, 302
    See also Overweight.
Obsession, 262, 279
    in sport, **158–159**
Obstacle course, *157*
Oligospermia, 216
Ophthalmologist, 172
Opium, 282
Orgasm
    female, 191
    male, 190
Orthodontics, 178
Osteopathy, **312–313**
Osteoporosis, 47, 209, 250
Ovaries, 186–187, 197, 208
Overweight
    in children, 74
    in menstruation, 205
    risk factors, 72
Ovulation, 215
Oxygen
    energy production and, 98–99
    in pregnancy, 215
    usage (aerobic system), 95, **98–99**,
        102

P

Painkillers
    acupuncture, 229, **318–319**
    in childbirth, 229
Pain relief
    hypnosis and, 331
Palmer, Daniel David, 312
Pangamic acid (pangamate), 59
Pankhurst, Emmeline, *43*
Pantothenic acid, 58
Papillary muscle, *96*
Parents, relationship with children,
    29–30, 33, 35–36, 200, 265
Pasternak, Boris, *48*
Pastries, calorie chart, *341*
Pectoral muscles. *See* Muscles;
    Strengthening.
Pedicure, 183
    See also Feet.
Pelvic tilt 140–141, 222, *223*
Pelvis
    floor muscle exercises, 222, 232
Penis, 190
    circumcision, 190
    disorders of, 216
Perkins, Frances, *46*
Personality, 21, **262–263**
    cigarette smoking and, 285
    driving and, 270, 272, *274*
    stress and, 22–23
    types of, 263
Pheromones, 166
Phobias, 262, 279, **334–335**
Phosphorus, in foods, 56, 60
Physiotherapy, 307
Pigmentation, 164
Pill, contraceptive, 196–197, *198–199*
    after childbirth, 231
    health risks and, 196–197, 206
Pituitary gland, 186–187
Placebo effect, 322, 327
Placenta, 219, 229
    delivery of, 228
    and smoking, 215
Planned Parenthood Association, 198
Plaque, 178
    See also Teeth and Gums.
Plastic surgery, 165
Podiatry, 183
Polysaccharides, 54
Postnatal well-being, **230–233**
    check-up, 231
    contraception, 231
    daily routine, 231
    depression, 231
    diet and weight, 230
    exercise, 34, 230, **232–233**
        crunches, *232*
        curl back, *232*
        elbow to knee, *232*
        leg lift, *232*
        leg and arm lift, *233*
        tricep tightener, *233*
    returning to work, 231
    sexual relations, 231
    weight, 230
Posture, *222*
    in yoga, **149–153**
Potassium, in foods, 60

Poultry
    calorie charts, *338*
    as protein, 56
Preconception well-being
    checklist, 215
    contraception, stopping, 214
    dental care, 215
    diet, *214*
    genetic abnormalities, 215
    health care, 214–215
    mumps, 214
    rubella (German measles), 214
        immunization, 214
Pre-eclampsia, 218
Pregnancy, **213–227**
    amniocentesis, 217
    antinausea medication, 220
    back problems, 138
    blood pressure, 218
    blood tests, 217
    breast changes, 206
    breathing techniques, 221, *225*
    calcium depletion, 221
    clothing, 221–222
    delivery date, 219
    dental care, 221
    detecting position of baby, *218*
    development of baby, *219*
    diet and, 35, *214*, 218, **220–221**
    drug addiction, 215
    ectopic, 197
    exercise and, 34, 215, 218
    genetic abnormalities (tests for), 215,
        219
    genetic counseling, 215
    inherited diseases, 215
    menstrual cycle, *215*
    miscarriage, 215–217
    pelvic floor exercises, *222–223*
    placenta, 215, *217*, 219
    routine tests in, 218
    sexual activity, 221
    smoking and alcohol, 215, 218
    sport and, 215
    termination, 219
    tests, 217
    twins, *217*
    ultrasound scan, 217
    vaginal infections, 220–221
    See also Childbirth; Postnatal well-
        being; Preconception well-being;
        Prenatal well-being.
Premature birth, 215
Premenstrual syndrome (PMS),
    202–203
    and crime, *202*
    and safety, *202*
    self-help plan, *203*
    symptoms, 202
    treatment, 202–203
Premenstrual tension (PMT). *See*
    Premenstrual syndrome (PMS).
Prenatal well-being
    care and checks, **217–219**
    exercise program, *220–227*
        cat position, *223*
        cat stretch, *225*
        chair sitting, *224*
        curl-up, *225*

deep twist, *227*
foot pedaling, *227*
hamstring stretch, *225*
head rolls, *223*
hip circles, *227*
pelvic tilt, *223*
posture, *222*
reach through, *226*
shoulder rolls, *223*
side twist, *222*
sitting side stretch, *226*
standing leg extension, *227*
standing side stretch, *224*
fitness, **220–221**
Progesterone, 186, 202, 208
Promiscuity, 189
Propionate, 64
Prostaglandin hormones, 203
Prostate gland, 190, 210, 216
Protein
constituents of, 54
in foods, 56
RDA, 54
Psoriasis, 170
Psychoanalysis, **332–333**
psychotherapies, 333
techniques of, 332
Psychopharmacology, 280
Puberty
boys, 187
girls, 187
Pulse rate, 12–13, 97, 108, 115, 117, 120, 122, 124
Pupil (eye), 172
stress and, 268
Push-ups, 122, *132–133*
Pyridoxine (vitamin B₆), 56, 58, 202

Q

Quadriceps muscles, 144

R

Racewalking, exercise program, *109*
Radiant heat, 303
Rahe, Dr. Richard, 23
Rank, Otto, 333
Rankin, Jeanette, *39*
Rapid eye movement (REM), *276*
Reality testing, 337
Recommended Dietary Allowances (RDA), 54, *58*, 59–60, *61*, 76, 80
Reflexology (zone therapy), **319**
points, *319*
Reich, Wilhelm, 316
Relationships
in crises, **296–297**
effect of alcohol on, 291
the elderly and, **248–249**
extramarital affairs, 201
family, 20, 28–31, 33–34, 36–37, 40, 43, 45, 200–201
homosexual, 192
identifying problems, 201
marriage, 33, 36, 38, 40, 42, *193*
middle age and, 209–211
overcoming stress in, *200*
parents and babies, 234
pressures in, **200–201**

sexual, 192, **194–195**
work and, 201
Relaxation, 33, 35, 37, 39 40, 45, 49, **272–273**
biofeedback, 326
pregnancy and, *220–221*, 228
sports and, 324–325
stress and, *273*
Relaxometer, 326
Respiratory system, 102, 112
Reticular activating system (RAS), *280*, *283*
Retired Senior Volunteer Program (RSVP), 246
Retirement, **240–249**
communities, **244–245**
developing new skills, 48, 50, *246–247*
education courses, 247
employment and volunteer work, 48, 51, 246–247
exercise routines, 252, *254–255*
financial matters, 49, 242–243
goals for, **48–51**
housing location, 49, *243*, 244–245
marital relationships, 248
physical activities, *245*
planning ahead for, 45, 47–48, 239, **242–243**
sexual relations, 249
social activities, 51, *248–249*
sporting activities, 247
younger generation, 249
See also Aging; Elderly people.
Rhesus factor, 218
Rheumatism, 251, 302, 307
Rhythm method, 198–199, 231
See also Contraception.
Riboflavin (vitamin B₂), 56, 58
Rolf, Dr. Ida P., 316
Rolfing, **316–317**
Roosevelt, Eleanor, *49*
Rosenman, Ray, 263
Rotator cuff tendonitis, *137*
Roughage. *See* Fiber, in foods.
Rowing
special stretch program, 128, 130–131
Rowing machines, 122, *123*
exercise program, *120*
Rubella (German measles), 204, 214–215, 218
Rudolph, Wilma, *34*
Ruminations, 279
Running, 108, **112–115**
interval training, **156**
marathon, *113*, 158
programs, *114–115*, 120
progress chart, **156**
shoes, 112, 115, *182–183*
special stretch program, 128–131
sprinting, *113*
tempo training, 99
See also Jogging.
Russian bath, *303*

S

Saccharin, 64
Sagan, Françoise, *31*

Salivary glands, and stress, 268
Salk, Jonas, *40*
Salt
daily consumption chart, *64*
reducing levels of, 65
tablets, 90
See also Sodium.
Samaritans, 295
Sauna, **304–305**
home sauna cabin, *305*
Schulz, Dr. J.K., 324
Sciatica, 302
Scrotum, 187, 190
Seaman, Elizabeth, *35*
Sebaceous glands, 162, 164
Selenium, in foods, 60
Self-esteem, 21, 263
Self-talk, 263, **272–273**, 274
Semen, 190, 193
analysis of, 216
seminal vesicles, 190, 216
Senility, 258
Senior Companion Program, 246
Serum alpha fetoprotein (AFP), 219
Service Corporation of Retired Executives (SCORE), 246
Sesame seeds, 89
Sex organs
female, 190–191
male, 188, 190
Sexual development, **186–189**
boys, 31, *187*, 187
girls, 31, 186–187
Sexual intercourse, 190–191, 195
Sexuality, **185–211**
body language, *190*
contraception, **196–199**
developing, 186–187
display and arousal, 191
the elderly, 249
improving your sex life, 103, **194–195**
libido, 191
menopause and, 209
middle age and, 47, 210–211
pregnancy and, 221
relationships, 192, 249
stress and, 269
See also Sexual problems.
Sexually transmitted diseases, 188, 193, 210
AIDS (Acquired Immune Deficiency Syndrome), 192–193
candidiasis (thrush), 193
genital herpes, 193
gonorrhea, 193
NSU (Nonspecific urethritis), 193
syphilis, 193
Sexual problems, 20, **194–195**, 264
in adolescence, 187–189
gynecological, 195
health and, 195
impotence, 195
psychological, 191, 195
self-help, 194–195
therapy, 194
Shelley, Mary, *34*
Shiatsu, 319, **320–321**
Shoulder exercises, **146–147**

"Show" (childbirth), 228
Sight. *See* Eyes.
Sit-up bench, 122, *123*
Sitz bath, 306
Skiing, special stretch program, 128–131
Skin, **162–167**
  aging and, 49, 164–165, 239
  care of, 162–163
  cosmetics and, 163
  disorders, treatment, 164–165
  facial, exercises, *165*
  functions of, 162
  pigmentation, 164
  plastic surgery, 165
  stress and, 268
  structure of, *162*
  sunshine and, 164, 166–167
  sweat glands, 162
  types of, *163*
  washing mitts, *164*
Skipping rope, exercise program, 29, *121*
Sleep, 31–32, 35, 48, 226
  back problems and, *139*
  cycle of, 271
  rapid eye movement (REM), *276*
  stages of, *276*
  stress and, **276–277**
  travel and, 270–271
Sleeping pills, 277
Slipped disk, 312
Smoking. *See* Cigarette smoking.
Snacking, *66*
  choice of foods, 42, *67*
Social goals
  adults, 32, 34–36
  children, 29
Sodium
  avoiding, 64
  in foods, 56, 60, 64
  low-sodium diet, *85*
  reducing intake, 64–65, 76–79, 203
Solvent-sniffing, 282
Soya sauce, 64
Soybeans, milk drink, 89
Sperm, 187, 190, 216
  oligospermia (low sperm count), 216
Spermicides, 198–199
  See also Contraception.
Spina bifida, 24, 215, 219
Spinal cord, 138–139, 312
Spine, 138, 139, 313
  sprain to, *137*
  See also Back.
Sponge, contraceptive, 196, 198–199, 231
  See also Contraception.
Sports
  adolescents and, *186*
  autogenics and, 324–325
  children and, 29–31, 36, **154–155**
  the elderly and, 247
  pregnancy and, 215, 222
  preparation and practice, 325
  pressures in, 325
  preventing injuries, **136–137**
  psychology of, **324–325**
  strength increasing, 132

stretch programs, **128–131**
  warm-up and cool-down exercises, **106–107**
  water loss in, *90*
Sports glasses, 174
Stair climbing, exercise program, *109*
Starch, 54
Steam cabinets, 302
Sterilization, 197
Steroid DES, 204, 214–215
Still, Dr. Andrew Taylor, 312
Stomach. *See* Abdomen.
Strengthening muscles, 95, 113, 122, **132–135**, 136
  equipment, **134–135**, 146
  training, 122, 136
  water exercise, 119
Stress, **260–299**
  Alexander Technique and, **314–315**
  autogenics and, 324–325
  biofeedback and, 263, 272, **326–327**
  body reactions to, 267, *268*, 269
  causes of, 267
  changing routine, 272
  coping with, 20, **22–23**, 267, **272–275**
  depression and, 278–279
  and digestive problems, 268–269, 278
  dreams and, 277
  drinking and, 272
  effects of, *266*
  exercise and, 272–273
  expectations and, 267
  illness and, **278–279**
  jet lag and, 270–271
  learning relaxation, *273*
  lifestyle, 275
  mental symptoms of, 269
  personal tests, **22–23**
  personality and, **262–263**
  physical symptoms of, 269
  prescribed drugs and, **280–281**
  problem solving and, 275
  self-esteem and, 263
  self-talk and, **272–273**, 274
  sleep and, **276–277**
  sweat glands and, 268
  thresholds, 266–267
  travel and, 270, *271*, 274
  yoga and, 272
Stretch (special) program, **128–131**, 136
Stretching, 113, **126–127**, 136
Styes, 173
Subluxations, 312
Sucrose, 64–65
Sugar, 64–65
  avoiding excess, 64
  effect on teeth, 178
Sulfur, in foods, 60
Sullivan, Harry Stack, 333
Sunglasses, 174
Sunlamps, 167
Sun protection factor (SPF), 167
Sun salutation (yoga), **152–153**
Sunshine
  children and, 167
  sunscreens, *166*, 167
  sunstroke, 167

Sweat glands, 166
  and stress, 268
Sweeteners (artificial), in foods, 65
Sweets, calorie chart, *341*
Swimming, 40, 108, **116–117**
  exercise programs, **116–118**
  pregnancy and, 215
  special stretch programs, 128–131
Syphilis, 193, 218
Syrups, 64
Systolic pressure. *See* Blood pressure.
Szewinska, Irena, *208*

T
T'ai Chi Ch'uan, *328–329*
Tampons, 196, 205
Tapotement (Swedish massage), 310
Tax Aid, 247
Teenagers. *See* Adolescence.
Teeth and gums, **178–179**
  care of, 33, 35–36, 39, 41, 43–44, 47, 49–50, 178–179
  children's, 28, 31, 178
  diet and, 178
  fluoride and, 178
  modern dentistry, 178
  in old age, 253
  orthodontics, 178
  plaque, 178
  in pregnancy, 221
  sugar and, 178
Temple, Shirley, *29*
Tempo training, 99
Tennis, special stretch program, 128–131
Tennis elbow, *137*
Teresa, Mother (of Calcutta), *49*
Tereshkova, Valentina, *38*
Testes, 187, 216.
Testicles. *See* Testes.
Testosterone, 187, 190–191
Thatcher, Margaret, *46*
Therapies. *See specific therapies.*
Thiamin (vitamin B_1), 56, 58
Thigh and knee machine, *135*
  See also Strengthening; Exercise programs.
Thinking, types of, *336*
Thrombosis
  contraceptive pill and, 196
  See also Heart disease.
Thrush (Candidiasis or Monilia), 193
Toenails, ingrown, 183
Tooth decay. *See* Dental problems; Teeth and gums.
Tortellier, Paul, 237
Toxic shock syndrome (TSS), 196, 205
Trace minerals, 56, 60
Trachea, 98
Training
  fitness record, **156**
  interval, 156
  obstacle course, *157*
Trampoline, 122, *123*
Tranquilizers, 195, 280–281
Travel, 18, 32, 35, 41
  stress and, 270, *271*
Treadmill, 122, *123*
  in fitness testing, *101*

Triangle exercise, yoga, *150*
Tricane, *257*
Triceps, 133
Trichomoniasis, 204
Tricuspid valve, 96
Tryptophan, 277
Tumor, benign, 206
Turkish bath, 303
Twins, *217*

U
Ultrasound scan, 217–218, *219*
Urethra, 190
Urine tests
   in pregnancy, 217–218
Uterus, 187, 190, 215–217, 229–230

V
Vacations, 19, 29, 35–36, 38, 41, 45, 48
Vagina
   examination of, 218
   hymen, 190
   infections of, 220–221
   labia, 190
   muscles, 195
   postnatal bleeding from, 230
Vaginal suppositories, 193
Valium, 280
Variable resistance equipment, 98, 134–135
Varicose veins, 216, 221, 302
Vas deferens, 41, 190, 197
Vasectomy, 41, 197
Vegetables
   calorie chart, *340*
   cruciferous, 56
   protein in, 54
   vitamins in, 56
Vegetarian diets, **86–89**
   children and, 86–87
   lacto-ovo, 86, 88–89
   pregnancy and, 87, 89
   protein content, 88
   semivegetarian, 86
   vegan, 86–89
Venereal diseases, 188, 192–193, 204, 210
Verruca, 183
Vertebral column. *See* Spine.
Vitamin A (retinol), 54, 56, 58
   for vegetarians, 89
Vitamin B_1 (thiamin), 56, 58
Vitamin B_2 (riboflavin), 56 58
Vitamin B_6 (pyridoxine), 56, 58, 202
Vitamin B_{12}, 56, 58
   and vegetarian diet, 59, 86, 88–89
Vitamin C (ascorbic acid), 56, 58
   for vegetarians, 87–88
Vitamin D (calciferol), 54–55, 58, 162
   for children, 59
   for vegetarians, 86, 88–89
Vitamin E (tocopherol), 54, 58
Vitamin K, 54, 58
Vitamins, **58–59**, 86–89, 202
   for alcoholics, 59
   for children, 59
   essential, *58*
   megadoses, 59
   over-the-counter, 59

RDA, 54, *58*, 59–61, 76, 80
   sources and role of, *58*
   supplements, 58–59
   for vegetarians, 59, 86–89
   See also specific vitamins.
VO_2 (max), 102–103
   See also Oxygen usage.
Volunteer Income Tax Assistance (VITA), 247
Volunteer work
   retirement and 246–247
   stress and, 272
Vulva, 190

W
Walking, **109**, 257
   exercise programs, 109
Warm-up exercises, **106–107**, 113, 128, 132, 134, 136, 140
Washington Medical School, 23
Water
   body loss and replacement of, *91*
   dieting and, 76, 90–91
   fluoride content of, 178
Water exercises
   clothing and equipment, 118
   for the disabled, 118
   jogging, *118*
   for nonswimmers, 199
   for the obese, 118
   programs, **118–119**
   stretching, 119
Wax baths, 303
Webster, Noah, *49*
Weight
   calories and, 78
   after childbirth, 230
   control of, **72–79**, 95
   exercise and, 78, 103
   frame size and, *75*
   loss of, 70, 72
   "pinch" test, 14, 72
   preconception and, 214
   pregnancy and, 214, 220
   tables of, *75*
   tips for losing, 77
Weight lifting, 98, 122
Weight training, 122
Weight Watchers, *79*
Whiplash (cervical spine sprain), *137*
Whirlpool bath, 302, 306, 307
Work, attitude to, 21
Working mothers, 231
Workouts, fitness record, 156
World Assembly on Aging, 240
Wrist weights, 98

X
X-rays, during pregnancy, 214

Y
Yeasts, nutritional, 89
Yin and yang, *319*
Yoga, **148–153**, 203
   alternate nostril breathing, *148*
   exercises
      back stretch, *151*
      child pose, *151*
      fish pose, *151*

front stretch, *151*
      full body stretch, *151*
      knee hug pose, *151*
      spinal roll, *151*
      sun salutation, *152–153*
      supported plow pose, *151*
      triangle pose, *151*
   practice, 150
Yogurt, 56

Z
Zanax, 280
Zen Buddhism, 328
Zen meditation, **328–329**
Zinc, in foods, 56, 60

CREDITS AND ACKNOWLEDGMENTS

l = left; *r* = right; *t* = top; *c* = center; *b* = bottom

3 W. Bokelberg/The Image Bank; 10 G & J Images/
The Image Bank; 26 R. Janeart/The Image Bank; 52
Syndication International; 63 Charlie Stebbings; 66
D&J Heaton/Colorific!; 74 Derek Berwin/The Image
Bank; 78 Paolo Curto/The Image Bank; 79*t* Michael
Yamashita/Colorific!; 79*b* Weight Watchers (UK) Ltd;
80 Charlie Stebbings; 86/87 Peter Myers; 90 David
Cannon/All-Sport; 92/93 Peter Myers; 94 T. McCarthy/
The Image Bank; 102 Michael Yamashita/Colorific!;
106/107 Peter Underwood; 112 R. Janeart/The Image
Bank; 113*l* Steve Dunnell/The Image Bank; 113*r* Dave
Cannon/All-Sport; 126/153 Peter Underwood; 154*t*
Peter Underwood; 154*b* W. Bokelberg/The Image
Bank; 155 Peter Underwood; 159 Vandystadt/All-
Sport; 160 Bensimon/Scoop/Transworld; 163 Marshall
Editions; 164 Silverstein/Scoop/Transworld; 166 T.
Frankell/All-Sport; 169*t* P. Pfander/The Image Bank;
169*c* David Vance/The Image Bank; 169*b* Novik/Vital
No3/Transworld; 170/171 Tony Stone Assoc.; 173 Tom
McCarthy/The Image Bank; 174 STC Business
Systems; 180 Chris Reinhardt/Scoop/Transworld; 184
G & J Images/The Image Bank; 186 All-Sport; 187 The
Photo Source; 188 Sally & Richard Greenhill; 189 Dave
Hogan/Rex Features; 190 Zao Longfield/The Image
Bank; 191 Nick Briggs; 192 Susan Griggs/Photofile;
193 Peter Correz/Tony Stone Assoc./194 Robert
Farber/The Image Bank; 200 Robin Forbes/The Image
Bank; 204 Sally & Richard Greenhill; 206 BUPA; 208
The Press Association; 211 Chris Bigg; 212 Tony
Stone Assoc.; 214 Gruner & Jahr AG & Co.; 218 Val
Wilmer/Format Photographers; 219 St. Bartholomew's
Hospital; 220/227 Peter Underwood; 228 Anthea
Sieveking/Zefa Picture Library; 229 Parents/Scoop/
Transworld; 230 Sandra Lousada/Susan Griggs
Agency; 232/233 Peter Underwood; 234*t* Peter
Underwood; 234*b* John Garrett; 235 Peter Underwood;
236 Lawrence Fried/The Image Bank; 238 Robin
Forbes/The Image Bank; 240 Sally & Richard
Greenhill; 243 Benn Mitchell/The Image Bank; 245
David Hurn/Magnum/The John Hillelson Agency; 246
W. Maehl/Zefa Picture Library; 247 David Hurn/
Magnum/The John Hillelson Agency; 248 Pat la Croix/
The Image Bank; 249 R. Phillips/The Image Bank; 250
Tony Stone Assoc.; 253 Western Morning News Co.
Ltd; 254/255 Peter Underwood; 259 Tom McCarthy/
The Image Bank; 260 Tony Stone Assoc.; 266*t* Barry
Lewis/Network; 266*b* Sally & Richard Greenhill; 274
Walter Bibikow/The Image Bank; 286 The Health
Education Council; 289 Cliff Feulner/The Image Bank;
300 Zao Grimberg/The Image Bank; 303 Feinblatt/
Scoop/Transworld; 306/307 David Brownell/The
Image Bank; 324 Tony Stone Assoc.; 327 Biofeedback
Systems; 330 David Parker/Science Photo Library;
334/335 Phillip Lee.

Artwork by
Malcolm Barter; John Davies; Karen Daws; Tony
Graham; Aziz Khan; Line and Line Ltd; Jim Robbins;
Les Smith.

Retouching: Roy Flooks.

The publishers would like to thank the following
people and organizations for their invaluable help: Liz
Anfield; Norman Ellis; Liv Lowrie; Peter McCullough;
Tim Newling; Bronwen Reynolds; Maggie Skiffington;
Mike Snell; Michelle Thompson; Alison Tomlinson;
Joan White; Jane Wilkie; Alison Williams; The BUPA
Medical Center; The Canada Fitness Survey; Central
Policy on Aging; Daltons Sports/Fitness Industries;
The Disabled Living Group; The Health Education
Council; Nautilus Fitness Center; Barbara Dale; Tony
Lycholat; Marina Chafelon; Fernando Calvino; Jonas
Øglaend Inc.